Community Health
Nursing Care Plans

Books of Related Interest

Ross: Ambulatory Care Organization and Management

Greene: Handbook of Adult Primary Care

Hogstel: Nursing Care of the Older Adult. Second edition.

Sands: A Guide to Arthritis Home Health Care

Snyder: Independent Nursing Interventions

Williams: How to Market Home Health Services. Second edition.

Woerner: Home Health

University of Missouri: In-Home Care: A Flexible Educational System for Quality Care

Community Health Nursing Care Plans

A Guide for Home Health Care Professionals
Second Edition

Susan L. Scherman, R.N.
Nurse Consultant, Risk Management
Bower & Gardner
New York, New York

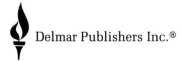

Delmar Publishers Inc.®

NOTICE TO THE READER

To the memory of my father, Everett H. Scherman

For information, address Delmar Publishers Inc.
2 Computer Drive West, Box 15-015
Albany, New York 12212

Delmar Staff

Executive Editor: Leslie Boyer
Associate Editor: Marjorie Bruce
Publications Coordinator: Karen Seebald
Design Coordinator: Susan Mathews

Printed in the United States of America
Published simultaneously in Canada
by Nelson Canada,
a division of The Thomson Corporation

10 9 8 7 6 5 4 3 2 1

Library of Congress Cataloging in Publication Data:

Scherman, Susan L.
    Community health nursing care plans : a guide for home health care
professionals / Susan L. Scherman. — 2nd ed.
        p.   cm.
    Includes bibliographical references.
    ISBN 0–8273–4357–4 (pbk.)
    1. Community health nursing—Outlines, syllabi, etc.   2. Home care
services—Outlines, syllabi, etc.   3. Nursing care plans—Outlines,
syllabi, etc.   I. Title.
    [DNLM: 1. Community Health Nursing—outlines.   2. Home Care
Services—outlines.   3. Nursing Process—outlines.   4. Patient Care
Planning—outlines.   WY 18 S326c]
RT96.S34   1990
610.73'43—dc20
DNLM/DLC
for Library of Congress   89–71432
                                                                      CIP

Care Plan Contents

Care Plan
Contents Cont'd

Care Plan
Contents Cont'd

Care Plan
Contents Cont'd

Care Plan
Contents Cont'd

Preface

Community Health Nursing Care Plans: A Guide for Home Health Care Professionals was written primarily for home health nurses who work in proprietary and official home health care agencies. It can also be used by community health nurses, public health nurses, hospital discharge planners, risk managers, and social workers and other health care professionals employed by state and local boards of health, ambulatory care units, quality assurance departments, and long-term care facilities.

The purpose of this book is to assist home health care nurses with the documentation of today's nursing process. Patient conditions are evaluated in terms of nursing diagnoses, behavioral objectives (short and long-term goals), outcome criteria, and nursing interventions. The book has been revised to include 106 care plans that present each of these five elements as related to a specific condition. The original nursing diagnoses in the first edition of this book were formulated from the North American Nursing Diagnosis Association, Sixth National Conference, April, 1984, but have been updated in this edition based on the Eighth National Conference, March, 1988.

Home health care nurses are usually required to document their records during the admission procedure in the home. Nurses may refer to or copy information directly from this book and transfer it onto the client plan of care in their records. If, for some reason, the home environment is not conducive to this process, nurses may photocopy each plan of care at a later date and place it on the client's record after circling the most applicable nursing diagnoses and causes, short- and long-term goals, outcome criteria, and nursing interventions. Nurses may circle more than one cause if necessary and may also add information listed under the "other" category for further clarification. Not all nursing interventions may be listed, so nurses are encouraged to list additional information, whenever necessary, onto each plan of care. Nurses may also wish to make certain headings more specific; for example, "Hypochromic" may be added to "Anemia Care Plan" for clarity to make a heading "Hypochromic Anemia Care Plan." Material contained in this book can be easily stored in computer systems and photocopied or transferred to other nursing units whenever continuity of care is necessary.

In response to the current popularity of and need for certain procedures that were once confined to the hospital but are now being introduced into the home, care plans for cancer chemotherapy, chest physiotherapy, home parenteral nutrition, nasogastric/enteric feeding, mechanical ventilation, hemodialysis, intravenous therapy, and transcutaneous electrical nerve stimulation (TENS) are also included in the book.

It appears that home health agencies differ in the parameters that they use for determining the number of visits that they are allotted by their major insurors. The number of visits specified in this text is in compliance with the requirements for reimbursement for major insurors such as Medicare and Blue Cross. If certain home health agencies prefer to expand their visits beyond the scope of these parameters, they may do so and add more visits to each of the short-term goals and nursing interventions. Some of the goals may seem ideal and unrealistic. However, caution is advised when agency reimbursement is at risk. Subsequent added visits may not be reimbursed. Additions, nevertheless, are left to the user's discretion.

Specific causes are not listed for a few of the knowledge deficit diagnoses in this book because of controversy over the cause at this time. An example is sudden infant death syndrome. Nurses must confine their diagnoses to those conditions that fall within the realm of nursing licensure as dictated by individual state practice acts. These diagnoses must not conflict with the client's medical diagnosis unless the condition is clear cut and no other diagnosis can be applied. Home health care nurses are advised to determine the extent of their authority by studying the nurse practice acts for their states carefully if a controversial nursing diagnosis should arise.

In conclusion, if nurses in a multitude of settings are to provide adequate client care, it should be reflected in thorough and efficient documentation, a process that it is hoped will be strengthened through the use of this book. In regard to risk management, discharging patients is now riskier than ever, especially when they are being sent home directly from intensive care units. Hospitals and home health personnel should minimize their liability through effective communication and documentation. It is common knowledge that federal budget restrictions and third-party payers encourage institutions to discharge patients as quickly as possible, and it is for this reason that liability is a key concern. To minimize the risks of client care, nurses should give certain areas special consideration. Some of these are medical record documentation, safety issues, issues of consent, laboratory testing, follow-up hospital discharge instructions, and admission to long-term care facilities. Attention should also be paid to timely placement and proper functioning of highly technologic medical equipment such as ventilators and hemodialysis machines. The best defense against liability is a well-documented medical record, and that is the major focus of this book.

I would like to thank the staff involved with the 1981 Framework for Action Training Workshop sponsored by the New Jersey State Department of Health, Northern Region Office, East Orange, New Jersey, for helping to clarify my own understanding of the formulation of the nursing process.

Susan L. Scherman

GENERAL GUIDELINES FOR THE USE OF THE NURSING CARE PLANS

1. When physicians orders are received for a client in the home health care agency, the nurse will review the medical diagnoses, medications, treatments, equipment, and additional therapists required. The Registered Professional Nurse usually makes the first visit to the client and supervises the plan of care.

2. Prior to the first visit the nurse may photocopy the pertinent care plans or bring this manual into the client's home for documentation and instructional purposes. The plan of care may then be completed at the bedside when time is limited and accuracy is required.

3. During the admission interview the nurse should begin to formulate the appropriate nursing diagnoses and thus, circle the nursing diagnosis/diagnoses, short- and long-term goals, outcome criteria and nursing interventions in each plan of care pertinent to the client's needs.

4. All nursing diagnoses, short- and long-term goals, outcome criteria, and nursing interventions in this text should be utilized as a reminder or model for the nurse when time is limited. This information should be added to the agency's preprinted forms, if necessary, for continuity of care for other caregivers and submission to major insurers. Please note that some agencies may prefer to add information to these care plans, such as additional diagnoses, visits, goals, outcome criteria and interventions; this is left to the nurse's discretion. Space has been provided for this purpose.

5. If major insurers require a care plan to be submitted prior to authorization of visits, these care plans may be photocopied with the appropriate circled information and then sent to the insurer. The original care plan may be kept in the client's home health chart. When concurrent review or utilization review is necessary and requested by insurers, then the nursing progress notes, which include dates and signatures, may also accompany the care plans.

6. These care plans may also be incorporated in pre-existing agency computer programs.

Health Care Personnel

M.D.	Medical doctor
R.N.	Registered nurse
H.H.A.	Home health aide
O.T.	Occupational therapist
P.T.	Physical therapist
R.T.	Respiratory therapist
S.T.	Speech therapist
M.S.W.	Medical social worker

Acquired Immune Deficiency Syndrome Care Plan

I. NURSING DIAGNOSIS

1. Anxiety related to:
   A. dying process.
   B. social isolation.
   C. other _____

   _____

2. Knowledge deficit related to:
   A. diagnoses within syndrome (e.g., oral candidiasis/Pneumocystis carinii pneumonia (viral: cytomegalovirus (CMV), Epstein-Barr virus, herpes simplex virus, and hepatitis B virus/bacterial: Mycobacterium avium, M. intracellulare, pulmonary nocardiasis, Salmonella, Shigella flexneri, Legionella pneumophila/protozoan: Toxoplasmosis gondii, cryptosporidium enteritis)/Kaposi's sarcoma.
   B. signs/symptoms.
   C. source of infection.
   D. isolation precautions.
   E. prevention/treatment of AIDS.
   F. medication administration (e.g., AZT)/adverse reactions.
   G. fluids/diet.
   H. postural drainage/chest physical therapy/incentive spirometry/ ultrasonic nebulizer/humidified air/supplemental oxygen/IPPB/ mechanical ventilation.
   I. position change.

    J. monogamous relationship.

    K. sexual precautions (e.g., use of a latex condom).

    L. proper hand-washing technique.

    M. skin breakdown/use of protective equipment (e.g., sheepskin/ heel bolsters/egg crate mattress).

    N. dressing change.

    O. immunizations for children and adults/precautions prior to administration.

    P. other _____

    _____

3. Ineffective breathing pattern related to:

    A. anxiety.

    B. retained secretions.

    C. difficulty with expectoration.

    D. poor positioning.

    E. deterioration of pulmonary functioning.

    F. other _____

    _____

4. Altered thought processes related to:

    A. high levels of anxiety.

    B. hallucinations.

    C. paresthesias.

    D. focal deficits.

    E. other _____

    _____

5. Impaired gas exchange related to:

    A. retained respiratory secretions.

    B. poor fluid/dietary intake.

    C. poor positioning.

    D. other _____

    _____

6. Impaired social interaction related to:

    A. severe malaise.

    B. mood swings.

    C. changes in sensorium.

    D. other _____

    _____

7. Potential for injury related to:

    A. mood swings.

    B. dizziness.

    C. potential for falling.

    D. poor vision.

    E. other _____

    _____

8. Altered patterns of urinary elimination (e.g., stress incontinence/ reflex incontinence/urge incontinence/functional incontinence/ total incontinence/urinary retention) related to:

    A. confusion.

    B. changes in sensorium.

    C. weakened musculature.

    D. other _____

    _____

9. Constipation/Diarrhea/Bowel incontinence related to:

    A. confusion.

    B. poor diet/inadequate fluids.

    C. changes in sensorium.

    D. other _____

    _____

10. Anticipatory/Dysfunctional grieving related to:

    A. fear of dying.

    B. rejection by significant others.

    C. dependence on others for care.

    D. alteration in body image.

    E. other _____

    _____

11. Impaired home maintenance management related to:

    A. excessive demands of caring for the sick.

    B. financial distress.

    C. partner/family discord.

    D. overwhelming family responsibilities.

    E. other _____

    _____

12. Impaired physical mobility related to:

    A. dependence on others for care.

    B. monoplegia.

    C. diplegia.

    D. paraplegia.

    E. hemiplegia.

    F. quadriplegia.
    G. dysarthria.
    H. athetosis.
    I. chorea.
    J. rigidity.
    K. dystonia.
    L. tremors.
    M. weakness.
    N. contractures.
    O. seizures.
    P. other _____

13. Noncompliance with therapy related to:
    A. denial.
    B. cost of medical care/poor insurance coverage.
    C. increasing demands on significant others for care.
    D. other _____

14. Altered nutrition: more than body requirements related to:
    A. dysphagia.
    B. vomiting.
    C. diarrhea.
    D. anorexia.
    E. fluid/electrolyte imbalances.
    F. other _____

15. Potential impaired skin integrity related to:
    A. decreased immune response.
    B. poor skin care.
    C. lesion formation.
    D. other _____

16. Sleep pattern disturbance related to:
    A. dry, hacking cough.
    B. shortness of breath.
    C. persistent diarrhea.
    D. night sweats.
    E. mood swings.

F. other _____

_____

17. Body image disturbance related to:
    A. changes in sensorium.
    B. lesion formation.
    C. weight loss.
    D. rejection by significant others.
    E. other _____

    _____

18. Sexual dysfunction related to:
    A. severe malaise.
    B. changes in sensorium.
    C. rejection by significant others.
    D. weakness.
    E. other _____

    _____

19. Impaired swallowing related to:
    A. oral/esophageal lesions.
    B. other _____

    _____

20. Altered parenting related to:
    A. changes in sensorium.
    B. weakness.
    C. dependence on others for care.
    D. other _____

    _____

21. Powerlessness related to:
    A. acquisition of a terminal illness.
    B. isolation.
    C. declining health/advance of disease process.
    D. impending death.
    E. other _____

    _____

22. Spiritual distress related to:
    A. guilt.
    B. abuse of drugs/deviant behavior.
    C. impending death.
    D. other _____

    _____

II. SHORT-TERM GOALS

1. Client/Contact/Family will immediately notify M.D. of/seek medical treatment for possible impending signs/symptoms of AIDS after 1 R.N. visit.
2. Client/Contact/Family will call National Gay Task Force's Crisis Hotline for additional information (recommended by Centers for Disease Control, Atlanta) after 1–2–3 R.N. visits.
3. Client/Contact/Family will administer prescribed medication as ordered after 1–2–3–4 R.N. visits.
4. Client/Family will immediately notify M.D. of adverse reactions to medications after 1–2–3 R.N. visits.
5. Client/Contact will isolate self from people with infectious diseases after 1 R.N. visit.
6. Client/Contact will consume nutritionally sound meals after 1–2–3 R.N. visits.
7. Client/Contact/Family will administer enteral feedings/ hyperalimentation as ordered after 1–2 R.N. visits.
8. Client/Contact/Family will follow prescribed physical therapy exercises after 1–2 R.N. visits.
9. Client/Contact/Family will verbalize fears, anxieties, and concerns after 1–2–3 R.N. visits.
10. Client/Contact will seek treatment for drug abuse after 1–2–3–4–5–6 R.N. visits.
11. Client/Contact will avoid nitrites and chemical abuse after 1–2–3 R.N. visits.
12. Client/Contact will maintain monogamous relationship after 1–2 R.N. visits.
13. Client/Contact will use latex condoms for sexual activity after 1–2 R.N. visits.

III. LONG-TERM GOALS

1. Monogamous sexual life-style will be sought in 6–8 weeks.
2. Drug addiction will be controlled in 6–12 months.
3. Independent activities of daily living will be resumed in 3–4 weeks.
4. All stages of death and dying will be resolved during course of disease.
5. Optimal level of health will be achieved in 6–12–24 months.

IV. OUTCOME CRITERIA

1. Vital signs are normal.
2. Lungs are clear.
3. Weight is appropriate.
4. Skin is clear, healthy, and intact.
5. Cardiovascular status is normal.
6. Neuromuscular tone is normal.
7. Appetite is normal.
8. Lymphatic system functions appropriately.
9. Bowel habits are normal.
10. Client is alert.
11. Client states he/she feels better.
12. Client seeks employment.

V. NURSING INTERVENTION/TREATMENT

1. R.N. will refer client/contact/family immediately to M.D. for any signs/symptoms of AIDS; will report to local board of health after confirmation of disease.
2. R.N. will determine number and location of contacts for notification and treatment.
3. R.N. will instruct client/family/contact/H.H.A. on:

   A. prevention and treatment of AIDS.

   B. signs, symptoms, and severity of disease.

   C. universal precautions (e.g., use of appropriate barriers, proper hand-washing technique before and after gloves are removed/ avoidance of injuries by needles, scalpels, and other sharp instruments or devices even though HIV transmission has not been seen in saliva/avoidance of emergency mouth-to-mouth resuscitation whenever possible, by using mouthpieces, resuscitation bags, and other ventilation devices/avoidance by workers with exudative lesions or weeping dermatitis of patient care and patient care equipment/precautions by pregnant health care workers to avoid perinatal infection).

   D. HIV/AIDS Related Complex testing via ELISA (EIA-enzyme-linked immunosorbent assay) and WB (Western blot, an additional more specific blood test for HIV antibody, used to validate seropositive reactions to EIA).

   E. use of barriers (e.g., masks/eye coverings/gloves/gowns).

   F. needle disposal (to prevent needlestick injuries, needles should not be recapped, bent, broken, or removed from disposable syringes or manipulated by hand). Place needles/syringes in a tin can, seal, and dispose.

G. laundry instructions/precautions.

H. prevention of transmission to family/friends (avoid sharing razor blades/toothbrushes/utensils/needles).

I. prevention of infection of client (e.g., client should avoid contact with infected persons/use pasteurized milk/eat washed fruits and vegetables/eat well-cooked meat/avoid infected animals).

J. importance of sexual abstinence/monogamous relationship/use of a latex condom/avoidance of anonymous partners/ substitution of high-risk acts with low-risk acts that minimize exchange of body fluids (e.g., cuddling, fondling, and fantasizing)/avoidance or minimal use of fisting, anal penetration, oral/genital sex, and oral/rectal sex).

K. avoidance of nitrites/chemicals/tobacco/alcohol/street drugs.

L. fluid/dietary regimen.

M. enteral feeding/hyperalimentation.

N. medication administration (e.g., AZT/Alpha Interferon/ Amligen/Anti-alpha interferon serum/AS-101, Gamma Interferon/Immune Globulin IG-IV/Imreg-I/Interleukin-II/ Isoprinosine/methionine-enkephalin/Thymopentin/ Thymostimuline)/adverse reactions (e.g., hematologic toxicity, including granulocytopenia and severe anemia requiring transfusions/severe headache/unresponsiveness/focal seizures). Coadministration of zidovudine with other drugs metabolized by glucuronidation should be avoided because combination may potentiate toxicity of either drug.

O. immediate notification of M.D. of adverse reactions or change in condition.

P. daily recording of intake and output.

Q. daily monitoring and recording of vital signs/weight.

R. exercise/rest as ordered.

S. disinfection of home/cleansing of spills of blood or body fluid/ drainage with freshly prepared solution of 1 part bleach and 10 parts water (i.e., a 1:10 solution).

T. precautions/immunizations for children/adults (see Immunization Care Plan).

U. chest physical therapy/postural drainage/IPPB/ultrasonic nebulizer/incentive spirometry/humidified air/supplemental oxygen/mechanical ventilation/cleansing of equipment.

    V. rehabilitation equipment (e.g., hospital bed/suction machine/ egg crate mattress/air mattress with pump/wheelchair/ disposable dishes/bedpan/commode/bath handrails/elevated toilet seat/sheepskin/disposable absorbent pads/bed trapeze).

    W. dressing care.

    X. mouth/skin care.

    Y. surgery/radiation.

    Z. organizations/hotline information/state task forces.

4. Health care personnel will take strict precautions to avoid contact with infected blood, blood products, secretions, excretions, and tissues from people with AIDS. Gloving is recommended for close contact with client and infected materials. Collected specimens and infected materials will be labeled appropriately (e.g., "contaminated material—AIDS") and double-wrapped for transport.

5. R.N. will provide M.D. with follow-up reports and discharge summary when case closes.

6. R.N. will notify client/contact/family/H.H.A./significant others when case will close.

Acute Abdomen
Care Plan

I. NURSING DIAGNOSIS

1. Anxiety related to:
   A. nausea/vomiting/indigestion/flatulence/anorexia.
   B. hematemesis.
   C. bleeding gums.
   D. weakness.
   E. change in bowel habits (e.g. diarrhea/constipation/bloody stools/ black, tarry stools).
   F. change in color and character of stools related to diet (red beans/ tomatoes/administration of iron preparations).
   G. abdominal pains (dull/sharp) (note location).
   H. jaundice.
   I. periumbilical/flank ecchymosis.
   J. other _____

2. Knowledge deficit related to:
   A. fluid/diet changes.
   B. abdominal distress.
   C. change in bowel habits.
   D. dyspnea.
   E. expanding midline mass.
   F. medication administration/adverse reactions.
   G. other _____

3. Decreased cardiac output related to:
   A. abdominal crisis.
   B. shock.
   C. hemorrhage.
   D. other _____

   _____

4. Pain related to:
   A. hemorrhage.
   B. shock.
   C. other _____

   _____

5. Ineffective individual/family coping related to:
   A. abdominal pain.
   B. dyspnea.
   C. nausea/vomiting.
   D. weakness.
   E. excessive demands of condition.
   F. other _____

   _____

6. Potential fluid volume deficit related to:
   A. anorexia.
   B. vomiting.
   C. abdominal pain.
   D. immobility.
   E. weakness.
   F. bleeding.
   G. other _____

   _____

7. Self-care deficit: feeding/bathing/grooming/dressing/ambulation/
   toileting related to:
   A. weakness.
   B. nausea/vomiting.
   C. confinement to bed.
   D. abdominal pain.
   E. dyspnea.
   F. other _____

   _____

8. Impaired home maintenance management related to:
   A. abdominal pain.

    B. weakness.

    C. nausea/vomiting.

    D. immobility.

    E. dyspnea.

    F. other _____

    _____

9. Constipation/Diarrhea/Melena related to:

    A. poor fluid intake.

    B. poor/inappropriate diet.

    C. anxiety.

    D. food poisoning.

    E. pain.

    F. other _____

    _____

10. Impaired physical mobility related to:

    A. nausea/vomiting.

    B. weakness.

    C. expanding midline abdominal mass.

    D. dyspnea.

    E. other _____

    _____

11. Noncompliance with therapy related to:

    A. denial.

    B. lack of support in home.

    C. intolerance of diet.

    D. immobility.

    E. other _____

    _____

12. Altered nutrition: less than body requirements related to:

    A. nausea/vomiting/indigestion.

    B. bleeding gums.

    C. weakness.

    D. malabsorption/intestinal obstruction.

    E. constipation/diarrhea.

    F. pain.

    G. fear of food poisoning.

    H. other _____

    _____

13. Potential for injury related to:
    A. delay in seeking medical treatment.
    B. food poisoning.
    C. hemorrhage.
    D. perforation.
    E. expanding midline mass.
    F. other _____

    _____

14. Ineffective breathing pattern related to:
    A. dyspnea.
    B. pain.
    C. other _____

    _____

15. Sleep pattern disturbance related to:
    A. pain.
    B. nausea/vomiting.
    C. hemorrhage.
    D. other _____

    _____

II. SHORT-TERM GOALS

1. Client/Family will seek medical attention for adverse GI symptoms after 1 R.N. visit.
2. Client/Family will take vital signs as ordered after 1–2–3 R.N. visits.
3. Client/Family will administer prescribed medication as ordered after 1–2–3 R.N. visits.
4. Client will consume fluids/diet as ordered after 1–2 R.N. visits.
5. Client/Family will perform appropriate skin care as ordered after 1–2 R.N. visits.
6. Client will exercise/rest/ambulate appropriately as ordered after 1–2 R.N. visits.
7. Client/Family will keep emergency phone numbers readily available after 1 R.N. visit.
8. Client/Family will change dressings as ordered after 1–2 R.N. visits.

III. LONG-TERM GOALS

1. GI tract will function normally in 1–2 weeks.

2. Independent activities of daily living will be resumed in 1–2 weeks.
3. Optimal level of health will be achieved in 1–2 weeks.

IV. OUTCOME CRITERIA

1. Vital signs are normal.
2. Swallowing is normal.
3. Skin/Mucous membrane is healthy and intact.
4. Stool is normal color and consistency.
5. Bowel habits remain normal.
6. Meals are appropriately digested.
7. Weight is normal.
8. Peristalsis is normal.
9. Pain is relieved.
10. Kidneys function normally.
11. Cardiovascular system functions normally.
12. Client states he/she feels better.

V. NURSING INTERVENTION/TREATMENT

1. R.N. will, through routine history and physical examination, assess GI status and vital signs, noting questionable abnormal signs/symptoms, and advance of condition; will determine if emergency exists.
2. R.N. will perform any testing in the home, if possible (e.g., stool for guaiac) and report to M.D. immediately.
3. For suspicious color of stool, R.N. will determine what client has been consuming that might be influencing color (e.g., red beans, tomatoes, iron preparations).
4. For overt abnormal signs/symptoms, R.N. will assess entire GI tract:
   A. mouth—for discoloration/bleeding gums/loose or missing teeth/sores/color and texture of tongue/anorexia/nausea/vomiting/dysphagia/dyspepsia/chalasia/pain.
   B. esophagus—for regurgitation/hiatus hernia.
   C. stomach–for ulcers/burning sensation/gnawing epigastric pain (note onset and location of pain)/hematemesis/gastroenteritis/food allergy/poisoning.
   D. gallbladder—for jaundice/sharp upper-right-quadrant pain, especially following a meal/nausea/vomiting/tenderness over

site/angina-like symptoms/stabbing, burning pain/tightening pressure around chest and back/shortness of breath/pain radiating to right shoulder and back/diaphoresis.

E. duodenum, jejunum, ileum, rectum, and anus—for burning/ pain/change in bowel habits (diarrhea, constipation, melena)/ obstruction/perforation/inflammation/peritonitis/appendicitis/ diverticulitis/fecal impaction/abcess formation/periumbilical ecchymosis/flank ecchymosis/subcutaneous emphysema/ ascites/expanding midline mass/rebound tenderness over McBurney's point/board-like abdomen/hemorrhoids/ abdominal pain.

5. R.N. will ask client to point to area in question. R.N. will first visually examine area in order to prevent possible further injury. If no distress is noted, palpation, percussion, or auscultation may be performed. Evidence of expanding midline mass could indicate abdominal aortic aneurysm; manipulation should not occur.

6. R.N. will administer prescribed medication or have client/family administer medication as ordered, with notation of side effects (1. R.N. will note side effects. 2. R.N. will explain side effects to client).

7. R.N. will immediately notify M.D. of adverse reactions or increasing signs/symptoms of distress.

8. R.N. will instruct client/family in dressing change.

9. R.N. will provide M.D. with follow-up reports and discharge summary when case closes.

10. R.N. will notify client/family/H.H.A./significant others when case will close.

Allergy
Care Plan

I. NURSING DIAGNOSIS

1. Knowledge deficit related to specific type of allergy, desensitization, and treatment.
2. Pain related to:
   A. biological agent(s).
   B. chemical agent(s).
   C. physical agent(s).
   D. psychological agent(s).
   E. other _____

   _____

3. Ineffective breathing patterns related to contact with:
   A. dust.
   B. pollen.
   C. emotional stress.
   D. animals (e.g., cats, dogs, horses, chickens).
   E. food (e.g., chocolate, fish, eggs, alcohol, strawberries, cheese, beef, orange juice).
   F. drugs (e.g., antibiotics, anesthetics, narcotics).
   G. plants (e.g., poison ivy, poison sumac, poison oak).
   H. cosmetics/perfumes/lotions.
   I. soaps, detergents/industrial chemicals.
   J. clothing (e.g., of wool, nylon, rayon fabric).
   K. exposure to sunlight.
   L. other _____

   _____

4. Altered nutrition: less than body requirements related to:
    A. gastrointestinal/pulmonary disturbances.
    B. other _____

    _____

5. Ineffective individual/family coping related to:
    A. skin rash.
    B. frequent sneezing.
    C. excessive lacrimation.
    D. rhinitus.
    E. coughing.
    F. dyspnea.
    G. pain.
    H. urticaria.
    I. other _____

    _____

6. Sleep pattern disturbance related to:
    A. skin rash.
    B. sneezing.
    C. excessive lacrimation.
    D. rhinitus.
    E. coughing.
    F. pain.
    G. urticaria.
    H. dyspnea.
    I. other _____

    _____

7. Self-care deficit: feeding/bathing/grooming/dressing related to:
    A. skin rash.
    B. dyspnea.
    C. pain.
    D. other _____

    _____

8. Impaired home maintenance management related to:
    A. skin rash.
    B. dyspnea.
    C. pain.
    D. other _____

    _____

9. Noncompliance with therapy related to:
    A. cost of medication/cost of therapy/poor insurance coverage.
    B. lengthy procedure for application/administration of medications.
    C. other _____
       _____

10. Potential impaired skin integrity related to:
    A. uncontrollable scratching/urticaria.
    B. bleeding.
    C. vesiculation.
    D. drying/cracking.
    E. other _____
       _____

II. SHORT-TERM GOALS

1. Client/Family will seek skin/laboratory testing after 1–2 R.N. visits.
2. Client/Family will state known or suspected allergen after 2–3 R.N. visits.
3. Client/Family will avoid known or suspected allergen after 2–3 R.N. visits.
4. Client/Family will apply lotions/ointments/solutions/sprays/ creams as ordered after 1–2 R.N. visits.
5. Client/Family will take antihistamines/cortisone preparations/ analgesics/tranquilizers as ordered after 1–2 R.N. visits.
6. Client/Family will visit M.D. regularly as ordered after 1–2 R.N. visits.
7. Client/Family will avoid emotional/job stress as ordered after 1–2 R.N. visits.
8. Client/Family will rest daily as ordered after 1–2 R.N. visits.
9. Client/Family will bathe as ordered by physician after 1–2 R.N. visits.
10. Client/Family will avoid extreme sunlight exposure as ordered after 1–2 R.N. visits.

III. LONG-TERM GOALS

1. Avoidance of allergen/irritant will result in normal GI respiratory/ skin integrity in 3–4 weeks.
2. Independent activities of daily living will be resumed in 2–3 weeks.
3. Optimal level of health will be achieved in 3–4 weeks.

IV. OUTCOME CRITERIA

1. Vital signs are normal.
2. Respiratory tract remains clear.
3. Edema has subsided.
4. Vomiting/Diarrhea has subsided.
5. Skin color and integrity remain normal.
6. Appetite remains normal.
7. Weight remains within normal limits.
8. Laboratory test results remain normal.
9. Client returns to school/work/play.
10. Client states he/she feels better.

V. NURSING INTERVENTION/TREATMENT

1. R.N. will encourage client/family to visit allergist as early as possible.
2. R.N. will assess possible irritant or allergen on initial history and physical examination in home; will determine location of home—industrial, suburban, or farm locale—for possible environmental etiology; will assess entire family history.
3. R.N. will instruct client/family on:
   A. avoidance of irritant or allergen.
   B. substitutions for irritant or allergen (drugs/food/clothing/pets).
   C. application/administration of oral medication/creams/ointments/solutions/lotions/sprays with special attention to side effects.
   D. immediate notification of M.D. of adverse reactions or change in condition.
   E. operation and cleaning of respiratory equipment (humidifiers/oxygen/IPPB).
   F. routine M.D. appointments, especially for desensitization.
   G. avoidance of immunization during acute period.
   H. avoidance of people with colds or infections.
   I. laboratory testing.
4. R.N. will refer client to lung associations/community groups for additional educational materials and further assistance.
5. R.N. will provide M.D. with follow-up reports and discharge summary when case closes.
6. R.N. will notify client/family/H.H.A./significant others when case will close.

Amputee
Care Plan

I. NURSING DIAGNOSIS

1. Anxiety related to:
   A. bandaging stump.
   B. dressing care.
   C. application of prosthesis.
   D. transfer exercises.
   E. stair climbing.
   F. range-of-motion exercise.
   G. crutch walking.
   H. other _____

2. Potential for disuse syndrome related to:
   A. phantom-limb sensation.
   B. impaired mobility.
   C. impaired healing.
   D. poor administration of medication.
   E. other _____

3. Ineffective individual/family coping related to:
   A. poor mobility.
   B. phantom-limb sensation.
   C. irritability.
   D. cost of medical care/poor insurance coverage.
   E. anger/hostility.
   F. delayed healing.

   G. difficulty using cane/walker/crutches/prosthesis/wheelchair.

   H. other _____

_____

4. Fear related to:
   A. ambulation.
   B. using a prosthetic device.
   C. rejection by significant others.
   D. other _____

_____

5. Grieving related to loss of a limb.
6. Impaired home maintenance management related to impaired mobility.
7. Knowledge deficit related to:
   A. bandaging stump.
   B. dressing care.
   C. application of prosthesis.
   D. transfer exercises.
   E. stair climbing.
   F. range-of-motion exercise.
   G. crutch walking.
   H. medication administration/adverse reactions.
   I. other _____

_____

8. Impaired physical mobility related to:
   A. amputation.
   B. delayed healing.
   C. noncompliance with exercise program.
   D. other _____

_____

9. Altered parenting related to immobility.
10. Temporary/Permanent self-care deficit: feeding/dressing/bathing/grooming/toileting related to immobility.
11. Self-esteem disturbance related to loss of a limb.
12. Sexual dysfunction related to:
    A. weakness.
    B. fear of rejection.
    C. impaired body image.
    D. other _____

_____

13. Potential impaired skin integrity related to:
    A. delayed healing at surgical site.
    B. poor dressing technique.
    C. other _____

    _____

14. Sleep pattern disturbance related to:
    A. pain.
    B. awkwardness in turning.
    C. restlessness.
    D. other _____

    _____

II. SHORT-TERM GOALS

1. Client will perform prescribed range-of-motion exercise as ordered after 1–2–3 R.N./P.T./O.T. visits.
2. Client will perform hyperextension exercises as ordered after 2–3 R.N./P.T./O.T. visits.
3. Client will transfer from bed to wheelchair/commode/chair after 2–3 R.N./P.T. visits.
4. Client will arise from bed/chair and stand after 3–4 R.N./P.T. visits.
5. Client will stand on toes while holding onto chair after 3–4 R.N./P.T. visits.
6. Client will balance on one leg without support after 4–5 R.N./P.T. visits.
7. Client will perform crutch walking as ordered after 5–6 R.N./P.T. visits.
8. Client/Family will bandage stump correctly after 1–2 R.N./P.T./O.T. visits.
9. Client/Family will change dressing as ordered after 1–2–3 R.N./P.T. visits.
10. Client will apply transcutaneous electrical nerve stimulation machine/heat, massage, whirlpool, or change position to counteract muscle spasm after 1–2 R.N./P.T. visits.
11. Family will protect stump with plastic wrap if client is incontinent after 1–2 R.N. visits.
12. Client will apply prosthetic device correctly after 8–10 R.N./P.T./O.T. visits.
13. Client will employ good skin care and personal hygiene measures to stump after 1–2 R.N. visits.

14. Client (arm amputee) will prepare food with one hand after 1–2–3–4 R.N./P.T./O.T. visits.
15. Client will perform independent activities of daily living after 1–2–3–4–5–6 R.N./P.T./O.T. visits.
16. Client will seek vocational skills counseling/job training after ambulation occurs after 6–12 R.N. visits.
17. Client/Family will administer medications as ordered after 1–2–3 R.N. visits.
18. Client/Family will state three adverse reactions to medications after 1–2 R.N. visits.
19. Client/Family will immediately notify M.D. of adverse reactions to medications/change in condition after 1–2 R.N. visits.
20. Client will seek laboratory testing/M.D. appointments after 1–2 R.N. visits.

III. LONG-TERM GOALS

1. Independent activities of daily living will be resumed in 1–2 weeks.
2. Optimal level of health will be achieved in 4–6 weeks.
3. Normal reintegration into community will occur in 4–6 weeks.

IV. OUTCOME CRITERIA

1. Vital signs are normal.
2. Granulation occurs.
3. Skin is healthy and intact.
4. Laboratory test results are normal.
5. Independent ambulation occurs.
6. Client is alert, oriented, sociable, and in good health.
7. Circulation is normal; pulses are equal and palpable.
8. Chest is clear.
9. Appetite is normal.
10. Bowel/Bladder control is normal.
11. Client states he/she feels better.
12. Client is employed.

V. NURSING INTERVENTION/TREATMENT

1. R.N. will communicate with hospital discharge planner about long-term and rehabilitation goals for client and equipment needed in home.

2. R.N. will arrange for all necessary equipment to be delivered to home upon hospital discharge.
3. R.N. will see that client obtains prescriptions/M.D. appointment before hospital discharge.
4. R.N. will instruct client/family/H.H.A. on:
   A. proper hand-washing technique/personal hygiene.
   B. dressing care.
   C. skin care.
   D. exercise/rest.
   E. fluid intake/dietary regimen prescribed.
   F. technique for bandaging stump.
   G. application of prosthetic device.
   H. crutch walking/use of cane/quad cane/walker.
   I. medication administration/adverse reactions.
   J. immediate notification of M.D. of adverse reactions or change in condition.
   K. medication administration/adverse reactions.
   L. literature on stump conditioning/ambulation/clubs/ organizations.
   M. laboratory testing/M.D. appointments.
5. R.N. will provide M.D. with follow-up reports and discharge summary when case closes.
6. R.N. will notify client/family/H.H.A./significant others when case will close.

Amyotrophic Lateral Sclerosis Care Plan (Progressive Spinal Muscular Atrophy)

I. NURSING DIAGNOSIS

1. Moderate/Severe anxiety related to:
   A. poor prognosis.
   B. dependence on others for care.
   C. immobility.
   D. loss of control.
   E. difficulty with mastication.
   F. dysphagia.
   G. difficulty speaking.
   H. other _____

2. Potential impaired skin integrity related to:
   A. muscle wasting.
   B. poor exercise tolerance.
   C. loss of control.
   D. difficulty with ambulation.
   E. poor positioning.
   F. other _____

3. Grieving related to:
   A. loss of control.

    B. dependence on others for care.

    C. progressive physical decline.

    D. fear of death.

    E. other _____

    _____

4. Ineffective individual/family coping related to:

    A. rejection by significant others.

    B. loss of control.

    C. progressive physical decline.

    D. poor prognosis.

    E. labile/inappropriate emotions.

    F. cost of medical care/poor insurance coverage.

    G. excessive physical care demands.

    H. other _____

    _____

5. Constipation/bowel incontinence/diarrhea related to:

    A. poor fluid/dietary intake.

    B. muscle wasting.

    C. loss of control.

    D. dysphagia.

    E. inability to prepare adequate meals.

    F. poor mobility.

    G. other _____

    _____

6. Potential fluid volume deficit related to:

    A. poor intake.

    B. dysphagia.

    C. other _____

    _____

7. Partial/Total self-care deficit: feeding/bathing/dressing/grooming/toileting related to:

    A. progressive decline in condition.

    B. extreme weakness.

    C. loss of control/spasticity.

    D. labile/inappropriate emotions.

    E. other _____

    _____

8. Impaired home maintenance management related to:

    A. labile/inappropriate emotions.

    B. loss of control/spasticity.

    C. progressive physical decline.

    D. rejection by significant others.

    E. excessive physical care demands.

    F. other _____

    _____

9. Knowledge deficit related to:

    A. disease process and general supportive therapy.

    B. progressive physical limitations/poor prognosis.

    C. other _____

    _____

10. Self-esteem disturbance related to loss of independence/ dependence on others for care.

11. Impaired physical mobility related to early weakness/spasticity/ atrophy of muscles.

12. Noncompliance with therapy related to:

    A. denial.

    B. lack of support in home.

    C. rejection by significant others.

    D. fear of death.

    E. other _____

    _____

13. Altered nutrition: potential for more than body requirements related to:

    A. dysphagia.

    B. difficulty with mastication.

    C. difficulty with meal selection/preparation.

    D. labile/inappropriate emotions.

    E. other _____

    _____

14. Altered parenting related to:

    A. immobility.

    B. extreme weakness.

    C. labile/inappropriate emotions.

    D. difficulty speaking.

    E. fatigue.

    F. other _____

    _____

15. Potential for injury related to:
    A. muscular weakness/atrophy of hands/arms/legs.
    B. loss of control.
    C. accidents.
    D. labile/inappropriate emotions.
    E. refusal to follow medical instructions.
    F. other _____
    _____

16. Ineffective airway clearance related to:
    A. dysphagia.
    B. obstruction of airway.
    C. potential for choking.
    D. ineffective suctioning of tracheostomy.
    E. inappropriate cough reflex.
    F. other _____
    _____

17. Sensory/Perceptual alterations related to:
    A. weakness/spasticity/atrophy of muscles.
    B. medication administration.
    C. other _____
    _____

18. Sexual dysfunction related to:
    A. weakness/spasticity/atrophy of muscles.
    B. labile/inappropriate emotions.
    C. apathy.
    D. rejection by significant others.
    E. other _____
    _____

19. Potential impaired skin integrity related to:
    A. immobility.
    B. poor nutritional habits.
    C. poor personal hygiene habits.
    D. lack of skilled assistance in home.
    E. other _____
    _____

20. Sleep pattern disturbances related to:
    A. restlessness.
    B. labile/inappropriate emotions.
    C. fear of loss of control.

    D. excessive noise in home/apartment.

    E. fear of death.

    F. other _____

_____

21. Impaired verbal communication related to:

    A. tracheostomy.

    B. weakness.

    C. other _____

_____

22. Social isolation related to:

    A. confinement to home.

    B. rejection by significant others.

    C. other _____

_____

II. SHORT-TERM GOALS

1. Client/Family will verbalize fears, questions, and concerns after 1–2–3–4 R.N. visits.

2. Client/Family will administer medication as ordered after 1–2–3 R.N. visits.

3. Client/Family will immediately contact M.D. about any adverse effects or signs/symptoms of complications of disease after 1–2 R.N. visits.

4. Client/Family will keep emergency phone numbers available at all times after 1 R.N. visit.

5. Client/Family will prepare and consume nutritionally sound meals after 1–2 R.N. visits.

6. Client/Family will provide tube feedings as ordered after 1–2–3 R.N. visits.

7. Client/Family will practice prescribed bowel regimen as ordered after 1–2 R.N. visits.

8. Client/Family will practice good oral/personal hygiene after 1–2 R.N. visits.

9. Client will exercise/rest as ordered after 1–2 R.N. visits.

10. Client will avoid fatigue as ordered after 1–2–3 R.N. visits.

11. Client/Family will practice good transfer technique from bed to wheelchair/commode/standing position after 1–2–3–4 R.N./P.T./O.T. visits.

12. Client will follow speech exercises as ordered after 1–2–3–4–5–6 R.N./S.T. visits.

13. Client/Family will follow respiratory therapy instructions as ordered for deep breathing/coughing/use of respiratory equipment after 1–2 R.N./R.T. visits.
14. Client/Family will clean and store respiratory equipment as ordered after 1–2 R.N./R.T. visits.
15. Client will wear/use braces/supportive devices as ordered after 1–2–3–4–5–6 R.N./P.T./O.T. visits.
16. Client/Family will clean inner cannula of tracheostomy tube correctly after 1–2–3–4 R.N. visits.
17. Client/Family will provide adequate catheter care as ordered after 1–2–3 R.N. visits.
18. Client/Family will change urinary drainage bag 1–2 times per month or as needed after 1–2–3 R.N. visits.
19. Client/Family will accurately record intake and output after 1–2 R.N. visits.
20. Client/Family will record weight daily after 1 R.N. visit.
21. Client/Family will seek diversional activities after 1–2 R.N. visits.
22. Client/Family will seek laboratory testing/M.D. appointments as ordered after 1–2 R.N. visits.

III. LONG-TERM GOALS

1. Preservation of muscle tone will be accomplished throughout course of disease.
2. Optimal nutritional status will be maintained throughout course of disease.
3. Adequate communication will be maintained throughout course of disease.
4. Independent activities of daily living will be resumed in 2–3 weeks.
5. Optimal level of health will be maintained throughout course of disease.

IV. OUTCOME CRITERIA

1. Vital signs are normal.
2. Appetite remains normal.
3. Nutritionally sound meals are consumed.
4. Swallowing reflex remains normal.
5. Adequate mastication is maintained.
6. Speech remains effective/unimpaired.

7. Emotional stability is maintained.

8. Range of motion is maintained in all four limbs.

9. Tongue control is normal.

10. Deep-tendon reflexes remain normal.

11. Chest remains clear; respirations are normal.

12. Laboratory test results are within normal limits.

13. Bowel/Bladder functioning remains normal.

14. Ambulation occurs normally.

15. Client states he/she feels better.

V. NURSING INTERVENTION/TREATMENT

1. R.N. will consult with hospital discharge planner about treatment, prognosis, insurance coverage, and rehabilitation goals for client.

2. All necessary medical equipment will be delivered to home before client's hospital discharge.

3. R.N. will instruct client/family/H.H.A. on:

   A. monitoring and recording of vital signs; if possible, R.N. will teach family member to monitor blood pressures.

   B. daily recording of intake and output.

   C. daily recording of weight.

   D. range-of-motion exercise/rest as ordered (avoidance of fatigue). R.N. will consult with P.T., if assigned, regarding types of exercises/weight bearing/transfer activities.

   E. application of splints/braces.

   F. deep-breathing exercises/chest physical therapy/operation, cleaning, and storage of respiratory equipment.

   G. aseptic technique.

   H. tracheostomy care/use of heated mist collar/ventilator care.

   I. catheter care as ordered.

   J. bowel regimen (use of laxatives/enemas/suppositories) as ordered/use of a fracture bedpan.

   K. fluid intake/dietary regimen/administration of tube feedings/ hyperalimentation as ordered/gastrostomy feedings.

   L. medication as ordered/adverse reactions.

   M. immediate notification of M.D. of adverse reactions or signs/ symptoms of complications of disease.

   N. oral and personal hygiene.

   O. skin care.

   P. turning or repositioning in bed every 2 hours.

Q. keeping emergency phone numbers available in home.

R. laboratory testing/M.D. appointments.

S. diversional activities.

T. speech activities/pharyngeal exercises/prosthetic equipment/ electronic communicator.

U. career/financial counseling.

4. R.N. will assign additional personnel to case if ordered (e.g., R.T., M.S.W., P.T., O.T., H.H.A., home attendant/homemaker/ housekeeper).

5. R.N. will provide client with names of resource personnel/ professional organizations/clubs for additional information.

6. R.N. will provide M.D. with follow-up reports and discharge summary when case closes.

7. R.N. will notify client/family/H.H.A./significant others when case will close.

Anemia
Care Plan

I. NURSING DIAGNOSIS

1. Knowledge deficit related to:
   A. signs/symptoms of anemia.
   B. laboratory testing.
   C. nutritional requirements.
   D. prevention/treatment of anemia.
   E. medication administration/adverse reactions.
   F. other _____
   _____

2. Fatigue related to:
   A. poor fluid/dietary intake.
   B. hemorrhaging.
   C. poor absorption of vitamin B_{12}.
   D. other _____
   _____

3. Altered nutrition: more than body requirements related to:
   A. poor meal preparation.
   B. poor fluid/dietary intake.
   C. other _____
   _____

4. Partial/Total self-care deficit: feeding/bathing/dressing/grooming/
   toileting related to:
   A. weakness/fatigue.

    B. dyspnea on exertion.

    C. hemorrhagic tendencies.

    D. bone and joint pain.

    E. fever.

    F. infection.

    G. anorexia/indigestion.

    H. constipation/diarrhea.

    I. sore mouth/beefy tongue.

    J. other _____

5. Noncompliance with therapy related to:

    A. denial.

    B. anger/hostility.

    C. grieving.

    D. fear.

    E. impending pain of injections.

    F. cost of testing/cost of therapy/poor insurance coverage.

    G. other _____

6. Potential for injury related to:

    A. weakness.

    B. sensitivity to cold.

    C. mental deterioration/changes in sensorium.

    D. drug therapy (e.g., radiation/antimicrobials/anticonvulsants/
       antithyroid drugs/antidiabetic agents/antihistamines/sedatives/
       analgesics).

    E. unsteady gait.

    F. other _____

7. Impaired physical mobility related to weakness/fatigue.

8. Impaired home maintenance management related to:

    A. weakness/fatigue.

    B. unsteadiness of gait/impaired mobility.

    C. hemorrhaging.

    D. dyspnea.

    E. pain.

    F. other _____

9. Impaired verbal communication related to changes in sensorium.

10. Ineffective breathing pattern related to dyspnea.
11. Decreased cardiac output related to:
    A. hypoxia.
    B. palpitations.
    C. chest pain.
    D. hemorrhaging.
    E. other _____

    _____

12. Impaired social interaction related to:
    A. pain.
    B. palpitations.
    C. weakness/fatigue.
    D. dyspnea.
    E. other _____

    _____

II. SHORT-TERM GOALS

1. Client/Family will obtain proper laboratory testing as ordered after 1–2 R.N. visits.
2. Client/Family will obtain prescribed medication after 1–2 R.N. visits.
3. Client will rest periodically throughout day as ordered after 1–2 R.N. visits.
4. Client/Family will perform mouth care as ordered after 1–2 R.N. visits.
5. Client will consume nutritionally sound meals after 1–2 R.N. visits.
6. Client/Family will elevate head of bed for dyspnea after 1–2 R.N. visits.
7. Client/Family will administer oxygen if needed after 1–2 R.N. visits.
8. Client/Family will verbalize fears, anxieties, and questions after 1–2 R.N. visits.
9. Client will refrain from unnecessary exertion after 1–2 R.N. visits.
10. Client/Family will maintain nonstressful environment after 1–2 R.N. visits.
11. Client/Family will record daily weights as ordered after 1–2 R.N. visits.
12. Client/Family will record intake and output daily after 1 R.N. visit.

13. Client will ambulate/exercise as ordered after 1–2 R.N. visits.
14. Client/Family will participate in diversional activities after 1–2 R.N. visits.
15. Client/Family will administer prescribed medication/injections after 1–2 R.N. visits.
16. Client/Family will keep M.D. appointments as scheduled after 1–2 R.N. visits.

III. LONG-TERM GOALS

1. Normal erythropoiesis will occur in 3–4 months.
2. Independent activities of daily living will be resumed in 1–2 weeks.
3. Adequate nutritional status will be achieved in 2–3 weeks.
4. Optimal level of health will be achieved in 3–4 weeks.

IV. OUTCOME CRITERIA

1. Vital signs remain normal.
2. Laboratory test results remain normal.
3. Skin color and integrity remain normal.
4. Mucous membrane remains healthy and intact.
5. EKG remains within normal sinus rhythm.
6. Chest remains clear.
7. Gait and ambulation remain steady.
8. Appetite remains normal.
9. Urine output remains clear, yellow, and in sufficient quantity.
10. Bowel elimination remains normal.
11. All stages of grief and grieving are worked through.
12. Client states he/she feels better.

V. NURSING INTERVENTION/TREATMENT

1. R.N. will instruct client/family/H.H.A. on:
   A. monitoring and recording of vital signs.
   B. daily recording of weight.
   C. fluid/dietary needs.
   D. strict recording of daily intake and output.
   E. ambulation/exercise/rest periods as ordered.
   F. avoidance of emotional stress.

G. diversional activities.

H. laboratory testing.

I. hemorrhagic tendencies.

J. oxygen administration/elevation of head of bed.

K. mouth and skin care.

L. breathing exercises.

M. administration of medications, especially IM injections of vitamins B_{12}, B_1, with specific attention to adverse effects; will encourage strict asepsis.

N. immediate notification of M.D. of hemorrhaging, sensorium changes, side effects of medication.

O. sensitivity to cold.

P. using footboards/bed cradles to avoid excessive weight on extremities.

Q. follow-up M.D. appointments.

2. R.N. will allow client to function independently whenever possible; will allow verbalization of all fears, anxieties, and concerns.

3. R.N. will provide additional services (e.g., P.T., medical, social services) whenever possible.

4. R.N. will provide M.D. with follow-up reports and discharge summary when case closes.

5. R.N. will notify client/family/H.H.A./significant others when case will close.

Arteriovenous Shunt Fistula/Graft Care Plan

I. NURSING DIAGNOSIS

1. Anxiety related to:
   - A. absence of thrill.
   - B. possible infection.
   - C. possible infiltration.
   - D. other _____

2. Potential impaired skin integrity related to:
   - A. poor positioning of needle.
   - B. repeated venipunctures.
   - C. poor aseptic technique.
   - D. clotting.
   - E. other _____

3. Potential for infection related to:
   - A. poor hand-washing technique.
   - B. poor aseptic technique.
   - C. poor dressing care.
   - D. scratching of skin.
   - E. other _____

4. Noncompliance with therapy related to:
   A. fear of hemorrhage.
   B. fear of infection.
   C. lack of understanding of procedure.
   D. other _____

5. Potential for injury: infection/hematoma/clotting related to:
   A. poor hand-washing technique.
   B. repeated venipunctures.
   C. weakening in vessel wall.
   D. poor injection technique.
   E. other _____

6. Impaired tissue integrity related to:
   A. hematoma formation.
   B. infiltration.
   C. clotting.
   D. infection.
   E. other _____

7. Knowledge deficit related to:
   A. palpation of thrill.
   B. prevention of infection.
   C. good hand-washing technique.
   D. dressing care.
   E. muscle-strengthening exercises.
   F. repeated venipuncture sites.
   G. hematoma formation/infiltration/clotting/hemorrhage.
   H. ingredients in over-the-counter medications (e.g., sugar, caffeine, sodium, potassium).
   I. other _____

8. Ineffective individual coping related to:
   A. constant complaints of pain/discomfort.
   B. rejection by significant others.
   C. numerous physician visits.
   D. financial insecurity.
   E. other _____

II. SHORT-TERM GOALS

1. Client/Family will verbalize fears, anxieties and concerns after 1–2–3 R.N. visits.
2. Client/Family will demonstrate proper hand-washing technique after 1–2–3 R.N. visits.
3. Client/Family will observe extremity for signs/symptoms of hematoma/infiltration/clotting/aneurysm/infection and will immediately report to M.D. after 1–2–3 R.N. visits.
4. Client/Family will demonstrate proper dressing care to site after 1–2–3 R.N. visits.
5. Client/Family will check "bruit" several times each day after 1–2–3 R.N. visits.
6. Client/Family will bathe site using antibacterial soap after 1–2–3 R.N. visits.
7. Client/Family will lubricate skin over fistula with cocoa butter, baby oil, or lanolin after 1–2–3 R.N. visits.
8. Client/Family will avoid taking blood pressure in designated arm after 1–2–3 R.N. visits.
9. Client/Family will avoid having blood samples taken in designated arm after 1–2–3 R.N. visits.
10. Client/Family will engage in prescribed exercises after 1–2–3 R.N. visits.

III. LONG-TERM GOALS

1. Access to the circulatory system for hemodialysis will occur in 1–4 weeks.
2. Regulation of the fluid balance of the body will occur in 1–4 weeks.
3. Removal of toxic substances and metabolic wastes from the body will occur in 1–4 weeks.
4. Independent activities of daily living will be resumed in 1–2 weeks.
5. Optimal level of health will be achieved in 3–4 weeks.

IV. OUTCOME CRITERIA

1. Skin is clear, intact, and healthy.
2. Thrill is palpated.
3. Bruit confirms normal blood flow.
4. Blood flow through shunt is bright red.

5. Shunt feels as warm as skin.

6. Forearm veins are enlarged and prominent.

7. Mobility is unimpaired to extremity.

8. Vital signs and blood pressure are normal.

V. NURSING INTERVENTION/TREATMENT

1. R.N. will confer with hospital discharge planner/M.D. for shunt/fistula/graft instructions.

2. R.N. will assess exit sites for signs of infection, hematoma, infiltration, poor blood flow, clotting, aneurysm, color of blood, skin temperature and bruit.

3. R.N. will instruct client/family/H.H.A. on:

   A. proper hand-washing technique.

   B. aseptic technique.

   C. cannulation (selection of venipuncture sites, types of gauge, fistula needles, etc.).

   D. dressing care/removal after 4–8 hours.

   E. troubleshooting complications such as bleeding, hematoma, infiltration, poor blood flow, clotting, aneurysm, infection, and absence of bruit.

   F. cleansing of site with antibacterial soap.

   G. lubrication of skin over fistula.

   H. avoidance of tourniquet application, except for dialysis.

   I. avoidance of blood pressure in affected arm.

   J. blood samples from appropriate sites.

   K. exercise (squeezing a rubber ball frequently during day and placing arm in warm water for 3–5 minutes, alternately opening and closing fist under water).

   L. rest.

   M. record keeping.

4. R.N. will provide M.D. with follow-up reports and discharge summary when case closes.

5. R.N. will notify client/family/H.H.A./significant others when case will close.

Asthma
Care Plan

I. NURSING DIAGNOSIS

1. Anxiety related to:
    A. airway obstruction/restriction.
    B. tightness in chest.
    C. dyspnea/shortness of breath.
    D. wheezing.
    E. diaphoresis.
    F. other _____

2. Knowledge deficit related to:
    A. humidification.
    B. medication administration/adverse reactions.
    C. oxygen therapy.
    D. positioning.
    E. allergens/etiology.
    F. emotional stress.
    G. infection.
    H. ingredients in over-the-counter medications (e.g., sugar, caffeine, sodium, potassium).
    I. other _____

3. Ineffective airway clearance related to:
    A. smooth-muscle spasm of bronchi/larger bronchioles.

B. edema of respiratory mucosa.
C. thick bronchiole secretions.
D. wheezing.
E. other ⸻
⸻

4. Ineffective breathing pattern related to:
A. smooth-muscle spasm of bronchi/larger bronchioles.
B. edema of respiratory mucosa.
C. thick bronchiole secretions.
D. wheezing.
E. other ⸻
⸻

5. Impaired gas exchange related to:
A. airway obstruction/restriction.
B. wheezing.
C. hypoxia.
D. rhonchi/rales.
E. hyperventilation.
F. other ⸻
⸻

6. Powerlessness related to:
A. airway obstruction/restriction.
B. hyperventilation.
C. other ⸻
⸻

7. Sleep pattern disturbance related to:
A. tightness in chest.
B. dyspnea/shortness of breath.
C. wheezing.
D. diaphoresis.
E. hyperventilation.
F. other ⸻
⸻

8. Ineffective individual/family coping related to:
A. increased demands of sick child/adult.
B. cost of medical care/poor insurance coverage.
C. absenteeism from school/work.
D. other ⸻
⸻

II. SHORT-TERM GOALS

1. Client/Family will verbalize all fears, anxieties, and concerns after 1–2 R.N. visits.
2. Client/Family will administer medication as ordered after 1–2 R.N. visits.
3. Client/Family will immediately notify M.D. of adverse reactions or change in condition after 1–2 R.N. visits.
4. Client/Family will contact M.D. at the first indication of a respiratory infection after 1–2 R.N. visits.
5. Client/Family will use respiratory equipment as ordered after 1–2 R.N. visits.
6. Client/Family will avoid smoking, pollutants, allergens after 1–2 R.N. visits.
7. Client/Family will avoid people with colds or infections after 1–2 R.N. visits.
8. Client/Family will prepare nutritionally balanced meals after 1–2 R.N. visits.
9. Client/Family will avoid emotional stress after 1–2 R.N. visits.
10. Client/Family will seek laboratory testing/M.D. appointments as ordered after 1–2 R.N. visits.

III. LONG-TERM GOALS

1. Adequate respiratory functioning will be achieved in 1–2 weeks.
2. Independent activities of daily living will be resumed in 1–2 weeks.
3. Optimal level of health will be achieved in 1–2 weeks.

IV. OUTCOME CRITERIA

1. Vital signs are normal.
2. Wheezing has ceased.
3. Airway is patent.
4. Respirations are normal.
5. Chest sounds clear.
6. Skin color is normal.
7. Laboratory test results are normal.
8. Client states he/she feels better.

V. NURSING INTERVENTION/TREATMENT

1. R.N. will assess general physical status on initial home visit.
2. R.N. will instruct client/family/H.H.A. on:
   A. proper hand-washing technique.
   B. monitoring and recording of vital signs.
   C. oral hygiene.
   D. adequate disposal of tissues and contaminated articles.
   E. fluid intake/diet.
   F. breathing exercises/respiratory therapy and care of equipment.
   G. positioning.
   H. oxygen therapy/precautions.
   I. rest/exercise.
   J. avoidance of allergens and etiologic agents.
   K. avoidance/limitation of smoking.
   L. medication administration/adverse reactions.
   M. immediate notification of M.D. of adverse reactions or change in condition.
   N. avoidance of emotional stress.
   O. laboratory testing/M.D. appointments.
   P. organizations/lung associations for further assistance.
3. R.N. will provide M.D. with follow-up reports and discharge summary when case closes.
4. R.N. will notify client/family/H.H.A./significant others when case will close.

Bowel Training Care Plan

I. NURSING DIAGNOSIS

1. Anxiety related to:
   A. diarrhea.
   B. constipation.
   C. pain.
   D. other _____

   _____

2. Constipation related to:
   A. laxative abuse.
   B. limited fiber in diet.
   C. poor fluid intake.
   D. impaction.
   E. other _____

   _____

3. Pain related to:
   A. improper diet.
   B. distention.
   C. diarrhea.
   D. constipation.
   E. hemorroids.
   F. anal irritation.
   G. other _____

   _____

4. Ineffective individual/family coping related to:
   A. irritability.
   B. pain/discomfort.
   C. incontinence.
   D. diarrhea.
   E. constipation.
   F. other _____

5. Knowledge deficit related to:
   A. fluid/dietary needs.
   B. medication administration/adverse reactions.
   C. enema administration.
   D. use of suppositories.
   E. avoidance of emotional stress.
   F. daily exercise/rest.
   G. other _____

II. SHORT-TERM GOALS

1. Client/Family will verbalize anxieties and concerns after 1–2 R.N. visits.
2. Client will drink 1–2 quarts of fluids daily as ordered after 1–2 R.N. visits.
3. Client will drink warm fluids in morning to stimulate peristalsis after 1–2 R.N. visits.
4. Client will take stool softener/laxatives as ordered after 1–2 R.N. visits.
5. Client will avoid large amounts of binding foods in diet (e.g., cheese, apples, bananas, rice, tea, and chocolate) after 1–2 R.N. visits.
6. Client will set up a daily routine for elimination after 1–2 R.N. visits.
7. Client will participate in physical exercise as ordered after 1–2 R.N. visits.
8. Client/Family will administer a purgative, carminative, anthelmintic, emollient, or medicated or nutritive enema as ordered after 1–2 R.N. visits.

III. LONG-TERM GOALS

1. Regular bowel elimination will be achieved in 1–2 weeks.
2. Adequate nutritional habits will be achieved in 1–2 weeks.
3. Independent activities of daily living will be resumed in 1–2 weeks.
4. Optimal level of health will be achieved in 1–2 weeks.

IV. OUTCOME CRITERIA

1. Vital signs are normal.
2. Daily bowel evacuation is normal.
3. Stool specimens remain normal.
4. Client states he/she feels better.

V. NURSING INTERVENTION/TREATMENT

1. R.N. will encourage client/family to assemble all equipment before visit.
2. R.N. will assess current bowel regimen to determine if modification of habits is necessary.
3. R.N. will instruct client/family/H.H.A. on:
   A. fluid intake/dietary regimen as ordered.
   B. medication administration/adverse reactions.
   C. ingredients in over-the-counter medications (e.g., sugar, caffeine, sodium, potassium).
   D. immediate notification of M.D. of adverse reactions or change in condition.
   E. enema administration and prevention of fecal impaction, and recording color, amount, consistency, and frequency of return.
   F. monitoring and recording of vital signs, especially if client has cardiopulmonary complications.
   G. use of bedpan/commode/rectal tube.
   H. obtaining stool specimens.
   I. laboratory testing/M.D. appointments.
4. R.N. will provide M.D. with follow-up reports and discharge summary when case closes.
5. R.N. will notify client/family/H.H.A./significant others when case will close.

Burn
Care Plan

I. NURSING DIAGNOSIS

1. Knowledge deficit related to:
   A. care of burns.
   B. medication administration/adverse reactions.
   C. prevention and disfigurement.
   D. rehabilitation.
   E. other _____

2. Ineffective breathing pattern related to:
   A. neurogenic shock.
   B. fluid-loss shock.
   C. infection.
   D. smoke inhalation.
   E. tracheal edema.
   F. hypoxia.
   G. obstructed tracheostomy tube.
   H. coma.
   I. other _____

3. Increased cardiac output related to:
   A. fluid loss.
   B. hypoxia.
   C. respiratory distress.
   D. increased metabolic demands.

    E. shock.

    F. poor renal functioning.

    G. electrolyte imbalance.

    H. other _____

    _____

4. Pain related to:

    A. poor healing.

    B. infection.

    C. skin grafting.

    D. wound debridement.

    E. other _____

    _____

5. Impaired verbal communication related to:

    A. extensive burns of neck and face.

    B. tracheostomy.

    C. other _____

    _____

6. Ineffective individual/family coping related to:

    A. severe pain.

    B. impaired body image (disfigurement).

    C. cost of medical care/poor insurance coverage.

    D. inability to work/loss of a job.

    E. other _____

    _____

7. Impaired social interaction related to:

    A. severe pain.

    B. immobility.

    C. poor vision.

    D. weakness.

    E. other _____

    _____

8. Fear related to:

    A. potential death.

    B. disfigurement.

    C. wound debridement.

    D. skin grafting.

    E. cost of medical care/poor insurance coverage.

    F. other _____

    _____

9. Actual/Potential fluid volume deficit related to:
    A. extensive area of burn/burns.
    B. poor tissue perfusion.
    C. shock.
    D. bleeding (hemoptysis/hematuria).
    E. inadequate fluid intake.
    F. other _____
    _____

10. Anticipatory grieving related to:
    A. fear of death.
    B. disfigurement.
    C. loss of a limb.
    D. feelings of guilt.
    E. other _____
    _____

11. Impaired home maintenance management related to:
    A. weakness.
    B. immobility.
    C. poor ambulation.
    D. dependence on others for care.
    E. other _____
    _____

12. Potential for injury related to:
    A. fire hazards in the home.
    B. secondary infection.
    C. refusal to comply with medical instructions.
    D. other _____
    _____

13. Impaired physical mobility related to:
    A. extensive area of burns.
    B. skin grafting.
    C. infection.
    D. other _____
    _____

14. Noncompliance with therapy related to:
    A. denial.
    B. fear.
    C. weakness.

     D. cost of medical treatment/cost of supplies/poor insurance
       coverage.

     E. other _____

     _____

15. Altered nutrition: more than body requirements related to:
     A. fluid loss.
     B. weight loss.
     C. formation of ulcers.
     D. psychologic stress.
     E. immobility.
     F. secondary infection.
     G. skin grafting.
     H. other _____

     _____

16. Altered parenting related to:
     A. immobility.
     B. weakness.
     C. difficulty ambulating.
     D. other _____

     _____

17. Self-care deficit: feeding/bathing/dressing/grooming related to:
     A. weakness.
     B. immobility.
     C. difficulty ambulating.
     D. dyspnea.
     E. secondary infections.
     F. skin grafting.
     G. other _____

     _____

18. Self-esteem disturbance related to:
     A. disfigurement.
     B. dependence on others for care.
     C. other _____

     _____

19. Sexual dysfunction related to:
     A. healing of burns.
     B. skin grafting.
     C. disfigurement.

  D. eschar formation.
  E. pain.
  F. other _____
  _____

20. Impaired skin integrity related to:
  A. burns.
  B. skin grafting.
  C. eschar removal.
  D. secondary skin infection.
  E. other _____
  _____

21. Sleep pattern disturbance related to:
  A. shock.
  B. impaired skin integrity.
  C. pain.
  D. secondary infection.
  E. skin grafting.
  F. other _____
  _____

22. Altered peripheral tissue perfusion related to:
  A. loss of fluids.
  B. stress.
  C. shock.
  D. extensive nature of burns.
  E. alteration in cardiac output.
  F. other _____
  _____

23. Altered patterns of urinary elimination related to:
  A. shock.
  B. oliguria.
  C. stress.
  D. poor tissue perfusion.
  E. poor fluid intake.
  F. other _____
  _____

24. Altered thought processes related to:
  A. shock.
  B. hypoxia.
  C. delirium.

D. changes in sensorium.

E. pyrexia.

F. other _____

_____

II. SHORT-TERM GOALS

1. Client/Family will verbalize fears, anxieties, and concerns after 1–2–3–4 R.N. visits.
2. Client/Family will administer/apply medication as ordered after 1–2 R.N. visits.
3. Client/Family will immediately notify M.D. of adverse reactions or changes in physical condition after 1–2 R.N. visits.
4. Client/Family will record weight daily after 1–2 R.N. visits.
5. Client/Family will record intake and output as ordered after 1–2 R.N. visits.
6. Client/Family will state 5 signs/symptoms of dehydration after 1–2 R.N. visits.
7. Client/Family will keep emergency phone numbers at bedside at all times after 1–2 R.N. visits.
8. Client/Family will wash hands properly after 1–2 R.N. visits.
9. Client/Family will elevate burned extremity as ordered after 1–2 R.N. visits.
10. Client/Family will change position/turn every 2 hours as ordered after 1 R.N. visit.
11. Client/Family will change dressings aseptically after 1–2 R.N. visits.
12. Client/Family will damp-dust room daily after 1–2 R.N. visits.
13. Client/Family will give frequent oral cleansing after 1 R.N. visit.
14. Client/Family will follow strict instructions for good personal hygiene after 1–2 R.N. visits.
15. Client will consume fluids/diet as ordered after 1–2 R.N. visits.
16. Client/Family will take vital signs as ordered after 1–2 R.N. visits.
17. Client/Family will provide tracheostomy care as ordered after 1–2–3 R.N. visits.
18. Client will perform breathing exercises/respiratory therapy as ordered after 1–2–3 R.N./R.T. visits.
19. Client will exercise/rest as ordered after 1–2 R.N. visits.
20. Client/Family will perform physical therapy/occupational therapy/speech therapy as ordered after 1–2 R.N./P.T./O.T./S.T. visits.

21. Client/Family will use medical equipment (e.g., hospital bed/air mattress/water bed/bed cradle/bed trapeze/splints) as ordered after 1–2–3–4 R.N. visits.
22. Client/Family will apply elastic bandages as ordered after 1–2 R.N. visits.
23. Client will use self-help devices for eating after 1–2 R.N./P.T./O.T. visits.
24. Client/Family will prevent accidents in the home after 1–2 R.N. visits.
25. Client/Family will seek laboratory testing/M.D. appointments as ordered after 1 R.N. visit.

III. LONG-TERM GOALS

1. Adequate rehabilitation of burn victim will be achieved in 2–3 months.
2. Independent activities of daily living will be resumed in 2–3 weeks.
3. Optimal level of health will be achieved in 2–3 months.

IV. OUTCOME CRITERIA

1. Vital signs are normal.
2. Granulation occurs.
3. Skin remains healthy and intact.
4. Weight is normal.
5. Gait is normal.
6. Vision is normal.
7. Intake and output are normal.
8. Laboratory test results are normal.
9. Neuromuscular system is normal.
10. GI system is normal.
11. Appetite is normal.
12. Nutritious meals are consumed.
13. Cardiovascular system is normal.
14. GU system is normal.
15. Client states he/she feels better.
16. Employment is sought.

V. NURSING INTERVENTION/TREATMENT

1. R.N. will consult with hospital discharge planner about treatment and rehabilitation goals; will make arrangements for medical equipment to be delivered to client's home upon discharge.
2. R.N. will instruct client/family/H.H.A. on:
   A. burn care and potential complications.
   B. proper hand-washing technique.
   C. monitoring and recording of vital signs.
   D. medication administration/adverse reactions.
   E. immediate notification of M.D. of adverse reactions or change in condition.
   F. placement of emergency phone numbers within reach at all times.
   G. daily recording of weight.
   H. recording of intake and output.
   I. laboratory testing/M.D. appointments.
   J. aseptic dressing change.
   K. skin care/care of graft sites/debridement procedures.
   L. turning/repositioning/exercise/rest as ordered.
   M. plans for P.T./S.T./O.T./H.H.A. services as ordered.
   N. tracheostomy care.
   O. use of medical equipment (e.g., hospital bed/air mattress with pump/bed trapeze/bed cradle/commode/elastic bandages/stockings/self-help devices for meal preparation).
   P. fluid intake/dietary regimen as ordered.
   Q. catheter care.
   R. quiet, restful, clean environment, free from dust, to prevent secondary infection while resistance is low.
   S. oral hygiene/personal hygiene.
   T. diversional activities.
3. R.N. will provide client/family with names of organizations for additional burn information/financial aid/housing/career counseling.
4. R.N. will provide M.D. with follow-up reports and discharge summary when case closes.
5. R.N. will notify client/family/H.H.A./significant others when case will close.

Cancer Chemotherapy Care Plan

I. NURSING DIAGNOSIS

1. Knowledge deficit related to:
   A. proper hand-washing technique.
   B. monitoring and recording of vital signs.
   C. medications/chemotherapeutic agents/adverse reactions (e.g., alopecia).
   D. sites for medications.
   E. monitoring and recording of intake and output.
   F. fluids/diet.
   G. urine testing for sugar, acetone, and occult blood.
   H. prevention of fractures.
   I. oral hygiene.
   J. methods of drug administration (e.g., infusion/long-term infusion, IV push/short-term infusion).
   K. operation of an ambulatory (outpatient) infusion pump (Auto Syringe pump, model AS2F from Auto Syringe, Inc., or The Cormed Pump from Travenol Laboratories).
   L. operation of an implantable vascular access system.
   M. biohazards of antineoplastics/sources of exposure/hand washing/drug preparation/drug administration/contaminated waste disposal guidelines.
   N. other _____

2. Constipation/Diarrhea related to toxic effects of chemotherapy.
3. Altered oral mucous membrane related to toxic effect of chemotherapy.

4. Ineffective individual/family coping related to toxic effects of chemotherapy.
5. Impaired social interaction related to toxic effects of chemotherapy.
6. Anxiety/Fear related to:
   A. numerous toxic reactions to chemotherapy.
   B. potential death.
   C. antidote administration.
   D. other _____

   _____

7. Potential fluid volume deficit related to:
   A. vomiting.
   B. fever.
   C. diarrhea.
   D. polyuria.
   E. bleeding.
   F. toxic effects of chemotherapy.
   G. other _____

   _____

8. Impaired home maintenance management related to toxic effects of chemotherapy.
9. Potential for injury related to toxic effects of chemotherapy.
10. Ineffective breathing pattern related to toxic effects of chemotherapy.
11. Impaired physical mobility related to toxic effects of chemotherapy.
12. Noncompliance with cancer treatment related to toxic effects of chemotherapy.
13. Altered nutrition: more than body requirements related to:
    A. nausea.
    B. vomiting.
    C. anorexia.
    D. abdominal cramping.
    E. diarrhea.
    F. constipation.
    G. GI bleeding.
    H. other _____

    _____

14. Altered parenting related to toxic effects of chemotherapy.
15. Sleep pattern disturbance related to toxic effects of chemotherapy.
16. Body image disturbance related to toxic effects of chemotherapy.

17. Self-esteem disturbance related to toxic effects of chemotherapy.
18. Personal identity disturbance related to toxic effects of chemotherapy.
19. Hopelessness related to terminal stages of cancer.
20. Sensory/Perceptual alterations related to:
    A. terminal stages of illness.
    B. toxic effects of chemotherapy.
    C. other _____

    _____

21. Pain related to:
    A. disease process.
    B. toxic reaction to chemotherapy.
    C. other _____

    _____

22. Diversional activity deficit related to:
    A. pain.
    B. nausea/vomiting.
    C. toxic effects of chemotherapy.
    D. weakness.
    E. other _____

    _____

23. Potential impaired skin integrity related to:
    A. breakdown of injection sites.
    B. extravasation.
    C. toxic effects of chemotherapy.
    D. other _____

    _____

24. Impaired skin integrity related to:
    A. breakdown of injection sites.
    B. extravasation.
    C. toxic effects of chemotherapy.
    D. other _____

    _____

25. Altered thought processes related to:
    A. incorrect dosage administration.
    B. toxic effects of chemotherapy.
    C. advance of disease process.
    D. other _____

    _____

26. Altered patterns of urinary elimination related to:
    A. toxic effects of chemotherapy.
    B. advance of disease process.
    C. stress.
    D. other _____

27. Feeding self-care deficit related to:
    A. weakness.
    B. toxic effects of chemotherapy.
    C. other _____

28. Impaired swallowing related to:
    A. advance of disease process.
    B. toxic effects of chemotherapy.
    C. other _____

29. Bathing/Hygiene self-care deficit related to:
    A. advance of disease process.
    B. toxic effects of chemotherapy.
    C. other _____

30. Dressing/Grooming self-care deficit related to:
    A. weakness.
    B. toxic effects of chemotherapy.
    C. advance of disease process.
    D. other _____

31. Toileting self-care deficit related to:
    A. pain.
    B. weakness.
    C. advance of disease process.
    D. toxic effects of chemotherapy.
    E. other _____

32. Altered growth and development related to:
    A. advance of disease process.
    B. toxic effects of chemotherapy.
    C. other _____

II. SHORT-TERM GOALS

1. Client/Family will administer medication as ordered to counteract toxic effects of chemotherapy after 1–2–3–4 R.N. visits.
2. Client/Family will report any adverse effects of medications/ change in condition/chemotherapy after 1–2–3–4 R.N. visits.
3. Client/Family will seek laboratory testing/M.D. appointments as ordered after 1–2 R.N. visits.
4. Client will take steroids with milk or antacids as ordered after 1–2 R.N. visits.
5. Client will practice good oral hygiene after 1–2 R.N. visits.
6. Client will force fluids as ordered after 1–2 R.N. visits.
7. Client will consume foods high in protein and calories as ordered after 1–2 R.N. visits.
8. Client will consume a ground, pureed, soft, or liquid diet as ordered after 1–2 R.N. visits.
9. Client/Family will administer enteral feedings/hyperalimentation as ordered after 1–2 R.N. visits.
10. Client/Family will administer feedings through an oral syringe after 1–2 R.N. visits.
11. Client will avoid tart, spicy, hot, and cold foods after 1–2 R.N. visits.
12. Client will rest appropriately after 1–2 R.N. visits.
13. Client will record daily weight after 1 R.N. visit.
14. Client will take stool softeners/laxatives as ordered after 1–2 R.N. visits.
15. Client/Family will record intake and output daily as ordered after 1–2 R.N. visits.
16. Client/Family will test urine for sugar/acetone/blood as ordered after 1–2 R.N. visits.
17. Client/Family will wash hands correctly after 1 R.N. visit.
18. Client/Family will guard against pathologic fractures as ordered after 1 R.N. visit.
19. Client/Family will take seizure precautions as ordered after 1–2 R.N. visits.
20. Client/Family will report any signs/symptoms of respiratory changes (e.g., cough, fever, rales, dyspnea, chest pain) after 1–2 R.N. visits.
21. Client will use a soft toothbrush for brushing teeth after 1–2 R.N. visits.
22. Client will avoid using aspirin-containing compounds after 1–2 R.N. visits.

23. Client will use warm, moist compresses for local irritation at IV sites after 1–2 R.N. visits.
24. Client/Family will supervise IV therapy in the home as ordered after 1–2 R.N. visits.
25. Client/Family will bring emesis basin and antiemetics to M.D. for routine chemotherapy injections in cases of vomiting after 1–2 R.N. visits.
26. Client/Family will operate an ambulatory infusion pump as ordered after 1–2–3–4 R.N. visits.
27. Client/Family will operate an implantable vascular access system as ordered after 1–2–3–4 R.N. visits.
28. Client/Family will administer antidote as ordered after 1–2–3–4 R.N. visits.

III. LONG-TERM GOALS

1. Remission of cancerous condition will occur in 6–12 months.
2. Independent activities of daily living will be resumed in 1–2 weeks.
3. Optimal level of health will be achieved in 3–4 weeks.
4. All stages of death and dying will be worked through in 6–12 months.

IV. OUTCOME CRITERIA

1. Metastasis is controlled/eradicated.
2. Vital signs are normal.
3. Visual response is normal.
4. Hair growth is normal/has returned to normal.
5. Pain is eliminated.
6. Ambulation is normal.
7. Breathing is clear.
8. Chest sounds are normal bilaterally.
9. Skin is clear, healthy, and intact.
10. Bowels function normally.
11. Urine output is normal.
12. Edema has subsided.
13. Weight is appropriate.
14. Mental outlook is healthy.
15. Client achieves goals and functions appropriately.
16. Client states he/she feels better.

V. NURSING INTERVENTION/TREATMENT

1. R.N. will visit client's home to assess complete history and physical condition. Hospital discharge planner will notify R.N. of prognosis and goals.

2. R.N. will instruct client/family/H.H.A. on:

   A. proper hand-washing technique.

   B. monitoring and recording of vital signs.

   C. intake and output as ordered.

   D. oral hygiene: avoidance of tart, spicy, hot, and cold foods; rinsing mouth after consuming milk and other dairy products; use of soft toothbrush.

   E. avoidance of aspirin products, to prevent bleeding.

   F. medication administration (e.g., administration of steroids with milk/antacids/antidote administration). Preparations for chemotherapy injections by M.D.

   G. immediate notification of M.D. of adverse reactions or change in condition.

   H. adverse medication reactions (e.g., stomatitis/oral moniliasis/ bleeding/bone marrow depression/hyperpigmentation of vein/ nausea/vomiting/alopecia/spinal cord compression).

   I. biohazards of antineoplastics/sources of exposure/hand-washing/drug preparation/drug administration/contaminated waste disposal guidelines.

   J. IV therapy in the home/standard criteria for client selection/ Heparin lock/implantable vascular access system(e.g., accessing port)/continuous infusion/medication administration/blood drawing/needle removal/refill schedules/troubleshooting/ avoiding activities which involve changes in temperature and pressure that can affect pump's infusion rate/IV push medications/short-term infusions/long-term infusions/safe operation of an ambulatory (outpatient) infusion pump (these external infusion pumps are worn in a pocket supported by either a shoulder harness or belt). Two available pumps are Auto Syringe Pump, Model AS2F, from Auto Syringe, Inc., or the Cormed Pump from Travenol Laboratories.

   K. enteral feedings/gastrostomy tube feedings/hyperalimentation.

   L. high-protein, high-calorie diet.

   M. adequate fluid intake.

   N. warm, moist compresses for local irritation at IV site.

   O. seizure precautions.

   P. daily recording of weight.

   Q. exercise/rest as ordered.
   R. laboratory testing/M.D. appointments.
   S. radiation/skin care/dressing care.
   T. prevention of pathologic fractures.
   U. urine testing at home for sugar/acetone/blood.
   V. breathing exercises/use of respiratory equipment.
   W. use of hairpiece/wig for alopecia.
   X. diversional activities.
   Y. socialization.
   Z. additional information to be obtained from nutritionists/cancer
      societies/research centers.
3. R.N. will assign additional personnel (e.g., P.T., O.T., S.T., M.S.W.)
   to case if ordered.
4. R.N. will provide M.D. with follow-up reports and discharge
   summary when case closes.
5. R.N. will notify client/M.D./H.H.A./P.T./O.T./S.T./M.S.W./
   significant others when case closes.
6. If death is imminent, R.N. will provide psychologic support/enlist
   support of clergy in final stages; will follow pronouncement of
   death procedures; will assist with funeral arrangements/cremation
   if necessary.

Cardiac
Care Plan

I. NURSING DIAGNOSIS

1. Anxiety related to:
   A. lack of support in the home.
   B. inability to perform activities of daily living.
   C. activity intolerance.
   D. possible death.
   E. other _____
   _____

2. Self-care deficit: feeding/bathing/dressing/grooming/ambulating/
   toileting related to:
   A. activity intolerance.
   B. dependence on others for care.
   C. other _____
   _____

3. Knowledge deficit related to:
   A. fluid/diet preparation.
   B. medication administration/adverse reactions (e.g., avoidance of
      sodium-containing laxatives/antacids)/(noting of ingredients in
      over-the-counter medications, e.g., sugar, caffeine, sodium,
      potassium).
   C. signs/symptoms of coronary insufficiency.
   D. exercise/rest.
   E. monitoring/recording of vital signs.
   F. avoidance of smoking/alcohol/caffeine.
   G. avoidance of excessive heat/cold.

H. avoidance of infection/crowded areas.
I. laboratory testing/M.D. appointments.
J. annual influenza vaccines.
K. sexual activity.
L. exercise stress testing/Holter monitoring.
M. other _____

_____

4. Decreased cardiac output related to:
   A. limited/excessive exercise.
   B. obesity.
   C. excessive hydration.
   D. stress intolerance.
   E. hypertension/hypotension.
   F. smoking.
   G. other _____

   _____

5. Ineffective breathing pattern related to:
   A. chest pain.
   B. shortness of breath/dyspnea.
   C. activity intolerance.
   D. excessive hydration.
   E. stress intolerance.
   F. smoking.
   G. other _____

   _____

6. Ineffective individual/family coping related to:
   A. dependence on others for care.
   B. cost of medical care/poor insurance coverage.
   C. unstable physical condition.
   D. other _____

   _____

7. Altered health maintenance related to:
   A. refusal to maintain M.D. appointments.
   B. mental confusion.
   C. impaired physical mobility/immobility.
   D. other _____

   _____

8. Sexual dysfunction related to:
   A. apathy.
   B. anxiety.
   C. fear of injury (MI/death).
   D. activity intolerance.
   E. other _____

9. Self-esteem disturbance related to:
   A. dependence on others for care.
   B. unemployment.
   C. other _____

10. Potential for injury related to:
    A. dizziness.
    B. overexertion.
    C. noncompliance with therapy.
    D. denial of severity of condition.
    E. smoking.
    F. other _____

11. Social isolation related to:
    A. activity intolerance.
    B. anger.
    C. dependence on others for care.
    D. rejection.
    E. other _____

12. Fear related to:
    A. death.
    B. dependence on others for care.
    C. other _____

13. Altered patterns of urinary elimination related to:
    A. medication administration/adverse reactions.
    B. limited exercise.
    C. other _____

14. Altered family processes related to:
    A. excessive client demands.
    B. mental confusion.
    C. dependence on others for care.
    D. cost of medical care/poor insurance coverage.
    E. other _____
       _____

15. Constipation/Diarrhea related to:
    A. poor fluid/dietary intake.
    B. dependence on others for assistance with toileting.
    C. limited exercise.
    D. medication toxicity.
    E. other _____
       _____

II. SHORT-TERM GOALS

1. Client/Family will verbalize fears, anxieties, and concerns after 1–2–3 R.N. visits.
2. Client/Family will administer medication as ordered after 1–2 R.N. visits.
3. Client/Family will immediately notify M.D. of adverse reactions or change in condition after 1–2 R.N. visits.
4. Client will limit fluid intake as ordered after 1–2 R.N. visits.
5. Client will avoid extremes in temperature of fluids/weather after 1–2 R.N. visits.
6. Client will drink in moderation or eliminate alcohol according to M.D. orders after 1–2 R.N. visits.
7. Client will begin weight reducing according to M.D. orders after 1–2 R.N. visits.
8. Client will engage in moderate/light exercise as ordered after 1–2 R.N. visits.
9. Client will ambulate slowly after 1–2 R.N. visits.
10. Client will reduce or eliminate smoking after 1–2 R.N. visits.
11. Client will substitute diversional activity for smoking after 1–2 R.N. visits.
12. Client/Family will seek laboratory testing/M.D. appointments after 1–2 R.N. visits.

III. LONG-TERM GOALS

1. Independent activities of daily living will be resumed in 1–2 weeks.
2. Normal cardiac functioning will be achieved in 3–4 weeks.
3. Optimum level of health will be achieved in 3–4 weeks.

IV. OUTCOME CRITERIA

1. Vital signs are normal.
2. CBC with differential remains normal.
3. Serum enzyme levels (SGOT, LDH, and CPK) are normal.
4. Chest is clear; breathing is normal.
5. Appetite is normal.
6. Weight is appropriate for height.
7. Intake and output are normal.
8. Peripheral pulses are normal.
9. Client is alert, oriented, and in good spirits.
10. Client states he/she feels better.

V. NURSING INTERVENTION/TREATMENT

1. R.N. will arrange to visit client's home.
2. R.N. will monitor apical and radial pulse rates and blood pressure; will seek laboratory testing (CBC with differential, electrolytes, digitalis level, prothrombin time, partial thromboplastin time, and sedimentation rate) as ordered by M.D.
3. R.N. will instruct client/family/H.H.A. on:
   A. disease process.
   B. monitoring and recording of vital signs, with emphasis on pulse (apical and radial, peripheral if necessary), along with monitoring and recording of temperature and respirations.
   C. medication administration/adverse reactions/(e.g., avoidance of sodium-containing laxatives/antacids)/(noting of ingredients in over-the-counter medications, e.g., sugar, caffeine, sodium, potassium).
   D. immediate notification of M.D. of adverse reactions or change in condition.
   E. emergency phone numbers to be kept at bedside.
   F. laboratory testing/M.D. appointments.
   G. exercise/stair climbing/lifting/daily rest periods as ordered.
   H. avoidance of air travel for 2–3 months as ordered by M.D.

    I. avoidance of temperature extremes.

    J. weight reduction/daily recording of weight.

    K. reduction/avoidance of smoking/caffeine/alcohol.

    L. recording of intake and output.

    M. bed rest/chair rest.

    N. fluids/diet (e.g., small, frequent high-protein, high-calorie meals supplying adequate bulk).

    O. exercise stress testing/Holter monitoring.

    P. pet ownership.

    Q. bowel regimen/avoidance of straining at stool.

    R. decreased work hours on return to work.

    S. diversional activities.

    T. sexual activity.

    U. financial assistance.

    V. rehabilitative housing with elevator.

    W. insurance coverage.

    X. employment.

4. R.N. will provide client/family with instructional literature and visual aids/organizations/clubs to contact for further assistance.

5. R.N. will assign additional personnel (e.g., M.S.W. or P.T.) to case if ordered.

6. R.N. will provide M.D. with follow-up reports and discharge summary when case closes.

7. R.N. will notify client/family/H.H.A./significant others when case will close.

Cast
Care Plan

I. NURSING DIAGNOSIS

1. Knowledge deficit related to:
   A. cast care.
   B. range-of-motion exercise/passive and active exercise/turning/repositioning.
   C. ambulation.
   D. medication administration/adverse reactions.
   E. pain management.
   F. other _____

2. Constipation related to:
   A. location of cast.
   B. poor fluid/dietary intake.
   C. other _____

3. Potential impaired skin integrity related to:
   A. location of cast.
   B. weight of cast.
   C. other _____

4. Ineffective individual/family coping related to:
   A. dependence on others for care.
   B. refusal to participate in care.
   C. irritability.
   D. immobility.

E. difficulty with turning/ambulation.

F. other _____

_____

5. Anxiety/Fear related to:

A. pain.

B. progressive mobility of body part.

C. falling.

D. other _____

_____

6. Potential for injury related to:

A. difficulty with ambulation.

B. poor mobility/difficulty with range-of-motion exercise.

C. frequent falling.

D. other _____

_____

7. Impaired physical mobility related to:

A. pain.

B. edema.

C. weight of cast.

D. location of cast.

E. other _____

_____

8. Powerlessness related to:

A. immobility.

B. pain.

C. dependence on others for care.

D. other _____

_____

9. Activity intolerance related to:

A. weight of cast.

B. location of cast.

C. other _____

_____

10. Self-care deficit: feeding/dressing/bathing/grooming/ambulating/ toileting related to:

A. immobility.

B. dependence on others for care.

C. pain.

D. edema.

E. other _____

_____

II. SHORT-TERM GOALS

1. Client/Family will verbalize all fears, concerns, and anxieties after 1–2 R.N. visits.
2. Client/Family/H.H.A. will keep cast clean, dry, and intact after 1 R.N. visit.
3. Client/Family/H.H.A. will support/elevate cast on pillows after 1 R.N. visit.
4. Client/Family/H.H.A. will administer prescribed medications after 1 R.N. visit.
5. Client/Family/H.H.A. will immediately notify M.D. of adverse reactions or change in condition after 1 R.N. visit.
6. Client/Family/H.H.A. will state signs/symptoms of impaired circulation after 1–2 R.N. visits.
7. Client will exercise fingers and toes (distal to cast) as ordered after 1 R.N. visit.
8. Client will use crutches/cane/quad cane/walker/wheelchair/commode correctly after 1–2 R.N. visits.

III. LONG-TERM GOALS

1. Bone healing will take place in 6–8 weeks.
2. Independent activities of daily living will be resumed in 1–2 weeks.
3. Optimal level of health will be achieved in 6–8 weeks.

IV. OUTCOME CRITERIA

1. Vital signs remain normal.
2. Pain/Edema is eliminated.
3. Circulation is normal.
4. Client achieves adequate mobility of body part.
5. Client states he/she feels better.

V. NURSING INTERVENTION/TREATMENT

1. R.N. will instruct client/family/H.H.A. on:
   A. signs/symptoms of circulatory or neurogenic impairment and need for immediate notification of M.D. of change in condition.

    B. monitoring and recording of vital signs.

    C. medication administration/adverse reactions and need for immediate notification of M.D.

    D. elevation/support of extremity when necessary.

    E. fluid/dietary needs.

    F. skin care/personal hygiene.

    G. turning/repositioning.

    H. exercise regimen (R.N. will confer with M.D. or P.T. when necessary).

    I. ambulation.

    J. use of assistive devices (crutches, cane, quad cane, walker, wheelchair, commode).

    K. application of sling.

    L. stair climbing.

    M. fine motor coordination (R.N. will confer with O.T. when necessary).

    N. follow-up M.D. appointments.

2. R.N. will refer client to additional community resources if necessary.

3. R.N. will provide M.D. with follow-up reports and discharge summary when case closes.

4. R.N. will notify client/family/H.H.A./P.T./O.T./significant others when case will close.

Cerebral Palsy Care Plan

I. NURSING DIAGNOSIS

1. Anxiety related to:
   A. loss of control.
   B. communication deficit.
   C. difficulty with self-care activities.
   D. dependence on others for care.
   E. poor financial resources.
   F. other _____

2. Knowledge deficit related to:
   A. signs/sympoms.
   B. medication administration/adverse reactions.
   C. nutritional requirements.
   D. bowel/bladder elimination.
   E. skin care.
   F. respiratory care.
   G. laboratory testing/M.D. appointments.
   H. insurance coverage.
   I. rehabilitation equipment.
   J. exercise.
   K. seizure control.
   L. socialization.
   M. other _____

3. Altered patterns of urinary elimination related to:
   A. medication administration.

    B. weakened musculature.

    C. poor sphincter control.

    D. other _____

    _____

4. Constipation/Diarrhea/Bowel incontinence related to:

    A. medication administration.

    B. fluids/diet administration.

    C. lack of exercise.

    D. fecal impaction.

    E. weakened musculature.

    F. other _____

    _____

5. Ineffective individual/family coping related to:

    A. excessive demands of caring for the sick.

    B. rejection by significant others.

    C. dependence on others for care.

    D. cost of medical care/poor insurance coverage.

    E. other _____

    _____

6. Fear related to:

    A. strabismus.

    B. history of falling.

    C. other _____

    _____

7. Potential fluid volume deficit related to:

    A. dysphagia.

    B. poor intake.

    C. other _____

    _____

8. Partial/Total self-care deficit: feeding/bathing/dressing/grooming/toileting/administration of medication/household chores related to:

    A. hemiplegia.

    B. paraplegia.

    C. quadriplegia.

    D. diplegia.

    E. dysarthria.

    F. monoplegia.

    G. athetosis.

    H. chorea.

I. rigidity.

J. dystonia.

K. tremors.

L. mental retardation.

M. strabismus.

N. other ——————————————————————

9. Anticipatory/Dysfunctional grieving related to:

A. loss of control.

B. rejection by significant others.

C. dependence on others for care.

D. alteration in body image.

E. other ——————————————————————

10. Impaired home maintenance management related to:

A. excessive demands of caring for the sick.

B. financial distress.

C. marital discord.

D. overwhelming family responsibilities.

E. other ——————————————————————

11. Impaired physical mobility related to:

A. monoplegia.

B. diplegia.

C. paraplegia.

D. hemiplegia.

E. quadriplegia.

F. dysarthria.

G. athetosis.

H. chorea.

I. rigidity.

J. dystonia.

K. tremors.

L. weakness.

M. contractures.

N. seizures.

O. dependence on others for care.

P. other ——————————————————————

12. Noncompliance with therapy related to:
    A. denial.
    B. cost of medical care/poor insurance coverage.
    C. poor comprehension of disease process and its treatment.
    D. demands on significant others for care.
    E. other _____

13. Altered nutrition: less than body requirements related to:
    A. dysphagia.
    B. athetosis.
    C. obesity.
    D. other _____

14. Activity intolerance related to:
    A. monoplegia.
    B. diplegia.
    C. hemiplegia.
    D. quadriplegia.
    E. dysarthria.
    F. athetosis.
    G. chorea.
    H. rigidity.
    I. dystonia.
    J. tremors.
    K. weakness.
    L. contractures.
    M. other _____

15. Altered parenting related to excessive demands of a sick child/adult.

16. Potential for injury related to:
    A. refusal to comply with medical instructions.
    B. accidents.
    C. difficulty with ambulation.
    D. secondary respiratory complications.
    E. poor adult supervision.
    F. other _____

17. Ineffective airway clearance related to:
    A. dysphagia.
    B. poor cough response.
    C. difficulty/absence of deep-breathing exercises.
    D. other _____

    _____

18. Self-esteem disturbance related to:
    A. tremors.
    B. spasticity.
    C. contractures.
    D. incontinence.
    E. abnormal gait.
    F. paralysis of upward gaze.
    G. strabismus.
    H. other _____

    _____

19. Sensory/Perceptual alterations related to:
    A. strabismus.
    B. mental retardation.
    C. other _____

    _____

20. Potential impaired skin integrity related to:
    A. immobility (formation of pressure sores).
    B. uncoordinatedness of arms/legs.
    C. accidents.
    D. overexposure to heat/cold.
    E. other _____

    _____

21. Sleep pattern disturbance related to:
    A. tremors.
    B. rigidity.
    C. seizures.
    D. incontinence.
    E. other _____

    _____

22. Altered thought processes related to mental retardation.

II. SHORT-TERM GOALS

1. Client/Family will verbalize fears, anxieties, and concerns after 1–2–3–4 R.N. visits.

2. Client/Family will administer prescribed medication after 1–2 R.N. visits.

3. Client/Family will immediately notify M.D. of adverse reactions of sign/symptoms of complications of disease after 1–2 R.N. visits.

4. Family will enroll infant in infant stimulation program as ordered after 1–2 R.N. visits.

5. Client/Family will obtain medical equipment (e.g., hospital bed/trapeze/wheelchair/cane/feeding devices/padding/helmet/splints/braces/crutches) as ordered after 1–2 R.N./P.T./O.T. visits.

6. Client/Family will allow sufficient time for feedings after 1–2–3 R.N. visits.

7. Client/Family will prepare concentrated feedings as ordered after 1–2 R.N. visits.

8. Client will consume small amounts of food 5–6 times daily after 1–2 R.N. visits.

9. Client/Family will follow prescribed fine-motor-coordination exercises for activities of daily living after 1 R.N./P.T./O.T. visit.

10. Client/Family will follow prescribed physical therapy exercises after 1 R.N. visit.

11. Client/Family will participate in breathing exercises/respiratory therapy as ordered after 1–2 R.N./R.T. visits.

12. Client/Family will turn/reposition every 2 hours as ordered after 1–2 R.N. visits.

13. Client/Family will follow prescribed bowel/bladder regimen after 1–2 R.N. visits.

14. Client/Family will practice good skin care/personal hygiene after 1–2 R.N. visits.

15. Client will wear corrective glasses for visual disturbances as ordered after 1–2 R.N. visits.

16. Client will wear hearing aid as ordered after 1–2 R.N. visits.

17. Client/Family will always keep a padded tongue blade within reach after 1–2 R.N. visits.

18. Family will record onset frequency and duration of seizures and report to M.D. after 1–2 R.N. visits.

19. Client/Family will follow prescribed speech therapy exercises after 1–2 R.N. visits.

20. Client/Family will keep laboratory/M.D. appointments as ordered after 1–2 R.N. visits.

21. Client/Family will seek adequate schooling after 1–2 R.N. visits.

22. Client will seek job counseling/rehabilitation after 1–2 R.N. visits.

III. LONG-TERM GOALS

1. Preservation of maximal level of functioning will be achieved in 3–6 months.
2. Independent activities of daily living will be achieved in 6–12 months.
3. Optimal level of health will be achieved in 6–12 months.

IV. OUTCOME CRITERIA

1. Vital signs are normal.
2. Voluntary muscle control is achieved.
3. Emotional stress is eliminated.
4. Swallowing reflex remains normal.
5. Client consumes nutritious meals.
6. Adequate ambulation/mobility occurs.
7. Chest is clear.
8. Speech is intelligible.
9. Hearing is normal.
10. Client demonstrates fine motor coordination.
11. Client attends infant stimulation program/adequate school program.
12. Seizures are controlled.
13. Laboratory test results are within normal limits.
14. Bowel/Bladder functions normally.
15. Client states he/she feels better.
16. Client seeks employment.

V. NURSING INTERVENTION/TREATMENT

1. R.N. will consult with hospital discharge planner about treatment and rehabilitation goals.
2. R.N. will instruct client/family/H.H.A. on:
   A. monitoring and recording of vital signs.
   B. oral hygiene/personal hygiene.
   C. skin care measures.
   D. medication administration/adverse reactions.
   E. immediate notification of M.D. of adverse reactions or change in condition.
   F. fluid intake/dietary regimen as ordered; including child/adult with family while dining. R.N. will encourage as normal a diet as possible (in concentrated form if possible) without increasing

bulk (increasing child's protein and calcium intake); will encourage child/adult to eat 5–6 small meals daily and understand feeding times may be lengthy; will encourage child/adult to eat finger foods or use special feeding devices for meals.

G. seizure precautions; maintaining padded tongue blade within reach.

H. visual testing/correction.

I. hearing and speech testing/correction.

J. turning/repositioning every 1–2 hours.

K. prescribed exercise/rest program (R.N. will consult with P.T./ O.T. about exercise tolerance, types of exercise).

L. application of splints/braces/helmet/additional padding as ordered.

M. use of incontinence aids (e.g., disposable pant liners, disposable drawsheets).

N. use of additional medical equipment (e.g., hospital bed/trapeze/ tub railing/padded side rails/sheepskin/Hoyer lift/commode/ wheelchair/raised toilet seat/crutches) as ordered.

O. remodeling of architectural barriers if affordable (organizations may be approached for financial aid for this purpose).

P. bowel/bladder regimen (administration of laxatives/ suppositories/enemas; catheter care).

Q. laboratory testing/M.D. appointments.

R. socialization with peers.

S. early enrollment in infant stimulation program/appropriate school/rehabilitation/vocational counseling/college.

T. institutionalization if recommended.

U. diversional activities.

V. adequate housing.

W. financial counseling.

X. employment.

3. R.N. will encourage client/family to request additional literature on cerebral palsy (acquired from cerebral palsy organizations, libraries, camps, schools, foundations).

4. R.N. will assign additional personnel (e.g., M.S.W., P.T., S.T., H.H.A., home attendant, homemaker, housekeeper) to case if ordered.

5. R.N. will provide M.D. with follow-up reports and discharge summary when case closes.

6. R.N. will notify client/family/H.H.A./significant others when case will close.

Cerebrovascular Accident Care Plan

I. NURSING DIAGNOSIS

1. Anxiety related to:
   A. potential falling/accidents.
   B. loss of control
   C. immobility.
   D. financial instability.
   E. cost of medical care/poor insurance coverage.
   F. other _____

2. Ineffective individual/family coping related to:
   A. difficulty with communication.
   B. cost of medical care/poor insurance coverage.
   C. excessive demands of condition.
   D. other _____

3. Self-care deficit: feeding/bathing/grooming/dressing/ambulating related to:
   A. hemiplegia.
   B. aphasia.
   C. loss of control.
   D. spasticity.
   E. other _____

4. Knowledge deficit related to:
   A. monitoring and recording of vital signs.
   B. feeding techniques/adaptive devices.

    C. enteral feedings/hyperalimentation.

    D. personal hygiene.

    E. medication administration/adverse reactions.

    F. exercise/rest/massage.

    G. sensory deficits—proprioceptive sensation (e.g., loss of sense of touch, movement, and position)/impaired hearing and vision (e.g., double vision and homonymous hemianopia [loss of sight in either the right or left half of the visual field])/hemianesthesia (e.g., loss of feeling on one side of the body)/loss of spatial sense.

    H. rehabilitative equipment (e.g., products from the AT&T National Special Needs Center).

    I. other _____

    _____

5. Impaired physical mobility related to:

    A. weakness.

    B. paralysis.

    C. other _____

    _____

6. Pain related to:

    A. severe muscle spasms.

    B. difficulty with weight bearing.

    C. poor exercise tolerance.

    D. other _____

    _____

7. Noncompliance with therapy related to:

    A. feelings of worthlessness.

    B. immobility.

    C. dependence on others for care.

    D. cost of medical care/poor insurance coverage.

    E. other _____

    _____

8. Impaired verbal communication related to:

    A. aphasia.

    B. alexia.

    C. aphonia.

    D. agnosia.

    E. apraxia.

    F. loss of motor power.

    G. other _____

    _____

9. Potential for injury related to:
    A. difficulty with ambulation.
    B. weakness.
    C. dizziness.
    D. confusion.
    E. poor coordination.
    F. other _____

10. Impaired home maintenance management related to:
    A. immobility/hemiplegia/paralysis.
    B. loss of control.
    C. refusal to participate in therapy.
    D. other _____

11. Constipation/Diarrhea/Bowel incontinence related to:
    A. poor fluid/dietary intake.
    B. immobility.
    C. refusal to administer laxatives/enemas/suppositories.
    D. other _____

12. Diversional activity deficit related to:
    A. generalized weakness.
    B. immobility.
    C. other _____

13. Sleep pattern disturbance related to:
    A. paralysis.
    B. incontinence.
    C. decubitus ulcer dressing changes.
    D. other _____

14. Self-esteem disturbance related to:
    A. altered body image.
    B. feelings of rejection by significant others.
    C. other _____

15. Sexual dysfunction related to:
    A. paralysis/hemiplegia.
    B. anger.

    C. hostility.

    D. disturbance in self-concept.

    E. other _____

_____

II. SHORT-TERM GOALS

1. Client/Family will verbalize fears, anxieties, and concerns after 1–2–3–4 R.N. visits.
2. Client/Family will administer medication as ordered after 1–2 R.N. visits.
3. Client/Family will notify M.D. immediately of adverse reactions or change in condition after 1–2 R.N. visits.
4. Client will feed self after 1–2–3 R.N./P.T./O.T. visits.
5. Client will assist with personal hygiene after 1–2–3 R.N./P.T./O.T. visits.
6. Client will speak one word after 4–5 R.N./S.T. visits.
7. Client will speak 3–5 words after 5–10 R.N./S.T. visits.
8. Client will dress himself/herself after 6–8 R.N./P.T./O.T. visits.
9. Client will transfer from bed to wheelchair and commode after 5–6 R.N./P.T. visits.
10. Client will ambulate with a cane after 6–10 R.N./P.T. visits.
11. Client will stand unassisted after 6–10 R.N./P.T. visits.
12. Client/Family will keep routine M.D. appointments as ordered after 1–2 R.N. visits.

III. LONG-TERM GOALS

1. Independent activities of daily living will be resumed in 1–2 weeks.
2. Independent ambulation will be achieved in 3–4 weeks.
3. Optimal level of health will be achieved in 3–4 weeks.

IV. OUTCOME CRITERIA

1. Vital signs are normal.
2. Skin remains healthy and intact.
3. Joint mobility is normal.
4. Chest remains clear.
5. Bowel/Bladder functions normally.
6. Laboratory test results are normal.

7. Client communicates verbally and in writing.

8. Client states he/she feels better.

V. NURSING INTERVENTION/TREATMENT

1. R.N. will contact discharge planner/M.D. to assess type of CVA sustained.

2. R.N. will arrange for P.T./O.T./S.T./M.S.W./H.H.A./home attendant/ homemaker/housekeeper to visit client, if ordered by M.D.

3. R.N. will instruct client/family/H.H.A. on:

   A. assessment of levels of consciousness.

   B. monitoring and recording of vital signs.

   C. fluid and dietary regimen, with restriction of sodium.

   D. use of feeding tubes/enteral feeding/pumps.

   E. recording of input and output.

   F. bowel and bladder training.

   G. turning/positioning in bed with flotation devices/pillows/air mattress with pump/sandbags.

   H. splinting of extremities.

   I. exercise (regularity of) in quadriceps setting/gluteal setting/ sitting balance/standing balance/massage/rest.

   J. use of hospital bed phone number to call in case of failure to operate.

   K. sexual activity with or without intercourse.

   L. medication administration/adverse reactions.

   M. immediate notification of M.D. of any adverse reactions to medications or change in condition.

   N. medication memory aids for forgetful clients (e.g., posters with pasted-on medications/colored dots on bottles which match dots on a chart/medication envelopes prepared in advance and labeled/partitioned boxes/preset medicated alarm boxes/vials.

   O. sensory deficits—proprioceptive sensation (e.g., loss of sense of touch, movement, and position)/impaired hearing and vision (double vision and homonymous hemianopia [loss of sight in either the right or left half of the visual field])/hemianesthesia (loss of feeling on one side of the body)/loss of spatial sense.

   P. rehabilitation equipment (e.g., splints/overhead bed trapeze/3–4 prong cane/wheelchair/ramps/grab rails/Hoyer lift/pulleys/raised toilet seat/environmental controls)/Ride-a-Stair electronic chair/ products from the AT&T National Special Needs Center.

   Q. breathing exercises/use of incentive spirometer/blow bottles/ blow toys/oxygen.

R. career counseling.

S. organizations for additional financial and educational assistance.

T. laboratory testing/M.D. appointments.

4. R.N. will confer with M.D./S.T./P.T./O.T./R.T./M.S.W. about all changes in therapies as progress is made.

5. R.N. will provide M.D. with follow-up reports and discharge summary when case closes.

6. R.N. will notify client/family/H.H.A./significant others when case will close.

Chest Physiotherapy Care Plan

I. NURSING DIAGNOSIS

1. Anxiety related to:
   A. infection.
   B. suture-line tenderness/edema.
   C. obstructed airway.
   D. frequent coughing/expectoration/wheezing.
   E. hemoptysis.
   F. pain.
   G. limited chest movement.
   H. turning/repositioning.
   I. breathing exercises.
   J. use of inhalation equipment/respirator.
   K. suctioning techniques/nasotracheal suctioning.
   L. percussion/huffing.
   M. smoking.
   N. other _____

2. Ineffective breathing patterns related to:
   A. pain.
   B. suture-line tenderness/edema.
   C. infection.
   D. limited mobility.
   E. unconsciousness.
   F. retained respiratory secretions.

    G. dyspnea.

    H. coughing/expectoration/wheezing.

    I. obstructed airway.

    J. activity intolerance.

    K. poor positioning/turning.

    L. frequent suctioning.

    M. nose/rib fracture.

    N. smoking.

    O. other _____

    _____

3. Pain related to:

    A. obstructed airway.

    B. frequent chest percussion/huffing.

    C. infection.

    D. frequent suctioning.

    E. nose/rib fracture.

    F. advanced disease process.

    G. other _____

    _____

4. Decreased cardiac output related to:

    A. chest percussion/huffing.

    B. suctioning.

    C. activity intolerance.

    D. obstructed airway.

    E. dyspnea.

    F. coughing/expectoration/wheezing.

    G. smoking.

    H. other _____

    _____

5. Impaired gas exchange related to:

    A. retained respiratory secretions.

    B. frequent suctioning.

    C. obstructed airway.

    D. infection.

    E. hemorrhage.

    F. poor cooperation in breathing exercises/inhalation therapy/ percussion/huffing.

    G. nose/rib fracture.

H. smoking.

I. other _____

_____

6. Noncompliance with therapy related to:

   A. fear.

   B. pain.

   C. dependence on others for care.

   D. cost of medical care/poor insurance coverage.

   E. smoking.

   F. other _____

_____

7. Self-care deficit: feeding/bathing/dressing/grooming/toileting/ administration of medication/household chores related to:

   A. limited mobility.

   B. pain.

   C. confusion.

   D. other _____

_____

8. Impaired home maintenance management related to:

   A. generalized weakness.

   B. lack of support in the home.

   C. dependence on others for care.

   D. activity intolerance.

   E. immobility.

   F. other _____

_____

9. Sleep pattern disturbance related to:

   A. coughing/expectoration/wheezing.

   B. dyspnea.

   C. congestion.

   D. frequent suctioning.

   E. frequent chest percussion/inhalation.

   F. frequent medication administration.

   G. other _____

_____

10. Self-esteem disturbance related to:

    A. activity intolerance.

    B. potential rejection by significant others.

    C. confusion.

    D. unemployment.

    E. other _____

    _____

II. SHORT-TERM GOALS

1. Client/Family will verbalize fears, anxieties, and concerns after 1–2 R.N. visits.
2. Client/Family will consume/administer fluids as ordered after 1–2 R.N. visits.
3. Client will cough 5–10 times each hour as ordered after 1–2 R.N. visits.
4. Client/Family will suction nose/throat/tracheostomy as necessary after 1–2 R.N. visits.
5. Client/Family will state signs/symptoms of infections after 1–2 R.N. visits.
6. Client will cough into a tissue and properly dispose of it after 1–2 R.N. visits.
7. Client/Family will maintain exercise while bedridden and thereafter as ordered after 1–2 R.N. visits.
8. Client/Family will administer medication as ordered after 1–2 R.N. visits.
9. Client/Family will immediately report to M.D. adverse reactions or change in condition after 1–2 R.N. visits.
10. Client will properly wash hands after expectorating/coughing after 1–2 R.N. visits.
11. Client/Family will demonstrate chest physical therapy/inhalation therapy/breathing exercises after 1–2 R.N. visits.
12. Client/Family will seek laboratory testing/M.D. appointments as ordered after 1–2 R.N. visits.

III. LONG-TERM GOALS

1. Independent activities of daily living will be resumed in 1–2 weeks.
2. Normal respiratory functioning will be achieved in 3–4 weeks.
3. Optimal level of health will be achieved in 3–4 weeks.

IV. OUTCOME CRITERIA

1. Vital signs are normal.

2. Chest is clear.

3. Breathing is normal.

4. Airway is patent.

5. Laboratory test results are normal.

6. Po_2 and Pco_2 are normal.

7. Appetite is normal.

8. Hydration is adequate.

9. Weight is appropriate for height.

10. Client states he/she feels better.

V. NURSING INTERVENTION/TREATMENT

1. R.N. will visit home and assess general physical status.

2. R.N. will allow client/family to verbalize fears, anxieties, and concerns.

3. R.N. will instruct client/family/H.H.A. on:

   A. proper hand-washing technique.

   B. monitoring and recording of vital signs.

   C. fluid intake/diet.

   D. positioning/turning every 2 hours.

   E. mouth care/personal hygiene.

   F. coughing/deep-breathing exercises.

   G. use of respiratory equipment (e.g., oxygen/inhalation equipment/humidification/blow bottles/spirometer/respirator).

   H. postural drainage/percussion/huffing/vibration/nasotracheal suctioning/aseptic suctioning technique if necessary.

   I. dressing care.

   J. avoidance/limitation of smoking.

   K. laboratory testing/sputum collections/x-rays.

   L. cleansing and storage of respiratory equipment.

   M. medication administration/adverse reactions.

   N. immediate notification of M.D. of adverse reactions or change in condition.

   O. exercise/rest.

   P. M.D. appointments.

4. R.N. will consult with respiratory equipment company for further instructions in management and operation of equipment while in home; will consult with R.T. for his/her instructions/ reports. R.N. will provide a description of services, benefits, and activities of the American Association for Respiratory Therapy, Dallas, Texas.

5. R.N. will provide follow-up reports and discharge summary to M.D. when case closes.
6. R.N. will notify client/family/H.H.A./significant others when case will close.

Chickenpox
Care Plan

I. NURSING DIAGNOSIS

    1. Ineffective thermoregulation related to:
- A. invasive nature of communicable disease.
- B. low resistance to infections.
- C. poor fluid/dietary intake.
- D. other _____

    2. Ineffective individual/family coping related to:
- A. confinement to bed.
- B. pruritus.
- C. malaise.
- D. lethargy.
- E. difficulty with mastication.
- F. positioning.
- G. difficulty sleeping.
- H. irritability.
- I. other _____

    3. Impaired social interaction related to:
- A. lethargy.
- B. malaise.
- C. irritability.
- D. pruritis.
- E. excessive scratching.

F. other _____

_____

4. Potential fluid volume deficit related to:
   A. anorexia.
   B. impairment of mucous membrane (oral lesions).
   C. lethargy.
   D. malaise.
   E. pyrexia.
   F. other _____

   _____

5. Potential for injury related to excessive scratching.
6. Knowledge deficit related to:
   A. proper hand-washing technique.
   B. medication administration/adverse reactions.
   C. prevention/isolation/treatment of chickenpox.
   D. skin care.
   E. other _____

   _____

7. Altered nutrition: potential for more than body requirements related to:
   A. anorexia.
   B. pyrexia.
   C. impaired mucous membrane.
   D. malaise.
   E. lethargy.
   F. other _____

   _____

8. Self-care deficit: feeding/dressing/bathing/grooming related to:
   A. lethargy.
   B. malaise.
   C. other _____

   _____

9. Impaired skin integrity related to:
   A. excessive scratching.
   B. macules/papules/vesicles/scabs.
   C. other _____

   _____

10. Sleep pattern disturbance related to:
    A. pruritus.

B. excessive scratching.

C. other _____

_____

II. SHORT-TERM GOALS

1. Client/Family will maintain strict isolation precautions after 1 R.N. visit.
2. Client/Family will force fluids after 1 R.N. visit.
3. Client will eat 5–6 small meals daily after 1 R.N. visit.
4. Client/Family will administer medication/apply lotions prescribed after 1 R.N. visit.
5. Client will rest periodically throughout day after 1 R.N. visit.
6. Client/Family will apply tepid tap water sponge after 1 R.N. visit.
7. Client/Family will participate in diversional activity after 1–2 R.N. visits.
8. Client/Family will visit M.D. as ordered after 1 R.N. visit.

III. LONG-TERM GOALS

1. Treatment of primary contacts in community will be established in 1–2 weeks.
2. Control of communicable disease will be established in 1–2 weeks.

IV. OUTCOME CRITERIA

1. Skin/Mucous membrane is healthy and intact.
2. Hydration/Normal weight is maintained.
3. Client states he/she feels better.
4. Client returns to play/school/work.

V. NURSING INTERVENTION/TREATMENT

1. R.N. will instruct client/family on:
   A. proper hand-washing technique/good personal hygiene/ laundering of personal care items.
   B. home isolation/bed rest.
   C. adequate fluid intake/diet in small, frequent amounts.
   D. medication administration/adverse reactions.
   E. application of lotions.
   F. proper disposal of tissues and garbage in community.

     G. daily rest periods.

     H. prevention of scratching/application of mittens.

     I. diversional activities.

     J. M.D. appointments.

2. R.N. will consult with M.D. about when client may return to play/school/work.

3. R.N. will provide M.D. with follow-up reports and discharge summary when case closes.

4. R.N. will notify client/family/significant others when case will close.

Cholecystectomy
Care Plan

I. NURSING DIAGNOSIS

1. Anxiety related to postoperative home care instructions.
2. Knowledge deficit related to:
   A. proper hand-washing technique.
   B. dressing care.
   C. skin care.
   D. medication administration/adverse reactions.
   E. fluid/dietary needs.
   F. postoperative cholangiogram with T-tube.
   G. other _____

3. Impaired gas exchange related to:
   A. failure to comply with medical orders.
   B. inconsistent breathing exercise.
   C. refusal to administer medication.
   D. inconsistent administration of medication.
   E. other _____

4. Ineffective individual/family coping related to:
   A. cost of medical care/poor insurance coverage.
   B. poor understanding of postoperative instructions.
   C. dependence on others for care.
   D. pain
   E. other _____

5. Diversional activity deficit related to:
   A. pain.
   B. dyspnea.
   C. respiratory congestion.
   D. other _____

   _____

6. Fear related to pain.
7. Potential fluid volume deficit related to:
   A. poor intake.
   B. vomiting.
   C. other _____

   _____

8. Impaired home maintenance management related to:
   A. dependence on others for care.
   B. pain.
   C. weakness.
   D. other _____

   _____

9. Potential for injury related to:
   A. poor supervision in the home.
   B. refusal to comply with medical instructions.
   C. other _____

   _____

10. Ineffective breathing pattern related to:
    A. postoperative pain.
    B. congestion.
    C. infection.
    D. other _____

    _____

11. Impaired physical mobility related to:
    A. weakness.
    B. abdominal pain.
    C. dyspnea.
    D. discomfort of abdominal suture line.
    E. other _____

    _____

12. Altered nutrition: potential for more than body requirements related to:
    A. anorexia.

 B. pain.

 C. obesity.

 D. low-fat diet.

 E. other _____
   _____

13. Altered parenting related to:

 A. pain.

 B. weakness.

 C. restriction of activity/heavy lifting.

 D. other _____
   _____

14. Self-care deficit: feeding/bathing/grooming/dressing/toileting related to:

 A. dependence on others for care.

 B. pain.

 C. weakness.

 D. other _____
   _____

15. Impaired skin integrity related to:

 A. abdominal drain.

 B. T-tube.

 C. suture line (sutures/staples).

 D. infection.

 E. other _____
   _____

II. SHORT-TERM GOALS

 1. Client/Family will verbalize fears, anxieties, and concerns after 1–2 R.N. visits.

 2. Client/Family will administer medication as ordered after 1 R.N. visit.

 3. Client/Family will immediately notify M.D. of adverse reactions or signs/symptoms of complications after 1 R.N. visit.

 4. Client/Family will properly wash hands after 1 R.N. visit.

 5. Client/Family will change abdominal dressing as ordered after 1–2 R.N. visits.

 6. Client/Family will clamp drainage tube/tubes as ordered 1 hour before and after each meal after 1–2 R.N. visits.

7. Client/Family will record color, amount, and consistency of bile every 24 hours as ordered after 1–2 R.N. visits.
8. Client/Family will follow breathing exercises/respiratory therapy as ordered after 1–2 R.N. visits.
9. Client will consume bile/bile preparations as ordered after 1–2 R.N. visits.
10. Client will consume fluids and low-fat diet as ordered after 1–2 R.N. visits.
11. Client will take vitamin K as ordered after 1 R.N. visit.
12. Client will exercise/rest as ordered after 1–2 R.N. visits.
13. Client/Family will apply abdominal binder as ordered after 1 R.N. visit.
14. Client will seek laboratory testing/M.D. appointments as ordered after 1 R.N. visit.

III. LONG-TERM GOALS

1. Normal digestion will be achieved in 2–4 weeks.
2. Independent activities of daily living will be resumed in 1–2 weeks.
3. Optimal level of health will be achieved in 2–4 weeks.

IV. OUTCOME CRITERIA

1. Vital signs are normal.
2. Weight remains normal.
3. Appetite is normal.
4. Chest is clear.
5. Skin is healthy and intact.
6. Ambulation is normal.
7. Laboratory results are within normal limits.
8. Client states he/she feels better.

V. NURSING INTERVENTION/TREATMENT

1. R.N. will consult with hospital discharge planner about treatment and rehabilitation goals.
2. R.N. will instruct client/family H.H.A. on:
   A. monitoring and recording of vital signs.
   B. proper hand washing.
   C. aseptic dressing change.

    D. clamping of drainage tube/tubes as ordered 1 hour before and after each meal.

    E. recording of color, amount, and consistency of bile every 24 hours.

    F. fluid intake/low-fat diet as ordered.

    G. recording of intake and output.

    H. daily recording of weight.

    I. weight reduction if ordered.

    J. good skin care measures.

    K. medication administration/adverse reactions.

    L. immediate notification of M.D. of adverse reactions or signs/symptoms of postoperative complications.

    M. postoperative cholangiogram with T-tube.

    N. breathing exercises/respiratory therapy (blow bottles, incentive spirometer, IPPB).

    O. exercise/rest as ordered.

    P. Vitamin K administration if ordered.

    Q. application of abdominal binder.

    R. diversional activities.

    S. laboratory testing/M.D. appointments.

3. R.N. will provide follow-up reports to M.D. and discharge summary when case closes.

4. R.N. will notify client/family/significant others/H.H.A. when case will close.

Chronic Obstructive Pulmonary Disease Care Plan

I. NURSING DIAGNOSIS

1. Anxiety related to:
   A. exertional dyspnea.
   B. breathlessness.
   C. chronic cough.
   D. difficulty with inspiration.
   E. wheezing.
   F. signs/symptoms of peptic ulcer formation.
   G. chest pain.
   H. hemoptysis.
   I. other _____

2. Knowledge deficit related to:
   A. signs/symptoms of COPD.
   B. medication administration/adverse reactions.
   C. laboratory testing/x-rays.
   D. rest/exercise.
   E. avoidance/limitation of smoking.
   F. fluid/dietary needs.
   G. signs/symptoms of peptic ulcer formation.
   H. treatment of peptic ulcer.
   I. breathing exercises/inhalation therapy/postural drainage/oxygen administration/chest physical therapy.

J. mouth care.

K. other _____

_____

3. Ineffective airway clearance related to:
    A. bronchospasm.
    B. exertional dyspnea.
    C. infection.
    D. smoking.
    E. other _____

_____

4. Impaired gas exchange related to:
    A. infection.
    B. smoking.
    C. breathlessness.
    D. difficulty with inspiration.
    E. other _____

_____

5. Ineffective individual/family coping related to:
    A. cigarette smoking.
    B. coughing.
    C. dependence on others for care.
    D. frequent hospitalizations.
    E. other _____

_____

6. Altered oral mucous membrane related to mouth breathing.
7. Impaired home maintenance management related to:
    A. activity intolerance.
    B. dependence on others for care.
    C. lack of support in the home.
    D. cost of medical care/poor insurance coverage.
    E. other _____

_____

8. Altered nutrition: potential for more than body requirements related to:
    A. anorexia.
    B. lack of support in the home.
    C. other _____

_____

9. Fear related to:
   A. dyspnea.
   B. poor prognosis.
   C. lack of support in the home.
   D. other _____

   _____

10. Altered thought processes related to:
    A. hypoxia.
    B. other _____

    _____

11. Ineffective breathing pattern related to:
    A. hyperpnea.
    B. hypoxia/shortness of breath.
    C. hemoptysis.
    D. chest pain/fatigue.
    E. inhibited cough response.
    F. limited chest movement postoperatively.
    G. poor positioning.
    H. obstructed airway.
    I. thick, retained secretions/wheezing.
    J. circulatory overload.
    K. other _____

    _____

12. Chest pain related to:
    A. difficulty expectorating.
    B. failure to cooperate with medical advice.
    C. refusal to take medication.
    D. inconsistent administration of medication.
    E. poor fluid/dietary intake.
    F. other _____

    _____

II. SHORT-TERM GOALS

1. Client/Family will verbalize all fears, anxieties, and concerns after 1–2 R.N. visits.
2. Client/Family will wash hands properly after handling respiratory equipment and contaminated materials after 1 R.N. visit.
3. Client will cough 5–10 times each hour after 1–2 R.N. visits.

4. Client/Family will administer medication as prescribed after 1–2 R.N. visits.
5. Client/Family will immediately notify M.D. of adverse reactions or change in condition after 1–2 R.N. visits.
6. Client/Family will avoid respiratory irritants (e.g., dust, pollen, smoking, temperature extremes, high altitudes, talcum, lint) after 1 R.N. visit.
7. Client/Family will use respiratory equipment (humidifier/incentive spirometer/blow bottles/toys/oxygen/suction) as ordered after 1–2 R.N. visits (in consultation with M.D. and R.T.).
8. Client/Family will perform postural drainage exercises as ordered after 1 R.N. visit.
9. Client will demonstrate breathing exercises as ordered after 1 R.N. visit.
10. Client will drink a warm beverage on arising for adequate expectoration after 1 R.N. visit.
11. Client will obtain adequate rest each day after 1 R.N. visit.
12. Client/Family will prepare small, frequent feedings to lessen pulmonary fatigue after 1 R.N. visit.
13. Client will exercise moderately after 1–2 R.N. visits.
14. Client/Family will seek laboratory testing/M.D. appointments as ordered after 1–2 R.N. visits.

III. LONG-TERM GOALS

1. Adequate respiratory functioning will be achieved in 3–4 weeks.
2. Independent activities of daily living will resume in 1–2 weeks.
3. Optimal level of health will be achieved in 3–4 weeks.

IV. OUTCOME CRITERIA

1. Vital signs are normal.
2. Skin color is normal.
3. Chest is clear.
4. Respirations are normal.
5. Airway is patent.
6. Laboratory test results are normal.
7. P_{O_2} and P_{CO_2} are normal.
8. Appetite is normal.
9. Weight is appropriate for height.
10. Hydration is appropriate.

11. Client is alert and oriented.

12. Client states he/she feels better.

V. NURSING INTERVENTION/TREATMENT

1. R.N. will assess general physical status on initial home visit.

2. R.N. will instruct client/family/H.H.A. on:

   A. proper hand-washing technique.

   B. monitoring and recording of vital signs.

   C. oral hygiene.

   D. adequate disposal of tissues and contaminated articles.

   E. breathing exercises/respiratory therapy and care of equipment.

   F. positioning.

   G. oxygen therapy/precautions.

   H. rest/exercise.

   I. avoidance of allergens and etiologic agents.

   J. avoidance/limitation of smoking.

   K. medication administration/adverse reactions.

   L. immediate notification of M.D. of adverse reactions or change in condition.

   M. avoidance of emotional stress.

   N. fluid intake/diet.

   O. laboratory testing/M.D. appointments.

3. R.N. will provide M.D. with follow-up reports and discharge summary when case closes.

4. R.N. will notify client/family/H.H.A./significant others when case will close.

5. R.N. will consult with respiratory equipment company about further instructions for managing and operating equipment while in the home; will also consult with R.T. for his/her instructions/report.

Cirrhosis
Care Plan

I. NURSING DIAGNOSIS

1. Knowledge deficit related to:
   A. prevention/treatment of cirrhosis.
   B. signs/symptoms.
   C. medication administration/adverse reactions.
   D. fluid/dietary needs.
   E. other _____

2. Altered nutrition: less than body requirements related to:
   A. anorexia.
   B. nausea/vomiting.
   C. chronic dyspepsia.
   D. poor meal preparation/consumption.
   E. hematemesis.
   F. other _____

3. Noncompliance with therapy related to:
   A. denial.
   B. alcoholism/drug abuse.
   C. confusion.
   D. lack of support in the home.
   E. other _____

4. Constipation/Diarrhea/Incontinence/Melena related to:
   A. confusion.
   B. poor fluid/dietary intake.
   C. poor administration of medication.
   D. inadequate exercise.
   E. other ⸺⸺⸺⸺⸺⸺⸺⸺⸺⸺⸺
   ⸺⸺⸺⸺⸺⸺⸺⸺⸺⸺⸺

5. Impaired verbal communication related to:
   A. confusion.
   B. disorientation.
   C. altered levels of consciousness.
   D. other ⸺⸺⸺⸺⸺⸺⸺⸺⸺⸺⸺
   ⸺⸺⸺⸺⸺⸺⸺⸺⸺⸺⸺

6. Potential for injury related to:
   A. increasing abdominal distention (ascites).
   B. increasing jaundice.
   C. excessive vomiting.
   D. dyspnea.
   E. fever.
   F. hemorrhagic manifestations (epistaxis/ecchymosis/petechiae/ bleeding gums).
   G. hematemesis.
   H. abdominal pain.
   I. weight loss.
   J. increasing stupor/mental changes.
   K. other ⸺⸺⸺⸺⸺⸺⸺⸺⸺⸺⸺
   ⸺⸺⸺⸺⸺⸺⸺⸺⸺⸺⸺

7. Fluid volume excess related to:
   A. ammonia intoxication.
   B. vitamin deficiency.
   C. poor fluid/dietary intake.
   D. hypovolemia.
   E. other ⸺⸺⸺⸺⸺⸺⸺⸺⸺⸺⸺
   ⸺⸺⸺⸺⸺⸺⸺⸺⸺⸺⸺

8. Fear related to:
   A. chronic nature of disease.
   B. death.
   C. other ⸺⸺⸺⸺⸺⸺⸺⸺⸺⸺⸺
   ⸺⸺⸺⸺⸺⸺⸺⸺⸺⸺⸺

9. Impaired physical mobility related to:
   A. ascites.
   B. nausea/vomiting.
   C. dyspnea.
   D. edema.
   E. diarrhea.
   F. fever.
   G. other _____

10. Self-care deficit: feeding/bathing/dressing/grooming/toileting/ ambulating related to:
    A. immobility.
    B. dyspnea.
    C. increasing stupor/mental changes.
    D. other _____

11. Impaired skin integrity related to:
    A. edema.
    B. hemorrhagic tendencies.
    C. other _____

12. Sleep pattern disturbance related to:
    A. restlessness.
    B. dyspnea.
    C. vomiting.
    D. diarrhea.
    E. mental changes.
    F. other _____

13. Altered gastrointestinal tissue perfusion related to:
    A. inadequate detoxification of the liver.
    B. ammonia intoxication.
    C. other _____

14. Altered thought processes related to:
    A. ammonia intoxication.
    B. coma.
    C. other _____

II. SHORT-TERM GOALS

1. Client/Family will seek immediate medical care after 1–2 R.N. visits.
2. Client/Family will keep strict intake and output records daily after 1–2–3 R.N. visits.
3. Client/Family will administer prescribed medication after 1–2 R.N. visits.
4. Client/Family will notify M.D. immediately for adverse reactions or change in condition after 1–2 R.N. visits.
5. Client/Family will seek prescribed laboratory testing after 1–2 R.N. visits.
6. Client will take vitamin therapy as ordered after 1 R.N. visit.
7. Client (nonedematous) will consume a high-protein diet as ordered after 1 R.N. visit.
8. Client will take small, frequent feedings instead of 3 large meals as ordered after 1–2 R.N. visits.
9. Client will take nourishment via tube feeding after 1–2–3 R.N. visits.
10. Client (with diarrhea) will take pancreatin as ordered after 1–2 R.N. visits.
11. Client (with edema/ascites) will restrict sodium to 200-500 mg daily as ordered after 1–2 R.N. visits.
12. Client will avoid table salt, salty foods, salted butter and margarine, and all canned and frozen foods as ordered after 1–2 R.N. visits.
13. Client will use salt substitutes such as lemon juice, oregano, and thyme.
14. Client will restrict fluid intake as ordered after 1–2 R.N. visits.
15. Client (experiencing impending/advanced coma) will consume a low-protein/protein-free diet as ordered after 1–2 R.N. visits.
16. Client will abstain from alcohol as ordered after 1–2–3–4 R.N. visits.
17. Client/Family will change position/turn every 2 hours after 1–2 R.N. visits.
18. Client will rest/exercise appropriately after 1–2 R.N. visits.
19. Client will seek aid of therapy groups/psychiatrist/organizations/religious advisor after 2–3 R.N. visits.
20. Client will seek employment as ordered by M.D. after 3–4 R.N. visits.

III. LONG-TERM GOALS

1. Independent activities of daily living will be resumed in 3–4 weeks.
2. Optimal level of health will be achieved in 6–8 weeks.

IV. OUTCOME CRITERIA

1. Vital signs are normal.
2. Skin/Mucous membrane is normal color and temperature, healthy, and intact.
3. Appetite is normal.
4. Weight is appropriate for height.
5. Circulatory status remains normal.
6. Bowel/Bladder functions normally.
7. Laboratory test results are normal.
8. Vision/Sclera is clear and normal.
9. Chest remains clear.
10. Alcohol is avoided.
11. Nutritious meals are consumed.
12. Client is alert, cooperative, and responsible.
13. Client states he/she feels better.
14. Client seeks employment.

V. NURSING INTERVENTION/TREATMENT

1. Before hospital discharge, R.N. will obtain explicit instructions about rehabilitation at home from hospital discharge planner.
2. R.N. will instruct client/family/H.H.A. on:
   A. monitoring and recording of vital signs; R.N. will, if possible, teach family member to take blood pressure.
   B. fluid restriction/sodium restriction/diet as ordered (normal protein, calorie, and vitamin intake). If coma is impending, client should receive a low-protein/protein-free diet high in calories.
   C. medication administration/adverse reactions.
   D. immediate notification of M.D. of adverse reactions or change in condition.
   E. skin care/personal hygiene.
   F. enteral feedings/hyperalimentation.
   G. IV therapy.

    H. exercise/rest.

    I. Foley catheter care.

    J. restriction of alcohol/illegal drugs.

    K. recording of intake and output.

    L. daily recording of weight.

    M. avoidance of constrictive clothing.

    N. collecting stool for guaiac testing.

    O. use of small-gauge needles for injections.

    P. avoidance of stress.

    Q. literature/organizations for additional assistance/hospice care.

    R. laboratory testing/M.D. appointments.

3. R.N. will provide M.D. with follow-up reports and discharge summary when case closes.

4. R.N. will notify client/family/H.H.A./significant others when case will close.

Colostomy/Ileostomy Care Plan

I. NURSING DIAGNOSIS

1. Anxiety related to:
   A. altered body image.
   B. contact with waste materials.
   C. actual/potential contamination of wound site.
   D. dressing care.
   E. other _____

2. Potential impaired skin integrity related to:
   A. leakage of fecal enzymes around stoma.
   B. allergic response to sealant.
   C. poor fit/poor application of bag.
   D. frequent changing of bag.
   E. other _____

3. Knowledge deficit related to:
   A. skin care/application of appliance.
   B. medication administration/adverse reactions.
   C. dressing care.
   D. signs/symptoms of infection.
   E. diet/fluids.
   F. enemas/bowel irrigations.
   G. signs/symptoms of infection/electrolyte imbalance.
   H. sexuality.

    I. other _____

_____

4. Constipation/Diarrhea related to:
    A. excessive fluid intake.
    B. hypovolemia.
    C. poor dietary habits.
    D. medication administration/adverse reactions.
    E. poor irrigation technique.
    F. inability to set up daily routine for evacuation.
    G. emotional stress.
    H. other _____

_____

5. Potential for infection related to:
    A. leakage of appliance.
    B. poor irrigation technique.
    C. allergic response to sealant.
    D. poor fluid/dietary intake.
    E. frequent changing of bag.
    F. other _____

_____

6. Ineffective individual/family coping related to:
    A. dependence on others for care.
    B. irritability.
    C. inadequate rest.
    D. cost of medical care/poor insurance coverage.
    E. other _____

_____

7. Noncompliance with therapy related to:
    A. denial.
    B. repulsion.
    C. weakness.
    D. other _____

_____

8. Fear related to:
    A. infection.
    B. potential/actual malignancy.
    C. rejection by others.
    D. other _____

_____

9. Sleep pattern disturbance related to:
    A. abdominal pain/discomfort.
    B. poor fit of appliance, resulting in leakage.
    C. anxiety.
    D. other _____

    _____

10. Social isolation related to:
    A. embarrassment.
    B. fear of rejection by others.
    C. other _____

    _____

11. Self-care deficit: feeding/bathing/dressing/grooming/colostomy care related to:
    A. weakness.
    B. repulsion.
    C. other _____

    _____

12. Situational low self-esteem related to:
    A. dependence on others for care.
    B. embarrassment.
    C. rejection by others.
    D. fear of death.
    E. other _____

    _____

II. SHORT-TERM GOALS

1. Client/Family will provide equipment in home after hospital discharge (after phone contact from community health nurse).
2. Client/Family will develop rapport with nurse after 1–2–3–4 R.N. visits.
3. Client/Family will verbalize fears, anxieties, and concerns after 1–2–3–4 R.N. visits.
4. Client/Family will demonstrate proper hand-washing technique after 1–2 R.N. visits.
5. Client/Family will remove appliance after 1–2 R.N. visits.
6. Client/Family will assemble all equipment after 1–2–3–4 R.N. visits.
7. Client/Family will change dressing/appliance as directed after 1–2–3–4 R.N. visits.

8. Client/Family will apply benzoin/karaya paste/stoma adhesive to create a level area for bag application after 1–2–3–4 R.N. visits.
9. Client/Family will learn to measure stoma opening and apply proper-fitting bag after 1–2–3–4 R.N. visits.
10. Client/Family will administer medication as ordered after 1–2 R.N. visits.
11. Client/Family will notify M.D. immediately of adverse reactions or change in condition after 1–2 R.N. visits.
12. Client/Family will seek laboratory testing/M.D. appointments as ordered after 1–2 R.N. visits.

III. LONG-TERM GOALS

1. Independent activities of daily living will be resumed in 1–2 weeks.
2. Optimal level of health will be achieved in 3–4 weeks.

IV. OUTCOME CRITERIA

1. Vital signs are normal.
2. Skin/Mucous membrane is healthy and intact.
3. Bowel elimination is normal.
4. Intake and output are normal.
5. Laboratory test results are normal.
6. Weight is appropriate for height.
7. Appetite is normal.
8. Client states he/she feels better.

V. NURSING INTERVENTION/TREATMENT

1. Before visiting home, R.N. will contact client/family to ensure proper supplies are present for instructions to be given.
2. R.N. will allow client/family to verbalize fears, anxieties, and concerns.
3. R.N. will assess prior instructions given to client and allow for redemonstration if necessary. R.N. will assess signs/symptoms of infection/fit of colostomy bag/color, amount, consistency, and frequency of stools.
4. R.N. will instruct client/family/H.H.A. on:
   A. proper hand-washing technique.
   B. dressing care/nonadhesive dressing (Telfa).

C. signs/symptoms of infection.

D. cleansing of skin and application of sealant and colostomy bag/ storage and cleaning of equipment.

E. fluid intake/diet as ordered.

F. medication administration/adverse reactions.

G. immediate notification of M.D. of adverse reactions or change in condition.

H. chemotherapy/radiation/adverse reactions

I. nonadhesive pouch (Perry Model 51 or Vance pouch).

J. sexuality.

K. enemas/bowel irrigations.

L. storage and cleaning of equipment.

M. monitoring of vital signs if necessary.

N. daily recording of weight.

O. laboratory testing/M.D. appointments.

P. exercise/rest.

Q. diversional activities.

5. R.N. will provide client with additional literature if necessary for colostomy care; will encourage client to join clubs or organizations/ speak with people who have had similar experience.

6. R.N. will provide M.D. with follow-up reports and discharge summary when case closes.

7. R.N. will notify client/family/H.H.A./significant others when case will close.

Colostomy Irrigation Care Plan

I. NURSING DIAGNOSIS

1. Anxiety related to:
   A. unfamiliarity with procedure.
   B. pain/discomfort.
   C. poor hospital discharge instructions.
   D. other _____
   _____

2. Pain related to:
   A. improper positioning of tubing.
   B. poor/improper dietary regimen.
   C. rapid administration of irrigation.
   D. insufficient lubrication of tubing.
   E. skin breakdown.
   F. inconsistent scheduling of daily irrigations.
   G. overdistention with fluid during irrigation.
   H. other _____
   _____

3. Self-care deficit; feeding/bathing/grooming/dressing/colostomy irrigations related to:
   A. pain/discomfort.
   B. confusion.
   C. dependence on others for care.
   D. poor hand grasp/weakness in upper/lower extremities.
   E. other _____
   _____

4. Potential for injury related to:
   A. poor hospital discharge instructions.
   B. use of inappropriate equipment.
   C. poor hand-washing technique.
   D. other _____

5. Knowledge deficit related to:
   A. fluid/dietary needs.
   B. medication administration/adverse reactions.
   C. irrigation technique.
   D. proper hand-washing technique.
   E. equipment needed.
   F. other _____

6. Social isolation related to:
   A. impaired body image.
   B. anger.
   C. fear of rejection by others.
   D. other _____

7. Ineffective individual/family coping related to:
   A. dependence on others for care.
   B. poor time scheduling for irrigations.
   C. cost of medical care/poor insurance coverage.
   D. other _____

8. Constipation/Diarrhea related to:
   A. inappropriate/inadequate fluid/dietary intake.
   B. emotional stress.
   C. poor time scheduling for irrigations.
   D. infection.
   E. inadequate exercise/rest.
   F. medication/adverse reactions.
   G. other _____

9. Situational low self-esteem related to:
   A. dependence on others for care.
   B. altered body image.

    C. rejection by others.

    D. other _____

_____

10. Noncompliance with therapy related to:

    A. denial.

    B. repulsion.

    C. dependence on others for care.

    D. other _____

_____

11. Impaired home maintenance management related to:

    A. numerous demands by family members.

    B. lengthy irrigation procedure.

    C. other _____

_____

12. Sexual dysfunction related to:

    A. rejection.

    B. anxiety.

    C. embarrassment.

    D. other _____

_____

II. SHORT-TERM GOALS

1. Client/Family will verbalize any fears, anxieties, and concerns after 1–2–3–4 R.N. visits.
2. Client/Family will assemble all equipment after 1–2–3 R.N. visits.
3. Client will position self comfortably in bathroom after 1–2 R.N. visits.
4. Client/Family will wash hands as directed after 1–2 R.N. visits.
5. Client/Family will clear tubing with water before administration after 1–2 R.N. visits.
6. Client/Family will lubricate tubing effectively after 1–2 R.N. visits.
7. Client/Family will control flow of solution by height of bag after 1–2–3–4 R.N. visits.
8. Client/Family will administer approximately 500-1000 cc according to tolerance and return (if necessary, increase fluid tolerance in increments of 50-200 cc) in 1–2–3–4 R.N. visits.
9. Client/Family will plan a comfortable daily/once-weekly/twice-weekly routine for irrigations after 3–4 R.N. visits.

10. Client/Family will apply appliance as ordered after 1–2–3–4 R.N. visits.
11. Client/Family will administer medication/creams/ointments as ordered after 1–2–3–4 R.N. visits.
12. Client/Family will immediately notify M.D. of adverse reactions or change in condition after 1–2 R.N. visits.

III. LONG-TERM GOALS

1. Independent activities of daily living will be resumed in 1–2 weeks.
2. Regular bowel regimen will be established in 1–2 weeks.
3. Optimal level of health will be achieved in 3–4 weeks.

IV. OUTCOME CRITERIA

1. Vital signs are normal.
2. Weight is appropriate for height.
3. Appetite is normal.
4. Skin/Mucous membrane is healthy and intact.
5. Laboratory test results are normal.
6. Bowel elimination is normal.
7. Intake and output are normal.
8. Client states he/she feels better.

V. NURSING INTERVENTION/TREATMENT

1. R.N. will allow client/family to verbalize all fears, anxieties, and concerns before start of procedure; will assess discharge planning instructions from hospital.
2. R.N. will instruct client/family/H.H.A. on:
   A. fluid intake/diet.
   B. hand-washing technique.
   C. skin cleansing, lubrication, insertion of tubing, amount of solution to flow through tubing and bag, height of bag, time allotment for return of intestinal contents, and cleaning of equipment.
   D. application of clean bag/storage and cleansing of equipment.
   E. daily bowel routine (once weekly/twice weekly/thrice weekly).
   F. medication administration/adverse reactions.
   G. monitoring and recording of vital signs.

      H. immediate notification of M.D. of adverse reactions or change in condition.

      I. laboratory testing/M.D. appointments.

3. R.N. will provide M.D. with follow-up reports and discharge summary when case closes.

4. R.N. will notify client/family/H.H.A./significant others when case will close.

Continuous Ambulatory Peritoneal Dialysis Care Plan

I. NURSING DIAGNOSIS

1. Anxiety related to:
    A. disturbed sleep pattern.
    B. nausea/vomiting.
    C. weight loss.
    D. unexpected fractures.
    E. potential infection.
    F. potential clotting of catheter.
    G. dislodgement of catheter.
    H. contamination.
    I. cost of treatment/supplies.
    J. other _____
    _____

2. Potential for infection related to:
    A. poor hand-washing technique.
    B. poor aseptic exchange technique.
    C. inappropriate bag change.
    D. poor dressing, catheter, and exit site technique.
    E. defective catheter.
    F. obstructed catheter.
    G. other _____
    _____

3. Altered renal tissue perfusion related to:
    A. too rapid infusion of dialysis solution.
    B. excessive suction during outflow phase.
    C. healing of incision.
    D. infection.
    E. fluid overload.
    F. increased removal and sodium from body.
    G. medication administration.
    H. poor diet.
    I. other _____

    _____

4. Ineffective breathing pattern related to:
    A. fluid overload.
    B. respiratory congestion.
    C. infection.
    D. strenuous exercise.
    E. other _____

    _____

5. Ineffective individual coping related to:
    A. cost of treatment/supplies.
    B. depression.
    C. lack of support in the home.
    D. rejection by significant others.
    E. necessity of daily dialysis routine.
    F. other _____

    _____

6. Fluid volume excess related to:
    A. infusion overload.
    B. excess sodium intake.
    C. poor dietary control.
    D. noncompliance with instructions.
    E. other _____

    _____

7. Potential fluid volume deficit related to:
    A. vomiting.

B. diarrhea.

C. dehydration.

D. inadequate fluid intake.

E. noncompliance with instructions.

F. strenuous exercise.

G. other _____

8. Constipation/Diarrhea related to:

A. medication administration.

B. fluids/diet.

C. emotional stress.

D. lack of exercise.

E. other _____

9. Impaired home maintenance management related to:

A. weakness.

B. fatigue.

C. dependence on others for care.

D. lack of support in the home.

E. cost of treatment/supplies.

F. other _____

10. Impaired physical mobility related to:

A. muscle spasms.

B. cramping of lower extremities.

C. back pain.

D. fractures.

E. other _____

11. Altered oral mucous membrane: dryness/ulcer formation/bleeding related to:

A. dehydration.

B. anemia.

C. other _____

12. Altered nutrition: less than body requirements related to:

A. sodium restriction.

B. potassium restriction.

    C. calcium/phosphate restriction.

    D. protein restriction.

    E. fluid restriction.

    F. other _____

    _____

13. Potential impaired skin integrity related to:

    A. poor hand-washing technique.

    B. poor dressing, catheter, and exit site technique.

    C. leakage around catheter.

    D. poor healing of incisional site.

    E. other _____

    _____

14. Knowledge deficit related to:

    A. disease process.

    B. signs/symptoms.

    C. prevention of complications (e.g., peritonitis)/injury.

    D. medication administration/adverse reactions.

    E. daily weights.

    F. fluids/diet/aluminum hydroxide (i.e., Dialume) recipes.

    G. vitamin therapy.

    H. daily recording of intake and output.

    I.   recording of vital signs, blood pressure, and edema.

    J. dressing care.

    K. skin care.

    L. catheter care.

    M. diabetic management.

    N. time schedule of fluid exchanges.

    O. environment for administration of dialysate solution.

    P. cost of treatment/equipment/supplies.

    Q. types of equipment/expiration dates of supplies/storage.

    R. recording of type and amount of fluid instilled and returned, duration of exchange, and medications added to dialysate.

    S. exercise/rest.

    T. laboratory testing/M.D. appointments/dental appointments.

    U. employment/vocational counseling/college.

    V. financial assistance.

    W. insurance.

    X. support groups/counseling/resources.

Y. recreation.

Z. other _____

_____

II. SHORT-TERM GOALS

1. Client/Family will verbalize fears, anxieties, and concerns after 1–2–3 R.N. visits.
2. Client/Family will administer prescribed medication after 1–2–3 R.N. visits.
3. Client/Family will notify M.D. immediately of adverse effects of medication or signs/symptoms of complications after 1–2–3 R.N. visits.
4. Client/Family will strictly record intake and output after 1–2 R.N. visits.
5. Client/Family will administer prescribed amount of fluids orally after 1–2–3 R.N. visits.
6. Client/Family will follow prescribed diet after 1–2–3 R.N. visits.
7. Client/Family will limit sodium, potassium, calcium, phosphorus, and protein in diet as ordered after 1–2–3 R.N. visits.
8. Client/Family will obtain teaching materials for CAPD after 1–2–3 R.N. visits.
9. Client/Family will record daily weight, vital signs, blood pressure, and signs/symptoms of edema before CAPD procedure after 1–2–3 R.N. visits.
10. Client will exercise/rest as ordered after 1–2–3 R.N. visits.
11. Client will avoid smoking/alcohol consumption after 1–2–3 R.N. visits.
12. Client/Family will obtain and properly store CAPD equipment/ supplies after 1–2 R.N. visits.
13. Client/Family will assemble CAPD supplies in safe, clean, well-lighted, environment after 1–2–3 R.N. visits.
14. Client/Family will wash hands properly after 1–2–3 R.N. visits.
15. Client will take showers and thoroughly rinse catheter site as ordered after 1–2–3 R.N. visits.
16. Client/Family will instruct other persons to wear masks if they approach within 10 feet of CAPD procedure after 1–2–3 R.N. visits.
17. Client will sit in a comfortable chair for procedure, in a room free from drafts, after 1–2–3 R.N. visits.
18. Client/Family will obtain a table/stand close to chair to hold supplies for procedure after 1–2 R.N. visits.

19. Client will have bladder emptied before procedure after 1–2–3 R.N. visits.
20. Client/Family will perform dialysis on time, according to daily schedule, after 4–5–6 R.N. visits.
21. Client/Family will warm solution as ordered after 1–2–3 R.N. visits.
22. Client/Family will perform catheter/dressing care using aseptic technique as ordered after 4–5–6 R.N. visits.
23. Client/Family will use germicidal exchange device as ordered after 4–5–6 R.N. visits.
24. Client/Family will attach bottle/plastic bag of sterile dialysis solution to catheter and raise the bag to shoulder level or higher after 4–5–6 R.N. visits.
25. Client/Family will take bag when empty and fold it under clothing after 4–5–6 R.N. visits.
26. Client/Family will unfold bag and lower it below abdomen for gravity drainage after prescribed time after 4–5–6 R.N. visits.
27. Client/Family will record type and amount of fluid instilled and returned, duration of exchange, and medications added after 4–5–6 R.N. visits.
28. Client/Family will discard used solution and attach a new bag as ordered after 4–5–6 R.N. visits.
29. Client will secure catheter to abdomen with tape and wear clean clothing every day after 1–2–3 R.N. visits.
30. Client/Family will seek employment, schooling, and recreation after 4–5–6 R.N. visits.

III. LONG-TERM GOALS

1. Regulation of the fluid balance of the body will occur in 1–4 weeks.
2. Removal of toxic substances and metabolic wastes from the body will occur in 1–4 weeks.
3. Independent activities of daily living will be resumed in 1–2 weeks.
4. Optimal level of health will be achieved in 3–4 weeks.

IV. OUTCOME CRITERIA

1. Vital signs are normal.
2. Blood pressure is normal.
3. Laboratory test results are normal.

4. Return dialysis solution is clear, free from infection and contamination.
5. Intake and output are within normal limits.
6. Appetite is normal.
7. Increased tolerance of different foods is normal.
8. Body weight is normal.
9. Exercise tolerance is normal.
10. Skin is improved in color, texture, and moisture.
11. Menses are normal.
12. Libido is normal.
13. Hair growth is normal.
14. Normal puberty is achieved.
15. Liver function tests are normal.
16. Diabetes is controlled.
17. Heart/Chest sounds are normal.
18. Chest x-ray and EKG are normal.
19. Bone growth is normal.
20. Mobility is normal.
21. Client is alert, sociable, and cooperative.
22. Client states he/she feels better.

V. NURSING INTERVENTIONS/TREATMENT

1. R.N. will contact hospital discharge planner for written instructions for CAPD.
2. R.N. will contact client/family to ensure proper supplies are present prior to home visit. R.N. will assess client/family level of understanding to estimate length of time needed for each training session.
3. R.N. will monitor vital signs, blood pressure, weight, color, and turgor of mucous membranes and skin, signs of bleeding, intake and output, and diabetic complications.
4. R.N. will contact M.D. for recent laboratory testing, fluids and diet, CAPD instructions, medications, etc.
5. R.N. will allow client/family to verbalize all fears, anxieties, and concerns about condition and procedures.
6. R.N. will instruct client/family/H.H.A. on:
   A. disease process and signs/symptoms.
   B. diabetic management, if applicable.
   C. complications of condition (e.g., peritonitis/cloudy effluent/

fever/abdominal pain and tenderness/nausea/vomiting) and
CAPD procedure (e.g., dialysis leak/bleeding/poor drainage/
respiratory distress/outflow problems/tunnel infection).

D. daily monitoring and recording of vital signs, including blood
pressure, weight, and edema.

E. medication administration (e.g., Heparin, antibiotics, iron
preparations, analgesics, androgen therapy, and insulin)/
adverse reactions/ingredients in over-the-counter medications.

F. immediate notification of M.D. of adverse reactions or change in
condition.

G. daily intake and output.

H. fluids/diet/Dialume recipes.

I. CAPD procedure: proper handwashing supplies/drainage and
infusion stand/dialysis solution containers/battery pack and
germicidal exchange device/AC adapter/soap/mask/transfer set/
medication/syringe/povidone-iodine swabs/outlet port clamp/
storage area/environment/avoidance of infection/aseptic
technique/skin care/central tunneled or central nontunneled
catheter and exit site care/tubing care/dressing care/operation of
germicidal exchange device/gravity drainage/removal of bag
from overpouch/height of equipment/hourly exchange process
as ordered and solution to be administered and discarded/
expiration dates of solutions/termination of dialysis.

J. types and storage of solutions.

K. CAPD home record: dates, times, weight, standing blood
pressure, solution (1.5%/2.5%/4.25%), drainage volume,
drainage condition (clear/cloudy), comments, and additives.

L. vitamin therapy/phosphate binders/calcium supplements.

M. bathing/showers.

N. types of clothing.

O. cost of treatment/equipment/supplies.

P. home care van delivery of supplies.

Q. exercise/rest.

R. employment.

S. vocational counseling.

T. college.

U. financial assistance.

V. insurance coverage.

W. support groups/home client networking program/education
programs/resources.

X. travel programs.

    Y. counseling.

    Z. recreation.

7. R.N. will provide M.D. with follow-up reports and discharge summary when case closes.

8. R.N. will notify client/family/H.H.A./significant others when case will close.

Continuous Cycler Peritoneal Dialysis Care Plan

I. NURSING DIAGNOSIS

1. Anxiety related to:
   A. disturbed sleep pattern.
   B. nausea/vomiting.
   C. weight loss.
   D. unexpected fractures.
   E. potential infection.
   F. potential clotting of catheter.
   G. dislodgement of catheter.
   H. contamination.
   I. cost of treatment/supplies.
   J. other _____

2. Potential for infection related to:
   A. poor hand-washing technique.
   B. poor aseptic exchange technique.
   C. inappropriate bag change.
   D. poor dressing, catheter, and exit site technique.
   E. defective catheter.
   F. obstructed catheter.
   G. other _____

3. Altered renal tissue perfusion related to:
   A. too rapid infusion of dialysis solution.
   B. excessive suction during outflow phase.
   C. healing of incision.
   D. infection.
   E. fluid overload.
   F. increased removal and sodium from body.
   G. medication administration.
   H. poor diet.
   I. other _____

4. Ineffective breathing pattern related to:
   A. fluid overload.
   B. respiratory congestion.
   C. infection.
   D. strenuous exercise.
   E. other _____

5. Ineffective individual coping related to:
   A. cost of treatment/supplies.
   B. depression.
   C. lack of support in the home.
   D. rejection by significant others.
   E. necessity of daily dialysis routine.
   F. other _____

6. Fluid volume excess related to:
   A. infusion overload.
   B. excess sodium intake.
   C. poor dietary control.
   D. noncompliance with instructions.
   E. other _____

7. Potential fluid volume deficit related to:
   A. vomiting
   B. diarrhea.
   C. dehydration.
   D. inadequate fluid intake.

    E. noncompliance with instructions.

    F. strenuous exercise.

    G. other _____

    _____

8. Constipation/Diarrhea related to:

    A. medication administration.

    B. fluids/diet.

    C. emotional stress.

    D. lack of exercise.

    E. other _____

    _____

9. Impaired home maintenance management related to:

    A. weakness.

    B. fatigue.

    C. dependence on others for care.

    D. lack of support in the home.

    E. cost of treatment/supplies.

    F. other _____

    _____

10. Impaired physical mobility related to:

    A. muscle spasms.

    B. cramping of lower extremities.

    C. back pain.

    D. fractures.

    E. other _____

    _____

11. Altered oral mucous membrane: dryness/ulcer formation/bleeding related to:

    A. dehydration.

    B. anemia.

    C. other _____

    _____

12. Altered nutrition: less than body requirements related to:

    A. sodium restriction.

    B. potassium restriction.

    C. calcium/phosphate restriction.

    D. protein restriction.

    E. fluid restriction.

F. other _____
_____

13. Potential impaired skin integrity related to:
    A. poor hand-washing technique.
    B. poor dressing, catheter, and exit site technique.
    C. leakage around catheter.
    D. poor healing of incisional site.
    E. other _____
    _____

14. Knowledge deficit related to:
    A. disease process.
    B. signs/symptoms.
    C. prevention of complications (e.g., peritonitis)/injury.
    D. medication administration/adverse reactions.
    E. daily weight.
    F. fluids/diet/aluminum hydroxide (i.e., Dialume) recipes.
    G. vitamin therapy.
    H. daily recording of intake and output.
    I. recording of vital signs, blood pressure, and edema.
    J. dressing care.
    K. skin care.
    L. catheter care.
    M. diabetic management.
    N. time schedule of fluid exchanges.
    O. environment for administration of dialysate solution.
    P. cost of treatment/equipment/supplies/expiration dates/storage.
    Q. operation of cycler machine/alarm system.
    R. recording of type and amount of fluid instilled and returned, duration of exchange, and medications added to dialysate.
    S. exercise/rest.
    T. laboratory testing/M.D. appointments/dental appointments.
    U. employment/vocational counseling/college.
    V. financial assistance.
    W. insurance.
    X. support groups/counseling/resources.
    Y. recreation.
    Z. other _____
    _____

II. SHORT-TERM GOALS

1. Client/Family will verbalize all fears, anxieties, and concerns after 1–2–3 R.N. visits.
2. Client/Family will administer prescribed medication after 1–2–3 R.N. visits.
3. Client/Family will notify M.D. immediately of adverse effects of medication or signs/symptoms of complications after 1–2–3 R.N. visits.
4. Client/Family will record intake and output after 1–2 R.N. visits.
5. Client/Family will administer prescribed amount of fluids orally after 1–2–3 R.N. visits.
6. Client/Family will follow prescribed diet after 1–2–3 R.N. visits.
7. Client/Family will limit sodium, potassium, calcium, phosphorus, and protein in diet as ordered after 1–2–3 R.N. visits.
8. Client/Family will obtain teaching materials for CCPD after 1–2–3 R.N. visits.
9. Client/Family will record daily weight, vital signs, blood pressure, and signs/symptoms of edema before CCPD procedure after 1–2–3 R.N. visits.
10. Client will exercise/rest as ordered after 1–2–3 R.N. visits.
11. Client will avoid smoking/alcohol consumption after 1–2–3 R.N. visits.
12. Client/Family will obtain and properly store CCPD equipment/ supplies after 1–2 R.N. visits.
13. Client/Family will assemble CCPD supplies in safe, clean, well-lighted environment after 1–2–3 R.N. visits.
14. Client/Family will wash hands properly after 1–2–3 R.N. visits.
15. Client will take showers and thoroughly rinse catheter site as ordered after 1–2–3 R.N. visits.
16. Client/Family will obtain a table/stand close to chair to hold supplies for procedure after 1–2 R.N. visits.
17. Client will have bladder emptied before procedure after 1–2–3 R.N. visits.
18. Client/Family will perform dialysis according to daily schedule, on time, after 4–5–6 R.N. visits.
19. Client/Family will verbally describe the 3 stages of dialysis: the inflow of solution, the dwell time, and the drain time, after 4–5–6 R.N. visits.
20. Client/Family will perform dialysis before sleep at night using continuous cycler as ordered after 1–2–3 R.N. visits.

21. Client/Family will perform combined programs of CAPD and CCPD as ordered after 1–2–3 R.N. visits.
22. Client/Family will perform CCPD only as ordered after 1–2–3 R.N. visits.
23. Client will secure catheter to abdomen with tape and wear clean clothing every day after 1–2–3 R.N. visits.
24. Client/Family will seek employment, schooling, and recreation after 4–5–6 R.N. visits.

III. LONG-TERM GOALS

1. Regulation of the fluid balance of the body will occur in 1–4 weeks.
2. Removal of toxic substances and metabolic wastes from the body will occur in 1–4 weeks.
3. Independent activities of daily living will be resumed in 1–2 weeks.
4. Optimal level of health will be achieved in 3–4 weeks.

IV. OUTCOME CRITERIA

1. Vital signs are normal.
2. Blood pressure is normal.
3. Laboratory test results are normal.
4. Return dialysis solution is clear and free from infection and contamination.
5. Intake and output are within normal limits.
6. Appetite is normal.
7. Increased tolerance of different foods is normal.
8. Body weight is normal.
9. Exercise tolerance is normal.
10. Skin is improved in color, texture, and moisture.
11. Menses are normal.
12. Libido is normal.
13. Hair growth is normal.
14. Normal puberty is achieved.
15. Liver function tests are normal.
16. Diabetes is controlled.
17. Heart/chest sounds are normal.
18. Chest x-ray and EKG are normal.

19. Bone growth is normal.
20. Mobility is normal.
21. Client is alert, sociable, and cooperative.
22. Client states he/she feels better.

V. NURSING INTERVENTIONS/TREATMENT

1. R.N. will contact hospital discharge planner for written instructions for CCPD.
2. R.N. will contact client/family to ensure proper supplies are present prior to home visit. R.N. will assess client/family level of understanding to estimate length of time needed for each training session.
3. R.N. will monitor vital signs, blood pressure, weight, color, and turgor of mucous membranes and skin, signs of bleeding, intake and output, and diabetic complications.
4. R.N. will contact M.D. for recent laboratory testing, fluids and diet, CCPD instructions, medications, etc.
5. R.N. will allow client/family to verbalize all fears, anxieties, and concerns about condition and procedures.
6. R.N. will instruct client/family/H.H.A. on:
   A. disease process and signs/symptoms.
   B. diabetic management, if applicable.
   C. complications of condition (e.g., peritonitis/cloudy effluent/ fever/abdominal pain and tenderness/nausea/vomiting) and CCPD procedure (e.g., dialysis leak/bleeding/poor drainage/ respiratory distress/outflow problems/tunnel infection).
   D. daily monitoring and recording of vital signs, including blood pressure, weight, and edema.
   E. medication administration (e.g., Heparin, antibiotics, iron preparations, analgesics, androgen therapy, and insulin)/ adverse reactions/ingredients in over-the-counter medications.
   F. immediate notification of M.D. of adverse reactions or change in condition.
   G. daily intake and output.
   H. fluids/diet/aluminum hydroxide (i.e., Dialume) recipes.
   I. CCPD procedure: proper handwashing/supplies/operation of automated peritoneal cycler with connector set, temperature alarm, drain alarm, systems drain alarm, nightly exchange process, gravity drainage; maintenance of cycler/area/ environment/avoidance of infection/aseptic technique/skin

care/tubing care/dressing care/solution to be administered and discarded/expiration dates of solutions and termination of dialysis.

J. central tunneled or central nontunneled catheter and exit site care.

K. types and storage of solutions.

L. CCPD home record: dates, times, weight, standing blood pressure, solution (1.5%, 2.5%, 4.25%), drainage volume, drainage condition (clear/cloudy), comments, and additives.

M. vitamin therapy/phosphate binders/calcium supplements.

N. bathing/showers.

O. types of clothing.

P. cost of treatment/equipment/supplies.

Q. exercise/rest.

R. employment.

S. home care van delivery of supplies.

T. vocational counseling/college.

U. financial assistance.

V. insurance coverage.

W. support groups/home client networking program/education programs/resources.

X. travel programs.

Y. counseling/psychiatric aid.

Z. recreation.

7. R.N. will provide M.D. with follow-up reports and discharge summary when case closes.

8. R.N. will notify client/family/H.H.A./significant others when case will close.

Cystic Fibrosis
Care Plan

I. NURSING DIAGNOSIS

1. Knowledge deficit related to:
   A. signs/symptoms.
   B. medication administration/adverse reactions.
   C. respiratory care.
   D. bowel management.
   E. fluid intake/diet management.
   F. laboratory testing.
   G. other _____

2. Ineffective airway clearance related to:
   A. retention of thick, tenacious, mucopurulent secretions.
   B. thickened bronchial walls.
   C. respiratory infection.
   D. dyspnea.
   E. allergies.
   F. other _____

3. Anxiety related to:
   A. severe, incurable, chronic nature of disease.
   B. complications of digestive and respiratory system.
   C. potential death.
   D. other _____

4. Constipation/Diarrhea related to:
   A. intestinal obstruction.
   B. lack of exercise.
   C. poor nutritional intake.
   D. failure to absorb fat-soluble vitamins.
   E. fecal impaction.
   F. other _____

5. Decreased cardiac output related to:
   A. electrolyte imbalance.
   B. poor medication administration.
   C. other _____

6. Fluid volume deficit related to:
   A. failure to absorb fat-soluble vitamins (A and D).
   B. increased viscous secretions of mucus-producing glands.
   C. allergies.
   D. respiratory infection.
   E. other _____

7. Ineffective family coping related to severe, incurable chronic nature of disease.

8. Potential fluid volume deficit related to:
   A. excessive respiratory secretions.
   B. watery stools.
   C. excessive sweat production.
   D. other _____

9. Impaired home maintenance management related to:
   A. increased demands concerning severe nature of disease.
   B. cost of disease/poor insurance coverage.
   C. other _____

10. Altered nutrition: more than body requirements related to:
    A. failure to absorb fat-soluble vitamins (A and D).
    B. lack/deficiency of pancreatic enzymes.
    C. increased viscous secretions of mucus-producing glands.
    D. irritability/listlessness of child.

    E. failure to gain weight.

    F. hearty appetite.

    G. other _____

_____

11. Altered parenting related to increased physical demands of a sick child.

12. Potential for injury related to:

    A. poor nutritional status.

    B. rectal prolapse.

    C. respiratory obstruction.

    D. immobility.

    E. other _____

_____

13. Impaired gas exchange related to:

    A. dyspnea.

    B. bronchial obstruction.

    C. respiratory infection.

    D. increased viscosity of pulmonary mucus.

    E. dry, unproductive cough.

    F. other _____

_____

14. Potential impaired skin integrity related to:

    A. excessive sodium in perspiration.

    B. watery stools/foul-smelling bulky stools.

    C. other _____

_____

15. Sleep pattern disturbance related to:

    A. respiratory distress.

    B. GI distress.

    C. irritability.

    D. other _____

_____

II. SHORT-TERM GOALS

1. Parent/Parents will arrange for M.D. appointments for accurate testing and treatment of disease after 1 R.N. visit.

2. Parent/Parents will join organizations that support cystic fibrosis after 1–2–3 R.N. visits.

3. Parent/Parents will carefully observe and record child's stools as ordered after 1–2–3–4 R.N. visits.

4. Parent/Parents will administer respiratory treatment as ordered after 1–2–3–4 R.N./R.T. visits.

5. Parent/Parents will assist child with postural drainage several times daily as ordered after 1–2–3–4 R.N./R.T. visits.

6. Parent/Parents will perform chest physical therapy over designated areas as ordered after 1–2–3–4 R.N./R.T. visits.

7. Parent/Parents will assist child with breathing exercises after 1–2–3–4 R.N./R.T. visits.

8. Parent/Parents will administer prescribed medication as ordered after 1–2–3 R.N. visits.

9. Parent/Parents will weigh child daily as ordered after 1–2 R.N. visits.

10. Parent/Parents will administer prescribed diet as ordered after 1–2–3 R.N. visits.

11. Parent/Parents will administer prescribed exercises as ordered after 1–2–3–4 R.N./P.T./O.T. visits.

12. Parent/Parents will administer appropriate skin care as ordered after 1–2–3 R.N. visits.

13. Parent/Parents will administer additional salt to child in hot weather as ordered after 1–2–3 R.N. visits.

14. Parent/Parents will obtain immunizations as ordered after 1–2 R.N. visits.

15. Parent/Parents will obtain additional laboratory testing as ordered after 1–2 R.N. visits.

16. Child will attend school as ordered after 1–2 R.N. visits.

III. LONG-TERM GOALS

1. Respiratory status will stabilize in 3–4 weeks.
2. Adequate nutrition will be maintained in 3–4 weeks.
3. Optimal level of health will be achieved in 6–12 months.

IV. OUTCOME CRITERIA

1. Vital signs are normal.
2. Chest is clear.
3. Stools are normal color and quantity sufficient.
4. Weight is normal for height.
5. Sodium and chloride levels are normal; sweat test result is normal.

6. Appetite is normal.
7. Child is alert, playful, sociable, and cooperative.
8. Muscle tone is normal.
9. Exocrine glands (e.g., pancreas, bronchial mucus glands, mixed and serous salivary and sweat glands) function normally.
10. Growth and development are appropriate for age.
11. Complete immunologic state is reached.
12. Child attends school.

V. NURSING INTERVENTION/TREATMENT

1. R.N. will make referral for child to visit M.D. when first signs and symptoms are observed.
2. R.N. will instruct family/H.H.A. on:
   A. monitoring and recording of vital signs.
   B. daily recording of weight.
   C. observation of respiratory status; administration of chest physical therapy over prescribed areas, postural drainage exercises, breathing exercises (diversional activities while these are occurring), and use of mist tent nebulization.
   D. administration of medication (antibiotics/expectorants/other)/adverse reactions.
   E. immediate notification of M.D. of adverse reactions or change in client's condition.
   F. vitamin therapy (vitamins A and D/multivitamins).
   G. fluid intake/diet (usually a high-calorie, high-protein diet with administration of pancreatic enzyme and total fat decreased).
   H. administration of pancreatic extract (usually given with food so child completes rest of meal).
   I. exercise/rest.
   J. skin care.
   K. laboratory testing/M.D. appointments.
   L. full participation in all childhood activities unless otherwise specified by M.D.
   M. genetic counseling of family.
   N. immunizations/TB testing.
   O. schooling.
   P. psychologic counseling of client and family if needed.
3. R.N. will provide M.D. with follow-up reports and discharge summary when case closes.

4. R.N. will assign additional personnel (e.g., M.S.W., P.T., O.T., R.T.) to case if ordered.
5. R.N. will notify client/family/H.H.A./significant others when case will close.

Cystitis
Care Plan

I. NURSING DIAGNOSIS

1. Anxiety related to:
    A. constant/intermittent bladder pain.
    B. dysuria.
    C. burning on urination.
    D. frequency of urination.
    E. pyuria.
    F. hematuria.
    G. pyrexia.
    H. back pain.
    I. urgency of need to urinate.
    J. other _____

2. Back pain related to:
    A. infection.
    B. inadequate fluid intake.
    C. other _____

3. Ineffective individual/family coping related to:
    A. pain.
    B. hematuria.
    C. fever.
    D. difficulty with ambulation.
    E. other _____

4. Diversional activity deficit related to:
   A. constant/intermittent bladder pain.
   B. weakness.
   C. back pain.
   D. frequency of urination.
   E. urgency of need to urinate.
   F. other _____

5. Fear related to:
   A. hematuria.
   B. pyuria.
   C. dysuria.
   D. constant/intermittent bladder pain.
   E. back pain.
   F. fever.
   G. weakness.
   H. impending surgery.
   I. other _____

6. Impaired home maintenance management related to:
   A. constant/intermittent bladder pain.
   B. fever.
   C. back pain.
   D. dependence on others for care.
   E. other _____

7. Knowledge deficit related to:
   A. prevention and treatment of cystitis.
   B. cystitis with stone formation.
   C. perineal care.
   D. good daily personal hygiene habits.
   E. medication administration/adverse reactions.
   F. other _____

8. Impaired physical mobility related to:
   A. fever.
   B. constant/intermittent bladder pain.
   C. back pain.

D. other _____

_____

9. Noncompliance with therapy related to:
A. denial.
B. promiscuity.
C. poor personal hygiene.
D. other _____

_____

10. Altered parenting related to:
A. fever.
B. immobility.
C. other _____

_____

11. Self-care deficit: feeding/bathing/dressing/toileting related to:
A. fever.
B. constant bladder/back pain.
C. immobility.
D. general malaise.
E. other _____

_____

12. Sexual dysfunction related to:
A. fever.
B. weakness.
C. constant bladder/back pain.
D. general malaise.
E. other _____

_____

13. Sleep pattern disturbance related to:
A. fever.
B. urgency of need to urinate.
C. frequency of urination.
D. constant/intermittent bladder pain.
E. back pain.
F. other _____

_____

14. Altered patterns of urinary elimination related to:
A. dysuria.
B. burning on urination.

C. frequency of urination.

D. pyuria.

E. hematuria.

F. urgency of need to urinate.

G. obstruction (stone formation).

H. inadequate fluid intake.

I. infection.

J. other _____

_____

II. SHORT-TERM GOALS

1. Client/Family will verbalize fears, anxieties, and concerns after 1–2 R.N. visits.
2. Client will take prescribed medication as ordered after 1 R.N. visit.
3. Client/Family will immediately notify M.D. of adverse reactions or change in condition after 1 R.N. visit.
4. Client will consume fluids/diet as ordered after 1 R.N. visit.
5. Client/Family will keep strict intake and output records after 1 R.N. visit.
6. Client will perform appropriate personal hygiene measures (perineal care) after 1 R.N. visit.
7. Client will wash hands properly after 1 R.N. visit.
8. Client will exercise/rest as ordered after 1 R.N. visit.
9. Client/Family will strain urine as ordered after 1 R.N. visit.
10. Client will perform self-catheterization properly after 1–2 R.N. visits.
11. Client will limit sexual partners as ordered after 1–2 R.N. visits.
12. Client will keep routine M.D. appointments after 1–2 R.N. visits.

III. LONG-TERM GOALS

1. Independent activities of daily living will be resumed in 1–2 weeks.
2. Optimal level of health will be achieved in 1–2 weeks.

IV. OUTCOME CRITERIA

1. Vital signs are normal.
2. Intake and output remain normal.

3. Urine is yellow, clear, and sufficient in quantity.
4. Laboratory test results are within normal limits.
5. Appetite is normal.
6. Kidneys, ureters, and bladder remain patent and function well.
7. Client is alert, sociable, and cooperative.
8. Client states he/she feels better.

V. NURSING INTERVENTION/TREATMENT

1. R.N. will instruct client/family/H.H.A. on:
   A. proper hand-washing technique.
   B. strict recording of intake and output.
   C. monitoring and recording of vital signs.
   D. medication administration/adverse reactions.
   E. immediate notification of M.D. of adverse reactions or advanced signs/symptoms of disease (pyuria/hematuria).
   F. forcing of fluids if ordered.
   G. diet prescribed.
   H. observation of urine, especially of renal calculi (crushing of clots; inspecting sides of urinal and bedpan for calculi).
   I. straining of urine through gauze.
   J. daily recording of weight.
   K. perineal care/good personal hygiene.
   L. laboratory testing/routine M.D. appointments.
   M. diversional activities.
   N. preoperative information.
2. R.N. will provide M.D. with follow-up reports and discharge summary when case closes.
3. R.N. will notify client/family/H.H.A./significant others when case will close.

Decubitus Ulcer Care Plan

I. NURSING DIAGNOSIS

1. Knowledge deficit related to:
   A. poor hand-washing technique.
   B. aseptic dressing technique.
   C. medication/cream/lotion/ointment/spray/gauze application/ adverse reactions.
   D. signs/symptoms of infection.
   E. wound irrigation.
   F. insertion of packing.
   G. heat lamp application.
   H. other _____

2. Impaired skin integrity related to:
   A. inappropriate turning/repositioning.
   B. poor dressing technique.
   C. poor hand-washing technique.
   D. tape excoriation/allergy.
   E. poor personal hygiene.
   F. other _____

3. Pain related to:
   A. immobility.
   B. poor dressing technique.
   C. poor turning/positioning.

D. other _____

_____

4. Altered nutrition: potential for more than body requirements related to wound healing.
5. Ineffective individual/family coping related to:
   A. poor/slow healing.
   B. discomfort.
   C. dependence on others for care.
   D. other _____

   _____

6. Self-care deficit: feeding/bathing/grooming/dressing/toileting/ dressing change related to:
   A. poor understanding of dressing care.
   B. weakness.
   C. dependence on others for care.
   D. other _____

   _____

7. Impaired home maintenance management related to:
   A. limited mobility/immobility.
   B. the need for frequent turning/repositioning.
   C. restricted exercise.
   D. dependence on others for care.
   E. other _____

   _____

8. Altered peripheral tissue perfusion related to:
   A. infrequent turning/repositioning.
   B. circulatory impairment.
   C. hyperglycemia/hypoglycemia.
   D. other _____

   _____

II. SHORT-TERM GOALS

1. Client/Family will verbalize fears, questions, and anxieties after 1–2 R.N. visits.
2. Client/Family/H.H.A. will maintain clean area for dressing change after 1–2 R.N. visits.
3. Client/Family/H.H.A. will dispose of contaminated materials and old dressings after 1–2 R.N. visits.

4. Client/Family/H.H.A. will store medication, ointments, creams, lotions, sprays, packing, bandages in clean, safe area after 1–2–3–4 R.N. visits.
5. Client/Family/H.H.A. will develop adequate hand-washing techniques after 1–2 R.N. visits.
6. Client/Family/H.H.A. will demonstrate aseptic technique after 1–2–3 R.N. visits.
7. Client/Family/H.H.A. will use nonallergic tape after 1–2 R.N. visits.
8. Client/Family/H.H.A. will cleanse wound appropriately after 1–2–3 R.N. visits.
9. Client/Family/H.H.A. will apply prescribed medication/ointments/creams/lotions/sprays to site after 1–2–3 R.N. visits.
10. Client/Family/H.H.A. will apply and secure appropriate dressing after 1–2–3–4 R.N. visits.
11. Client/Family/H.H.A. will notify M.D. immediately of adverse effects or changes at wound site after 1–2 R.N. visits.
12. Client/Family will keep routine M.D. appointments after 1 R.N. visit.
13. Client/Family/H.H.A. will obtain air mattress after 1–2–3 R.N. visits.
14. Client/Family/H.H.A. will secure sheepskin/heel pads/leg bolsters/flotation pads to areas of greatest pressure after 1–2–3–4 R.N. visits.
15. Client/Family/H.H.A. will assist with range-of-motion exercise to all extremities after 1–2–3–4 R.N. visits.
16. Client/Family/H.H.A. will assist in turning/repositioning every 1–2 hours after 1–2 R.N. visits.
17. Client/Family/H.H.A. will assist with massage of body part with cream/lotion if intact and unbroken after 1–2 R.N. visits.

III. LONG-TERM GOAL

1. Adequate wound healing will occur in 2–3 weeks.

IV. OUTCOME CRITERIA

1. Client/Family/H.H.A. performs appropriate skin care daily.
2. Granulation occurs normally.
3. Wound heals appropriately.
4. Skin remains healthy and intact.

5. Vital signs remain normal.
6. Client states he/she feels better.

V. NURSING INTERVENTION/TREATMENT

1. R.N. will call client's home before visiting to ensure that proper supplies are present for instructions in application.
2. R.N. will allow client/family to verbalize any questions or concerns and will provide answers.
3. R.N. will instruct client/family/H.H.A. on:
   A. monitoring and recording of vital signs.
   B. fluid intake/dietary regimen as ordered.
   C. good personal hygiene.
   D. proper hand-washing techniques.
   E. observation of signs/symptoms of infection.
   F. aseptic dressing technique.
   G. importance of clean living environment.
   H. adequate disposal of contaminated materials and old dressings.
   I. medication administration/adverse reactions.
   J. immediate notification of M.D. of adverse reactions or signs/symptoms of complications.
   K. heat lamp application.
   L. preparation of medication/ointments/vitamins/honey-sugar preparation/yogurt/milk of magnesia and merthiolate to wound, if ordered.
   M. recording of color, amount, consistency of drainage, and size of decubitus ulcer. R.N. will perform culture and sensitivity tests on wound if necessary and ordered by M.D.
   N. cleansing of wound (normal saline/peroxide/Betadine).
   O. packing of wound (with gauze/Kerlix/Kling)/Op Site/dry sterile dressing.
   P. turning/repositioning of client every 1–2 hours.
   Q. massaging unbroken areas of skin with lotion every 1–2 hours.
   R. application of air mattress/water bed/heel pads/sheepskin/elbow protectors/splints/Restons/leg bolsters/flotation pads.
   S. range-of-motion/active and passive exercises/splinting.
   T. good body mechanics for lifting, turning, repositioning.
   U. powdering bedpad before use.
   V. M.D. appointments.

4. R.N. will provide M.D. with follow-up reports and discharge summary when case closes.
5. R.N. will notify client/family/H.H.A. when case will close.
6. R.N. will make further community referral for long-term care if necessary.

Dermatitis
Care Plan

I. NURSING DIAGNOSIS

1. Anxiety related to:
   A. uncontrolled spread of rash.
   B. urticaria.
   C. social isolation.
   D. other _____

2. Powerlessness related to spread of rash.
3. Potential for infection related to:
   A. lesion formation: macules/papules/vesicles/crusts.
   B. poor skin care.
   C. excessive scratching.
   D. other _____

4. Knowledge deficit related to:
   A. avoidance of allergens/desensitization.
   B. testing/treatment.
   C. medication administration/adverse reactions.
   D. other _____

5. Social isolation related to spread of rash.
6. Pain related to:
   A. biologic agents.
   B. chemical agents.

C. physical agents.

D. psychologic agents.

E. other _____

_____

II. SHORT-TERM GOALS

1. Client/Family will seek skin testing/desensitization after 1–2 R.N. visits.
2. Client/Family/H.H.A. will wash hands appropriately after 1 R.N. visit.
3. Client/Family will limit/avoid allergens after 1–2 R.N. visits.
4. Client/Family will administer medication/creams/lotions/ ointments/emollients after 1–2 R.N. visits.
5. Client/Family will take/administer medicated baths as ordered after 1–2 R.N. visits.
6. Client/Family will administer inhalation therapy as ordered by M.D. after 1–2 R.N. visits.
7. Client/Family will avoid/prevent scratching and rubbing the affected region after 1–2 R.N. visits.
8. Client/Family/H.H.A. will prepare an elimination diet as ordered after 1–2 R.N. visits.
9. Client/Family/H.H.A. will launder clothing and bed linens using appropriate soap/detergent after 1–2 R.N. visits.
10. Client/Family will seek ultraviolet therapy as ordered by M.D. after 1–2 R.N. visits.
11. Client/Family will immediately notify M.D. of adverse reactions to medications/change in condition after 1–2 R.N. visits.
12. Client will seek laboratory testing/M.D. appointments as ordered after 1–2 R.N. visits.

III. LONG-TERM GOALS

1. Normal skin integrity will be achieved in 1–2 weeks.
2. Optimal level of health will be achieved in 1–2 weeks.

IV. OUTCOME CRITERIA

1. Skin is clear, healthy, and intact.
2. Vital signs are normal.
3. Weight is within normal limits.
4. Edema has subsided.

V. NURSING INTERVENTION/TREATMENT

1. R.N. will instruct client/family/H.H.A. on:
   A. proper hand-washing techniques.
   B. administration of medication/creams/lotions/ointments/ emollients/adverse reactions.
   C. medicated shampoos/baths.
   D. monitoring and recording of vital signs.
   E. avoidance of scratching and rubbing.
   F. avoidance of allergens.
   G. recommended skin testing/desensitization.
   H. nail care/application of gloves/mittens.
   I. fluid intake/dietary regimen as ordered; elimination diet if ordered.
   J. laundering of clothing and bed linens.
   K. follow-up M.D. appointments.
2. R.N. will provide M.D. with follow-up reports and discharge summary when case closes.
3. R.N. will notify client/family/H.H.A./significant others when case will close.

Diabetes
Care Plan

I. NURSING DIAGNOSIS

1. Anxiety related to:
   A. poor understanding of diabetes and its treatment.
   B. skin breakdown/poor healing.
   C. weight loss.
   D. blurred vision.
   E. muscle cramps.
   F. weakness.
   G. glycosuria.
   H. self-administration of injections.
   I. other _____

2. Knowledge deficit related to:
   A. diabetes (e.g., diabetes mellitus/diabetes insipidus/juvenile diabetes/novel-syndrome diabetes/adult-onset diabetes)/ overview of treatment.
   B. meal preparation/diet restrictions/exchange lists.
   C. skin care.
   D. aseptic technique.
   E. injection therapy/rotation of injection sites.
   F. external insulin pump therapy/complications/cost.
   G. operation of a portable blood glucose monitor.
   H. urine testing.
   I. ingredients in over-the-counter medications (i.e., sugar, caffeine, sodium, and potassium).

    J. wearable insulin pump with standard supply of insulin.

    K. medication administration/adverse reactions.

    L. vision testing.

    M. avoidance of emotional stress.

    N. adequate rest/exercise.

    O. hyperglycemia/hypoglycemia/ketoacidosis/coma.

    P. control of infection.

    Q. laboratory testing.

    R. other _____

    _____

3. Ineffective individual/family coping related to:

    A. denial.

    B. alcoholism/drug abuse.

    C. poor understanding of disease and its treatment.

    D. large amount of subject material to be learned.

    E. reluctance to administer injections.

    F. dietary restrictions.

    G. weight control.

    H. dependence on others for care.

    I. other _____

    _____

4. Pain related to:

    A. hyperglycemia.

    B. hypoglycemia.

    C. wound debridement.

    D. poor fluid/dietary intake.

    E. poor medication administration.

    F. poor skin care.

    G. refusal to seek adequate medical care.

    H. other _____

    _____

5. Ineffective breathing pattern related to:

    A. hyperglycemia.

    B. hypoglycemia.

    C. convulsions.

    D. ketoacidosis.

    E. other _____

    _____

6. Impaired verbal communication related to:
    A. drowsiness.
    B. faintness.
    C. slurred speech.
    D. irrational behavior.
    E. convulsions.
    F. coma.
    G. other _____

7. Fear related to:
    A. skin breakdown/poor healing.
    B. tachycardia.
    C. tremors.
    D. faintness.
    E. abdominal pain.
    F. convulsions.
    G. loss of control.
    H. dependence on others for care.
    I. other _____

8. Potential fluid volume deficit related to:
    A. poor intake.
    B. vomiting.
    C. sweating.
    D. polyuria.
    E. other _____

9. Impaired home maintenance management related to:
    A. dependence on others for care.
    B. overwhelming family responsibilities.
    C. irrational behavior.
    D. amputation/poor mobility.
    E. faintness/extreme weakness.
    F. abdominal pain.
    G. convulsions.
    H. coma.
    I. other _____

10. Potential for injury related to:
    A. denial.

B. refusal to comply with medical advice.
C. skin breakdown.
D. poor aseptic technique.
E. advance of gangrene.
F. poor understanding of treatment.
G. other _____

11. Impaired physical mobility related to:
A. abdominal pain.
B. faintness.
C. convulsions.
D. coma.
E. other _____

12. Noncompliance with therapy related to:
A. fear/reluctance to self-administer injections.
B. denial.
C. alcoholism/drug abuse.
D. other _____

13. Altered nutrition: potential for less than body requirements related to:
A. polydipsia.
B. polyphagia.
C. anorexia.
D. restlessness.
E. vomiting.
F. abdominal pain.
G. refusal to comply with medical advice.
H. dietary control/restrictions.
I. convulsions.
J. coma.
K. other _____

14. Altered parenting related to:
A. weakness.
B. restriction of spontaneous/strenuous activity.
C. nervousness.

D. drowsiness.

E. faintness.

F. slurred speech.

G. irrational behavior.

H. convulsions.

I. coma.

J. other _____

15. Self-care deficit: feeding/bathing/grooming/dressing/toileting/self-administration of medication/testing urine related to:

A. dependence on others for care.

B. fear/reluctance/denial.

C. faintness.

D. irrational behavior.

E. convulsions.

F. coma.

G. other _____

16. Sensory/Perceptual alterations related to:

A. faintness.

B. drowsiness.

C. irrational behavior.

D. convulsions.

E. weakness.

F. coma.

G. neuropathy.

H. other _____

17. Potential impaired skin integrity related to:

A. poor injection technique.

B. infection.

C. poor foot care.

D. gangrene.

E. amputation.

F. other _____

18. Sleep pattern disturbance related to:

A. restlessness.

   B. thirst.
   C. vomiting.
   D. abdominal pain.
   E. faintness.
   F. diaphoresis.
   G. tachycardia.
   H. convulsions.
   I. other _____

   _____

19. Altered patterns of urinary elimination related to:
   A. poor fluid intake.
   B. vomiting.
   C. infection.
   D. stress.
   E. altered metabolism.
   F. other _____

   _____

20. Altered peripheral tissue perfusion related to:
   A. hyperglycemia.
   B. hypoglycemia.
   C. ketoacidosis.
   D. other _____

   _____

II. SHORT-TERM GOALS

   1. Client/Family will verbalize questions, fears, and anxieties about diabetic condition after 1–2–3–4 R.N. visits.
   2. Client will avoid sugar, candy, honey, jam, pie, cake, syrup, cookies, condensed milk, soft drinks as ordered after 1–2 R.N. visits.
   3. Client/Family will state 3 foods from each diet exchange list after 1–2–3 R.N. visits.
   4. Client/Family will state 10 foods from each diet exchange list after 2–3–4–5–6 R.N. visits.
   5. Client will consume diabetic diet as ordered after 1–2–3 R.N. visits.
   6. Client/Family will demonstrate aseptic technique correctly after 1–2 R.N. visits.

7. Client/Family will prepare and administer insulin after 1–2–3–4 R.N. visits.
8. Client/Family will alternate injection sites after 1–2–3 R.N. visits.
9. Client/Family will administer medication as ordered after 1–2–3–4 R.N. visits.
10. Client/Family will immediately notify M.D. of signs/symptoms of adverse reactions/change in condition after 1 R.N. visit.
11. Client/Family will avoid people with infections and communicable diseases after 1 R.N. visit.
12. Client/Family will seek routine eye examinations after 1–2 R.N. visits.
13. Client will exercise routinely each day as ordered after 1–2 R.N. visits.
14. Client will purchase comfortable shoes after 1–2 R.N. visits.
15. Client/Family will perform foot care as ordered after 1–2 R.N. visits.
16. Client/Family will state signs/symptoms of ketoacidosis and hypoglycemia after 3–4 R.N. visits.
17. Client/Family will test urine for sugar and acetone (bid/tid/qid) upon arising and prior to each meal after 1–2–3 R.N. visits.
18. Client/Family will change dressings as ordered after 1–2–3–4 R.N. visits.
19. Client will wear/carry emergency ID card/bracelet/necklace after 1 R.N. visit.
20. Client/Family will request literature/join clubs/organizations concerned with management of diabetes after 1–2 R.N. visits.
21. Client/Family will safely operate external infusion pump after 1–2–3–4 R.N. visits.
22. Client/Family will safely operate a portable blood glucose monitor after 1–2–3–4 R.N. visits.
23. Client/Family will safely operate a wearable insulin pump after 1–2–3–4 R.N. visits.
24. Client/Family will avoid over-the-counter medications that include sugar, caffeine, sodium, and potassium as ordered after 1–2–3 R.N. visits.

III. LONG-TERM GOALS

1. Independent activities of daily living will be resumed in 1–2 weeks.
2. Optimal health maintenance level will be restored in 3–4 weeks.

IV. OUTCOME CRITERIA

1. Vital signs remain normal.
2. Weight is appropriate.
3. Skin remains healthy and intact.
4. Vision is clear and normal.
5. Neuromuscular system functions normally.
6. Intake and output are normal.
7. Urine is clear, yellow, and sufficient in quantity.
8. Pain is relieved.
9. Ambulation occurs normally.
10. Laboratory test results are within normal limits.
11. Client cooperates in following directions.
12. Client maintains positive outlook toward prognosis.
13. Client follows prescribed insulin regimen.
14. Client returns to play/school/work.
15. Client states he/she feels better.

V. NURSING INTERVENTION/TREATMENT

1. R.N. will consult with hospital discharge planner about previous teaching done with client and possible further teaching that must be done in home.
2. R.N. will allow client to redemonstrate what he/she has been taught in the hospital.
3. R.N. will instruct client/family/H.H.A. on:
   A. diabetes (e.g., diabetes mellitus/diabetes insipidus/juvenile diabetes/novel-syndrome diabetes/adult-onset diabetes)/ overview of treatment.
   B. fluid intake/dietary regimen as ordered; always having a hard piece of candy or orange juice to offset insulin reaction.
   C. signs/symptoms of hyperglycemia and hypoglycemia.
   D. medication administration/adverse reactions.
   E. immediate notification of M.D. of adverse reactions or signs/ symptoms of complications of disease.
   F. rest/exercise as ordered; regulation of activity essential.
   G. insulin administration, aseptic technique, rotation of sites.
   H. operation of a portable blood glucose monitor.
   I. ingredients in over-the-counter medications (i.e., sugar, caffeine, sodium, and potassium).

J. wearable insulin pump with standard supply of insulin.

K. oral hypoglycemic agents.

L. recording of intake and output.

M. daily recording of weight.

N. vision testing.

O. dressing care.

P. skin care, foot care, prevention of gangrene.

Q. local allergic reactions (e.g., insulin lumps, fat tissue and muscle tissue atrophy, local abcess of fat necrosis).

R. emergency medical identification (ID card/bracelet/necklace).

S. urine testing bid/tid/qid.

T. prevention and control of vaginal infections.

U. stump care.

V. application of prosthesis.

W. laboratory testing/M.D. appointments.

4. R.N. will assign additional personnel (e.g., M.S.W., P.T., podiatrist, O.T., H.H.A., home attendant, homemaker, housekeeper) to case if ordered.

5. R.N. will provide M.D. with follow-up reports and discharge summary when case closes.

6. R.N. will notify client/family/H.H.A./significant others when case will close.

7. R.N. will notify client/family of additional educational materials from clubs/organizations.

8. R.N. will notify client/family of employment opportunities/career counseling.

Diverticulitis
Care Plan

I. NURSING DIAGNOSIS

1. Anxiety related to:
   A. crampy abdominal pain.
   B. flatulence.
   C. nausea.
   D. irregular bowel habits.
   E. general malaise.
   F. other _____

2. Ineffective breathing pattern related to abdominal pain.
3. Abdominal pain related to:
   A. refusal to adhere to low-roughage diet.
   B. refusal to seek adequate medical care.
   C. poor administration of medication.
   D. inadequate fluid intake.
   E. irregular bowel habits.
   F. other _____

4. Knowledge deficit related to:
   A. fluid intake/dietary instructions.
   B. meal preparation.
   C. prescribed medication/adverse reactions.
   D. administration of laxatives/enemas.
   E. bowel regularity.

F. other _____

_____

5. Impaired physical mobility related to:
   A. crampy abdominal pain.
   B. weakness.
   C. other _____

   _____

6. Noncompliance with therapy related to:
   A. denial.
   B. refusal to cooperate with therapy.
   C. other _____

   _____

7. Altered nutrition: potential for more than body requirements related to:
   A. dietary change.
   B. elimination of coarser cereals and vegetables.
   C. low-residue diet.
   D. other _____

   _____

8. Sleep pattern disturbance related to:
   A. crampy abdominal pain.
   B. nausea.
   C. flatulence.
   D. general malaise.
   E. other _____

   _____

9. Constipation/Diarrhea related to:
   A. poor fluid/dietary intake.
   B. lack of exercise.
   C. emotional stress.
   D. other _____

   _____

10. Sexual dysfunction related to:
    A. crampy abdominal pain.
    B. weakness.
    C. other _____

    _____

II. SHORT-TERM GOALS

1. Client/Family will verbalize fears, anxieties, and questions after 1–2 R.N. visits.
2. Client will take prescribed medication as ordered after 1–2 R.N. visits.
3. Client will take laxatives as ordered after 1–2 R.N. visits.
4. Client/Family will notify M.D. of adverse reactions to medication or additional signs/symptoms of disease after 1–2 R.N. visits.
5. Client/Family will administer enemas as ordered after 1–2 R.N. visits.
6. Client will consume a low-residue diet after 1–2 R.N. visits.
7. Client will avoid roughage, such as coarser cereals and vegetables, after 1–2 R.N. visits.
8. Client will seek laboratory testing/M.D. appointments as ordered after 1–2 R.N. visits.

III. LONG-TERM GOALS

1. Regular bowel habits will be achieved in 1–2 weeks.
2. Optimal level of health will be achieved in 2–3 weeks.

IV. OUTCOME CRITERIA

1. Vital signs remain normal.
2. Client consumes low-residue diet.
3. Appetite is normal.
4. Client avoids roughage in diet.
5. Peristalsis is normal.
6. Intestinal mucosa remains healthy and intact.
7. Circulatory status remains normal.
8. Skin remains healthy and intact.
9. Client is in good spirits and free from pain.
10. Client states he/she feels better.

V. NURSING INTERVENTION/TREATMENT

1. R.N. will arrange to visit home for history and physical assessment.
2. R.N. will instruct client/family/H.H.A. on:
   A. monitoring and recording of vital signs.
   B. daily recording of weight.

    C. fluid intake/dietary regimen as ordered; low-residue diet; elimination of coarser cereals and vegetables.

    D. laboratory testing/M.D. appointments.

    E. medication administration/adverse reactions.

    F. enema administration.

    G. preoperative teaching if necessary.

    H. exercise/rest as ordered.

    I. diversional activities.

3. R.N. will provide M.D. with follow-up reports and discharge summary when case closes.

4. R.N. will notify client/family/H.H.A./significant others when case will close.

Dressing
Care Plan

I. NURSING DIAGNOSIS

1. Anxiety related to:
   A. inexperience with dressing change.
   B. poor understanding of aseptic technique.
   C. fear of contamination of site.
   D. other _____

2. Potential impaired skin integrity related to:
   A. poor hand-washing technique.
   B. break in aseptic technique.
   C. history of diabetes/other metabolic disorders.
   D. poor understanding of dressing technique.
   E. tape excoriation/allergy.
   F. poor personal hygiene.
   G. other _____

3. Pain related to:
   A. poor/slow healing of wound site.
   B. skin allergy to tape.
   C. poor application/administration of medication.
   D. poor hand-washing technique.
   E. other _____

4. Ineffective individual/family coping related to:
   A. poor/slow healing.
   B. discomfort.

   C. dependence on others for care.

   D. other _____

   _____

5. Self-care deficit: feeding/bathing/grooming/dressing/toileting/
dressing care related to:

   A. refusal to obtain adequate supplies.

   B. weakness/fatigue/general malaise.

   C. dependence on others for care.

   D. paraplegia/hemiplegia/quadriplegia.

   E. other _____

   _____

6. Impaired home maintenance management related to:

   A. limited mobility/immobility.

   B. restricted activity.

   C. restricted exercise.

   D. dependence on others for care.

   E. other _____

   _____

7. Noncompliance with dressing technique related to:

   A. poor personal hygiene.

   B. other _____

   _____

8. Knowledge deficit related to:

   A. poor hand-washing technique.

   B. aseptic dressing technique.

   C. medication/cream/lotion/ointment/spray application/adverse
reactions.

   D. signs/symptoms of infection.

   E. wound irrigation.

   F. other _____

   _____

9. Potential for injury (i.e., infection, gangrene, etc.) related to:

   A. poor personal hygiene.

   B. refusal to change dressings as ordered.

   C. poor comprehension of aseptic technique.

   D. other _____

   _____

10. Altered peripheral tissue perfusion related to:

   A. circulatory impairment.

B. poor metabolism.

C. other _____

_____

11. Altered nutrition: potential for more than body requirements related to:

A. slow granulation.

B. infection.

C. normal wound healing.

D. other _____

_____

12. Sleep pattern disturbance related to:

A. pain.

B. location of dressing.

C. other _____

_____

II. SHORT-TERM GOALS

1. Client/Family will verbalize fears, questions, and anxieties after 1–2–3 R.N. visits.

2. Client/Family will maintain a clear area for dressing change after 1–2 R.N. visits.

3. Client/Family will dispose of contaminated materials and old dressings after 1–2 R.N. visits.

4. Client/Family will store medication, ointments, creams, lotions, sprays in a clean, safe area after 1–2 R.N. visits.

5. Client/Family will develop adequate hand-washing techniques after 1–2 R.N. visits.

6. Client/Family will demonstrate aseptic technique after 1–2 R.N. visits.

7. Client/Family will use nonallergic tape after 1–2 R.N. visits.

8. Client/Family will cleanse wound appropriately after 1–2 R.N. visits.

9. Client/Family will apply prescribed medication/ointment lotions/sprays to site after 1–2–3 R.N. visits.

10. Client/Family will notify M.D. immediately of ad changes at wound site after 1–2–3 R.N. visits.

11. Client/Family will apply and secure appropriate 1–2–3 R.N. visits.

12. Client/Family will keep routine M.D. appointm visit.

III. LONG-TERM GOALS

1. Adequate wound healing will occur in 1–2 weeks.
2. Independent activities of daily living will be resumed in 1 week.
3. Optimal level of health will be achieved in 1–2 weeks.

IV. OUTCOME CRITERIA

1. Vital signs remain normal.
2. Client is able to apply his/her own dressings.
3. Wound heals appropriately.
4. Granulation occurs normally.
5. Skin remains healthy and intact.
6. Client states he/she feels better.

V. NURSING INTERVENTION/TREATMENT

1. R.N. will call client's home before visiting to ensure that proper supplies are present for instruction in application.
2. R.N. will allow client/family to verbalize questions or concerns and will provide answers.
3. R.N. will check wound for cleanliness, odor, suture line, signs/symptoms of infection.
4. R.N. will instruct client/family/H.H.A. on:
   A. monitoring and recording of vital signs.
   B. fluid intake/dietary regimen as ordered.
   C. good personal hygiene.
   D. importance of clean living environment.
   E. proper hand-washing technique.
   F. observation of signs/symptoms of infection.
   G. aseptic dressing technique.
   H. adequate disposal of contaminated materials and old dressings.
   I. medication administration/adverse reactions.
   J. immediate notification of M.D. of adverse reactions or change in condition.
5. R.N. will provide M.D. with follow-up reports and discharge summary when case closes.
6. R.N. will notify client/family/H.H.A./significant others when case will close.

Epistaxis
Care Plan

I. NURSING DIAGNOSIS

1. Ineffective airway clearance related to:
   A. epistaxis.
   B. dysphagia.
   C. other _____

2. Ineffective breathing pattern related to:
   A. epistaxis.
   B. insertion of nasal packing.
   C. dysphagia.
   D. other _____

3. Pain related to:
   A. insertion of nasal packing.
   B. previous injury.
   C. noncompliance with medication administration.
   D. other _____

4. Ineffective individual/family coping related to:
   A. frequent bleeding.
   B. restriction of alcohol.
   C. restriction of smoking.
   D. avoidance of stressful activity.
   E. other _____

5. Diversional activity deficit related to:
   A. discomfort of nasal packing.
   B. restriction of contact sports/strenuous exercise.
   C. other _____

6. Fear related to frequent episodes of bleeding.
7. Knowledge deficit related to:
   A. management of nosebleeds.
   B. prevention of nosebleeds.
   C. medication administration/adverse reactions.
   D. oral hygiene.
   E. fluid intake/dietary regimen as ordered.
   F. bowel elimination (i.e., avoidance of straining at stools).
   G. use of respiratory equipment.
   H. other _____

8. Impaired physical mobility related to:
   A. dizziness/light-headedness.
   B. weakness.
   C. other _____

9. Altered nutrition: potential for more than body requirements related to:
   A. potential for bleeding.
   B. nonconsumption of adequate fluids and small, soft, frequent meals.
   C. reduced appetite.
   D. alcoholism.
   E. terminal illness.
   F. other _____

10. Noncompliance with therapy related to:
    A. denial.
    B. confusion.
    C. fear.
    D. other _____

11. Altered parenting related to:
    A. activity intolerance.

     B. potential for injury during play.

     C. other _____

     _____

12. Self-care deficit: feeding/bathing/dressing/grooming related to:
     A. weakness.
     B. vomiting.
     C. fainting.
     D. other _____

     _____

13. Altered cerebral tissue perfusion related to:
     A. metabolic disorders.
     B. adverse reactions to medication/chemotherapy.
     C. alcoholism.
     D. other _____

     _____

14. Sleep pattern disturbance related to:
     A. nasal bleeding.
     B. dysphagia.
     C. swallowing blood.
     D. vomiting.
     E. discomfort of nasal packing.
     F. other _____

     _____

II. SHORT-TERM GOALS

1. Client/Family will contact M.D. immediately about signs/symptoms of bleeding after 1 R.N. visit.
2. Client/Family will take prescribed medication as ordered after 1 R.N. visit.
3. Client/Family will notify M.D. immediately of signs/symptoms of adverse reactions after 1 R.N. visit.
4. Client will limit coughing as much as possible after 1–2 R.N. visits.
5. Client will limit/avoid smoking after 1–2 R.N. visits.
6. Client will avoid sneezing after 1–2 R.N. visits.
7. Client will refrain from picking, rubbing, or inserting foreign objects into nose after 1–2 R.N. visits.
8. Client/Family will obtain laboratory testing as ordered after 1–2 R.N. visits.

9. Client will avoid blowing nose forcefully after 1 R.N. visit.

10. After nasal packing, client will avoid physical exertion for first 24 hours after 1 R.N. visit.

11. After nasal packing, client will avoid drinking alcohol for 1 week after 1 R.N. visit.

12. After nasal packing, client will avoid taking aspirin for at least 1 week after 1 R.N. visit.

13. After nasal packing, client will avoid drinking hot liquids for 1 week after 1 R.N. visit.

14. Client will avoid strenuous activity/play after 1 R.N. visit.

15. Client will consume small, frequent, soft meals with a high-fiber content after 1–2 R.N. visits.

16. Client/Family will use respiratory equipment as ordered after 1–2 R.N. visits.

17. Client/Family will administer appropriate mouth care as ordered after 1 R.N. visit.

18. Client will take stool softeners/laxatives as ordered to avoid straining at stool after 1 R.N. visit.

III. LONG-TERM GOALS

1. Nasal bleeding will be identified, treated, and prevented in 1–2 weeks.

2. Optimal level of health will be achieved in 1–2 weeks.

IV. OUTCOME CRITERIA

1. Airway is clear.

2. Breathing is normal.

3. Vital signs are normal.

4. Circulatory status is normal.

5. Chest is clear.

6. Laboratory test results are normal.

7. Skin/Mucous membrane is normal, healthy, and intact.

8. Appetite is normal.

9. Client consumes nutritious meals.

10. Intake and output are normal.

11. Sense of smell is normal.

12. Client states he/she feels better.

V. NURSING INTERVENTION/TREATMENT

1. R.N. will assess cause, location, and type of nosebleed through history and physical examination; will assess need for anterior or posterior nasal packing (note anterior bleeding usually results from trauma; posterior bleeding may be indicative of blood dyscrasias, leukemia, vitamin deficiency, chemotherapy, chronic renal or liver disease, arteriosclerosis, or tumors).

2. R.N. will instruct client/family/H.H.A. on:

   A. good oral hygiene/mouth breathing.

   B. monitoring and recording of vital signs.

   C. avoidance of coughing, sneezing, bumping, picking, or inserting a foreign object in nose.

   D. current medication regimen/adverse reactions possible with any additional medication ordered/immediate notification of M.D. of adverse reactions or change in condition.

   E. avoidance of smoking/alcohol.

   F. avoidance of emotional stress.

   G. avoidance of physical exertion/contact sports as ordered.

   H. restriction of aspirin as ordered.

   I. restriction on drinking hot beverages as ordered.

   J. sufficient fluids/small, frequent, soft-food meals with high-fiber content as ordered to prevent straining at stool.

   K. mild laxatives/stool softener if ordered.

   L. for child who picks nose compulsively, trimmed nails or diversional activity as substitute for habit.

   M. laboratory testing/follow-up M.D. appointments.

3. For initial emergency measures, R.N. will:

   A. calm client.

   B. assess cause, location, and type of nosebleed.

   C. place client in a sitting position with head forward over basin; prevent backflow of blood down throat by preventing client from placing head backward.

   D. check vital signs and blood pressure.

   E. encourage client to gently blow nose to allow for possible better visualization.

   F. check nose with bright light. If bleeding is anterior, insert a wet, cool cotton ball (well wrung-out) into bleeding nostril. Pinch both nostrils together with steady pressure. After approximately 5 minutes, remove cotton ball. Ice can also be applied to outside of nose for 5 minutes.

G. contact M.D. for persistent bleeding.

H. encourage mouth breathing and have client avoid talking.

I. measure or estimate blood loss.

J. arrange for immediate transport to emergency room.

4. R.N. will provide follow-up reports and discharge summary when case closes.

5. R.N. will notify client/family/H.H.A./significant others when case will close.

Fetal Alcohol Syndrome Care Plan

I. NURSING DIAGNOSIS

1. Anxiety related to:
   A. developmental delay.
   B. anomalies.
   C. low birth weight.
   D. tremors.
   E. cost of medical care/poor insurance coverage.
   F. other _____
   _____

2. Knowledge deficit related to:
   A. prevention/treatment of fetal alcohol syndrome.
   B. medication administration/adverse reactions.
   C. seizure control/precautions.
   D. infant stimulation/special education.
   E. other _____
   _____

3. Ineffective individual/family coping related to:
   A. alcoholism.
   B. anomalies.
   C. overwhelming demands of the sick child.
   D. marital discord.
   E. prematurity.
   F. retardation.
   G. other _____
   _____

4. Impaired physical mobility related to:
   A. limited joint movement.
   B. tremors.
   C. other _____

   _____

5. Decreased cardiac output related to:
   A. prematurity.
   B. other _____

   _____

6. Sleep pattern disturbance related to:
   A. high-pitched cry.
   B. tremors.
   C. other _____

   _____

7. Altered patterns of urinary elimination related to:
   A. genital malformations.
   B. poor fluid intake.
   C. other _____

   _____

8. Potential for injury related to:
   A. tremors.
   B. ineffective airway clearance.
   C. other _____

   _____

9. Altered parenting related to:
   A. alcoholism.
   B. overwhelming demands of the sick child.
   C. single parenthood.
   D. separation/divorce.
   E. other _____

   _____

10. Sensory/Perceptual alterations related to:
    A. microophthalmia.
    B. ptosis.
    C. microcephaly.
    D. blindness.
    E. other _____

    _____

11. Altered nutrition: potential for more than body requirements related to:
    A. delayed feeding.
    B. poor intake.
    C. vomiting.
    D. prematurity.
    E. other _____
    _____

12. Noncompliance with therapy related to:
    A. alcoholism.
    B. denial.
    C. peer pressure.
    D. other _____
    _____

II. SHORT-TERM GOALS

1. Mother/Father will verbalize fears, concerns, and anxieties after 1–2–3–4 R.N. visits.
2. Parents will enroll infant in infant stimulation program after 1–2 R.N. visits.
3. Parents will practice prescribed exercises after 1–2 R.N. visits.
4. Infant will consume appropriate feedings after 1–2 R.N. visits.
5. Parents will treat infant as normally as possible after 1–2 R.N. visits.
6. Mother/Father will seek professional counseling for alcoholism after 3–4–5–6 R.N. visits.
7. Siblings will be encouraged to interact with infant after 1–2 R.N. visits.
8. Parents will administer prescribed medication after 1–2–3 R.N. visits.
9. Infant will sleep appropriately after 1–2 R.N. visits.
10. Infant will urinate/defecate after 1–2 R.N. visits.
11. Infant will receive appropriate immunizations after 1–2 R.N. visits.
12. Parents will seek laboratory testing/M.D. appointments for infant after 1–2 R.N. visits.

III. LONG-TERM GOALS

1. Normal growth and development will occur in 6–12 months.
2. Normal socialization will occur in 6–12 months.

3. Adequate nutritional status will be achieved in 6–12 months.
4. Adequate mental status will be achieved in 6–12 months.
5. Optimal level of health will be achieved in 6–12 months.

IV. OUTCOME CRITERIA

1. Vital signs are normal.
2. Cardiac output is normal.
3. Bladder/Bowel elimination is normal.
4. Laboratory test results remain normal.
5. Weight is appropriate for age.
6. Length is appropriate for age.
7. Developmental milestones are reached.
8. Socialization is appropriate.
9. Parents love and accept child.
10. Siblings love and accept child.
11. Child consumes nutritious meals.
12. Nervous system functions normally.
13. Child adapts well to new situations and strangers.
14. Child attends school.

V. NURSING INTERVENTION/TREATMENT

1. R.N. will answer all questions and respond to anxieties raised by parents.
2. R.N. will instruct family/H.H.A. on:
    A. feeding schedule and formula preparation.
    B. normal newborn care (i.e., bathing/diapering/skin care).
    C. prescribed medication (i.e., anticonvulsants/antibiotics/ sedatives/adverse reactions).
    D. infant stimulation programs.
    E. exercise/rest.
    F. play activity.
    G. laboratory testing.
    H. counseling groups/pediatric and adult mental health units.
3. R.N. will provide M.D. with follow-up reports and discharge summary when case closes.
4. R.N. will notify family/H.H.A./significant others when case will close.

Gastrostomy
Care Plan

I. NURSING DIAGNOSIS

1. Anxiety related to:
   A. skin care.
   B. dressing care.
   C. inexperience with administration of feedings.
   D. prescribed exercise/rest.
   E. medication administration/adverse reactions.
   F. fear of metastasis.
   G. other _____

2. Self-care deficit: feeding/bathing/grooming/dressing/toileting related to:
   A. dependence on others for care.
   B. generalized weakness.
   C. fear.
   D. poor technique.
   E. paralysis.
   F. abdominal pain.
   G. other _____

3. Knowledge deficit related to:
   A. skin care.
   B. dressing care.
   C. medication administration/adverse reactions.
   D. percutaneous endoscopic gastrostomy.
   E. use of infusion pump.

F. intake and output.

G. gastrostomy feedings.

H. presence of bowel sounds.

I. exercise/rest.

J. other _____

_____

4. Potential for injury related to:

A. poor hand-washing technique.

B. too rapid induction of fluid into gastrostomy tube.

C. introduction of too cold/too hot fluids into tube.

D. poor dressing care.

E. other _____

_____

5. Fluid volume deficit/excess related to:

A. limited/excessive intake.

B. vomiting.

C. diarrhea.

D. other _____

_____

6. Sexual dysfunction related to altered body image.

7. Noncompliance with feeding related to:

A. dependence on others for care.

B. lack of support in home.

C. fatigue/lethargy.

D. altered levels of consciousness.

E. other _____

_____

8. Social isolation related to:

A. altered body image.

B. confinement to bed.

C. weakness/fatigue.

D. other _____

_____

9. Potential impaired skin integrity related to:

A. poor hand-washing technique.

B. poor dressing care.

C. tape allergy.

D. wound seepage.

E. other _____

_____

10. Altered nutrition: potential for more than body requirements related to:
    A. anorexia.
    B. poor preparation of feedings.
    C. food allergy (i.e., diarrhea/constipation).
    D. abdominal pain.
    E. vomiting.
    F. other _____
       _____

II. SHORT-TERM GOALS

1. Client/Family will assemble all equipment in home before initial R.N. visit.
2. Client/Family will verbalize all fears, anxieties, and concerns after 1–2–3–4 R.N. visits.
3. Client/Family will wash hands before procedure after 1 R.N. visit.
4. Client/Family will prepare and measure fluids and blenderized feedings after 1–2–3 R.N. visits.
5. Client/Family will warm feedings or allow feeding to warm to room temperature before introduction into stomach after 1–2–3–4 R.N. visits.
6. Client/Family will weigh self/client daily on rising after 1–2–3 R.N. visits.
7. Client/Family will administer medication as prescribed and feedings as prescribed through gastrostomy tube using clean technique after 1–2–3 R.N. visits.
8. Client/Family will follow feedings with 50 cc water to flush tubing after 1–2–3 R.N. visits.
9. Client/Family will clean equipment after 1–2 R.N. visits.
10. Client/Family will apply prescribed cream/paste if leakage should occur around stoma after 1–2–3–4 R.N. visits.
11. Client/Family will immediately notify M.D. of adverse reactions or change in condition after 1–2 R.N. visits.
12. Client/Family will state signs/symptoms of infection after 1–2–3 R.N. visits.
13. Client/Family will record color, amount, consistency, and frequency of loose stools after 1–2 R.N. visits.
14. Client/Family will demonstrate dressing changes after 1–2–3–4 R.N. visits.
15. Client/Family will safely operate infusion pump after 1–2–3 R.N. visits.

16. Client/Family will check for presence of bowel sounds prior to feedings after 1–2–3–4 R.N. visits.
17. Client/Family will record daily intake and output as ordered after 1–2–3–4 R.N. visits.
18. Client/Family will seek laboratory testing/M.D. appointments as ordered after 1–2 R.N. visits.

III. LONG-TERM GOALS

1. Adequate nutritional status will be achieved in 1–2 weeks.
2. Independent activities of daily living will be resumed in 1–2 weeks.
3. Optimal level of health will be achieved in 2–3 weeks.

IV. OUTCOME CRITERIA

1. Vital signs are normal.
2. Skin is healthy, intact, and clear.
3. Nutritional status remains normal.
4. Mental health is normal.
5. Laboratory test results are normal.
6. Weight is appropriate for height.
7. Sleep pattern is normal.
8. Client states he/she feels better.

V. NURSING INTERVENTION/TREATMENT

1. During initial visit, R.N. will assess instructions in feeding techniques before being given notice of client's hospital discharge.
2. R.N. will allow client to express feelings about altered body image and will answer all questions about care.
3. R.N. will instruct client/family/H.H.A. on:
    A. proper hand-washing technique.
    B. skin care/clean dressing technique/use of nonallergic tape.
    C. monitoring and recording of vital signs/signs and symptoms of infection or change in condition.
    D. medication administration/adverse reactions.
    E. immediate notification of M.D. of adverse reactions or change in condition.
    F. presence of bowel sounds prior to feeding.

    G. before each feeding, unclamping tubing, checking residual gastric contents from previous feeding, and administering feeding via tube; following feeding with 30-50 cc water to clear tubing; allowing water to flow via gravity drainage.

    H. administration of feeding/clamping of tubing/cleansing of equipment/operation of an infusion pump.

    I. daily recording of intake and output.

    J. daily recording of weight.

    K. culture and sensitivity testing of site, if necessary and ordered by M.D.

    L. laboratory testing/M.D. appointments.

4. R.N. will allow for appropriate redemonstration of feeding.

5. R.N. will encourage client/family/H.H.A. to measure fluids and introduce them at room temperature slowly, without introducing air into stomach.

6. R.N. will provide client/family with additional instructional material/visual aids/information on organizations/clubs/introduce people with same procedure.

7. R.N. will provide M.D. with follow-up reports and discharge summary when case closes.

8. R.N. will notify client/family/H.H.A./significant others when case will close.

Genital Herpes
Simplex Virus
Care Plan

I. NURSING DIAGNOSIS

    1. Knowledge deficit related to:
   - A. poor understanding of disease process.
   - B. prevention/treatment of genital herpes.
   - C. medication administration/adverse reactions.
   - D. sexual abstinence.
   - E. other _____

    2. Pain related to:
   - A. blister formation.
   - B. poor administration of prescribed medication.
   - C. noncompliance with medication administration.
   - D. other _____

    3. Ineffective individual/marital coping related to:
   - A. pain/discomfort.
   - B. sexual abstinence.
   - C. other _____

    4. Diversional activity deficit related to pain.
    5. Noncompliance with therapy related to:
   - A. cost of medical care/cost of medication/poor insurance coverage.
   - B. refusal to abstain from sexual relations as ordered.
   - C. other _____

6. Self-esteem disturbance related to:
   A. acquisition/transmission of communicable disease.
   B. rejection by significant others.
   C. infidelity.
   D. sexual abstinence.
   E. anger.
   F. other _____

   _____

7. Potential impaired skin integrity related to painful blister formation.
8. Altered patterns of urinary elimination related to painful blister formation.
9. Sexual dysfunction related to:
   A. painful blister formation.
   B. sexual abstinence.
   C. other _____

   _____

10. Sleep pattern disturbance related to painful blister formation.
11. Potential injury (blindness in newborn) related to genital herpes.
12. Activity intolerance related to painful lesions.

II. SHORT-TERM GOALS

1. Client will abstain from sexual relations until medical clearance is given after 1–2 R.N. visits.
2. Client will visit M.D./appropriate diagnostic facility for confirmation and treatment of genital herpes after 1–2 R.N. visits.
3. Client will purchase prescribed medication after 1 R.N. visit.
4. Client will inform and refer all possible sexual contacts for testing and treatment after 1 R.N. visit.
5. Client will immediately notify M.D. of adverse reactions or change in condition after 1–2 R.N. visits.
6. Client will seek laboratory/routine M.D. appointments after 1–2 R.N. visits.

III. LONG-TERM GOALS

1. Communicable disease will be controlled in 1–2 weeks.
2. Optimal level of health will be achieved in 1–2 weeks.

IV. OUTCOME CRITERIA

1. Vital signs are normal.
2. Skin remains clear, healthy, and intact.
3. Sexual abstinence is practiced during exacerbation.
4. Mental status remains normal.
5. Client states he/she feels better.

V. NURSING INTERVENTION/TREATMENT

1. R.N. will instruct client/contact on:
    A. proper hand-washing technique.
    B. sexual abstinence according to M.D.'s orders.
    C. reading material on genital herpes.
    D. laboratory testing/M.D. appointments.
    E. medication administration/adverse reactions. Usual prescription is for acyclovir ointment 5% to all lesions every 3 hours, 6 times daily for 7 days to reduce viral shedding and duration of disease. Exacerbations are not preventable at this time.
    F. condom application.
    G. yearly Pap tests/importance of stressing history of genital herpes to M.D. early in pregnancy.
    H. possible cesarean section for active genital herpes infection at onset of labor.
    I. counseling groups/psychotherapy.
2. R.N. will provide M.D. with follow-up reports and discharge summary when case closes.
3. R.N. will notify client/contact/significant others when case will close.

Glaucoma Care Plan

I. NURSING DIAGNOSIS

1. Knowledge deficit related to:
   A. prevention/treatment of glaucoma.
   B. signs/symptoms.
   C. medication administration/adverse reactions.
   D. use of contact lenses.
   E. argon laser trabeculoplasty/trabeculectomy.
   F. other_____

2. Severe pain in/around eye related to:
   A. refusal to seek medical advice.
   B. poor administration of medication.
   C. advance of condition.
   D. other_____

3. Anxiety related to:
   A. medication instillation.
   B. potential blindness.
   C. accidents.
   D. other_____

4. Ineffective individual/family coping related to:
   A. cloudy, blurred vision.
   B. severe eye pain.

C. nausea/vomiting.

D. other⎯⎯⎯⎯⎯⎯⎯⎯⎯⎯⎯⎯⎯⎯⎯⎯⎯⎯⎯⎯⎯⎯⎯⎯⎯⎯

⎯⎯⎯⎯⎯⎯⎯⎯⎯⎯⎯⎯⎯⎯⎯⎯⎯⎯⎯⎯⎯⎯⎯⎯⎯⎯⎯⎯⎯⎯⎯

5. Altered parenting related to:

A. cloudy, blurred vision.

B. blindness.

C. other⎯⎯⎯⎯⎯⎯⎯⎯⎯⎯⎯⎯⎯⎯⎯⎯⎯⎯⎯⎯⎯⎯⎯⎯⎯⎯⎯

⎯⎯⎯⎯⎯⎯⎯⎯⎯⎯⎯⎯⎯⎯⎯⎯⎯⎯⎯⎯⎯⎯⎯⎯⎯⎯⎯⎯⎯⎯⎯

6. Self-care deficit: feeding/bathing/grooming/dressing/toileting related to:

A. cloudy, blurred vision.

B. severe eye pain.

C. nausea/vomiting.

D. other⎯⎯⎯⎯⎯⎯⎯⎯⎯⎯⎯⎯⎯⎯⎯⎯⎯⎯⎯⎯⎯⎯⎯⎯⎯⎯

⎯⎯⎯⎯⎯⎯⎯⎯⎯⎯⎯⎯⎯⎯⎯⎯⎯⎯⎯⎯⎯⎯⎯⎯⎯⎯⎯⎯⎯⎯⎯

7. Impaired home maintenance management related to:

A. cloudy, blurred vision/blindness.

B. severe eye pain.

C. cost of medical care/poor insurance coverage.

D. other⎯⎯⎯⎯⎯⎯⎯⎯⎯⎯⎯⎯⎯⎯⎯⎯⎯⎯⎯⎯⎯⎯⎯⎯⎯⎯

⎯⎯⎯⎯⎯⎯⎯⎯⎯⎯⎯⎯⎯⎯⎯⎯⎯⎯⎯⎯⎯⎯⎯⎯⎯⎯⎯⎯⎯⎯⎯

8. Potential for injury related to:

A. emotional stress.

B. omission of medication.

C. failure to report adverse reactions or change in condition to M.D.

D. other⎯⎯⎯⎯⎯⎯⎯⎯⎯⎯⎯⎯⎯⎯⎯⎯⎯⎯⎯⎯⎯⎯⎯⎯⎯⎯

⎯⎯⎯⎯⎯⎯⎯⎯⎯⎯⎯⎯⎯⎯⎯⎯⎯⎯⎯⎯⎯⎯⎯⎯⎯⎯⎯⎯⎯⎯⎯

9. Potential fluid volume deficit related to vomiting.

10. Altered nutrition: potential for more than body requirements related to:

A. anorexia.

B. nausea/vomiting.

C. other⎯⎯⎯⎯⎯⎯⎯⎯⎯⎯⎯⎯⎯⎯⎯⎯⎯⎯⎯⎯⎯⎯⎯⎯⎯⎯

⎯⎯⎯⎯⎯⎯⎯⎯⎯⎯⎯⎯⎯⎯⎯⎯⎯⎯⎯⎯⎯⎯⎯⎯⎯⎯⎯⎯⎯⎯⎯

11. Self-esteem disturbance related to:

A. cloudy, blurred vision.

B. blindness.

C. inability to perform activities of daily living.

D. unemployment.

E. other_____

_____

12. Noncompliance with therapy related to:

A. denial.

B. confusion.

C. other_____

_____

13. Sleep pattern disturbance related to:

A. nausea/vomiting.

B. severe eye pain.

C. other_____

_____

14. Impaired home maintenance management related to:

A. lack of continuity in M.D. appointments.

B. denial.

C. confusion.

D. dependence on others for care.

E. other_____

_____

15. Social isolation related to:

A. anger.

B. fear of ambulating outdoors.

C. confusion.

D. blindness.

E. dependence on others for care.

F. other_____

_____

II. SHORT-TERM GOALS

1. Client/Family will seek laboratory testing/M.D. appointments as ordered after 1–2 R.N. visits.

2. Client/Family will obtain prescribed medication after 1–2 R.N. visits.

3. Client/Family will correctly administer prescribed medication after 1–2 R.N. visits.

4. Client/Family will notify M.D. of adverse reactions or change in condition after 1–2 R.N. visits.

5. Client/Family will change eye dressings as ordered after 1–2–3 R.N. visits.
6. Client will wear corrective glasses if ordered after 1–2 R.N. visits.
7. Client/Family will wash hands correctly before and after instillation or removal of contact lenses after 1–2 R.N. visits.
8. Client/Family will insert or remove contact lenses, if prescribed, after 1–2 R.N. visits.
9. Client/Family will wash hands correctly before and after instillation of eye medication after 1–2 R.N. visits.
10. Client/Family will cleanse and store contact lenses appropriately after 1–2 R.N. visits.
11. Client will avoid emotional stress (e.g., worry, fear, anger, and excitement) after 1–2 R.N. visits.
12. Client will refrain from wearing tight clothing (e.g., girdles, collars, belts, and pants) after 1–2 R.N. visits.
13. Client will avoid straining at stool after 1-2 R.N. visits.
14. Client will avoid heavy lifting of objects after 1–2 R.N. visits.
15. Client will avoid drinking excessive fluids as ordered after 1–2 R.N. visits.
16. Client will read in moderation as ordered after 1–2 R.N. visits.
17. Client will exercise moderately as ordered after 1–2 R.N. visits.
18. Client will carry medical information at all times after 1–2 R.N. visits.
19. Client will undergo argon laser trabeculoplasty/trabeculectomy after 1–2–3 R.N./M.D. visits.

III. LONG-TERM GOALS

1. Normal, corrected vision will be achieved in 3–4 weeks.
2. Independent activities of daily living will be resumed in 3–4 weeks.
3. Optimal level of health will be achieved in 3–4 weeks.

IV. OUTCOME CRITERIA

1. Vision is clear.
2. Pain is relieved.
3. Vital signs are normal.
4. Appetite is normal.
5. Fluid and electrolyte balance is normal.
6. Client states he/she feels better.

V. NURSING INTERVENTION/TREATMENT

1. R.N. will arrange for initial home visit and general physical assessment.
2. R.N. will instruct client/family/H.H.A. on:
   A. prevention and treatment of glaucoma.
   B. proper hand-washing technique.
   C. medication administration/adverse reactions.
   D. immediate notification of M.D. of adverse reactions or change in condition.
   E. care of glasses, with specific directions for usage.
   F. installation, removal, cleansing, and storage of contact lenses.
   G. avoidance of emotional stress.
   H. proper wearing apparel (avoidance of constrictive clothing, e.g., girdles, collars, belts, pants) to prevent increase in intraocular pressure.
   I. proper bowel regimen/avoidance of straining at stool.
   J. avoidance of heavy lifting as ordered.
   K. fluid intake/dietary regimen as ordered (avoidance of excessive fluids).
   L. moderate reading as ordered.
   M. moderate exercise as ordered.
   N. medical identification (bracelet/wallet ID card/necklace).
   O. dressing care/aseptic technique.
   P. laboratory testing/M.D. appointments.
   Q. argon laser trabeculoplasty/trabeculectomy.
3. R.N. will arrange for additional personnel if ordered (e.g., M.S.W. to assist with services for the blind).
4. R.N. will provide follow-up reports and discharge summary to M.D. when case closes.
5. R.N. will notify client/family/H.H.A./significant others when case will close.

Glomerulonephritis Care Plan

I. NURSING DIAGNOSIS

1. Anxiety related to:
   A. alteration in urination.
   B. weakness.
   C. visual changes.
   D. hemorrhage.
   E. potential death.
   F. other_____

2. Potential fluid volume deficit related to:
   A. epistaxis.
   B. vomiting.
   C. polyuria.
   D. other_____

3. Fear related to:
   A. alteration in urination.
   B. weakness.
   C. visual changes.
   D. hemorrhage.
   E. the dying process.
   F. other_____

4. Ineffective individual/family coping related to:
   A. hemorrhage.
   B. vomiting.
   C. poor visual response.
   D. weakness.
   E. dependence on others for care.
   F. other_____

5. Pain related to:
   A. altered kidney function.
   B. alteration in blood flow to the brain.
   C. poor mobility.
   D. fluid loss.
   E. infection.
   F. other_____

6. Diversional activity deficit related to:
   A. weakness.
   B. headache.
   C. vomiting.
   D. hemorrhage.
   E. dyspnea.
   F. polyuria.
   G. dizziness.
   H. general malaise.
   I. seizures.
   J. other_____

7. Individual/Family grieving related to fear of death.
8. Impaired home maintenance management related to:
   A. weakness.
   B. dependence on others for care.
   C. impaired mobility.
   D. other_____

9. Potential for injury related to:
   A. possible chronic, progressive nature of disease.
   B. poor supervision in the home.

    C. alteration in thought process.

    D. other_____

---

10. Knowledge deficit related to:

    A. nature of disease.

    B. medication administration/adverse reactions.

    C. intake and output.

    D. fluid intake/dietary instructions.

    E. seizures.

    F. advance of disease.

    G. other_____

---

11. Noncompliance with therapy related to:

    A. denial.

    B. anger.

    C. changes in mental status.

    D. cost of medical care/poor insurance coverage.

    E. dependence on others for care.

    F. other_____

---

12. Impaired physical mobility related to:

    A. pitting/dependent edema.

    B. weakness.

    C. dizziness.

    D. dyspnea.

    E. shortness of breath.

    F. changes in visual response.

    G. other_____

---

13. Altered nutrition: potential for more than body requirements related to:

    A. nausea/vomiting.

    B. weakness.

    C. fever.

    D. poor mobility.

    E. changes in mental status.

    F. dependence on others for care.

    G. general malaise.

H. other_____

_____

14. Altered parenting related to:
    A. weakness.
    B. changes in mental status.
    C. difficulty in ambulation.
    D. dependence on others for care.
    E. other_____

    _____

15. Self-care deficit: feeding/bathing/grooming/dressing/toileting/
    ambulating related to:
    A. weakness.
    B. changes in mental status.
    C. difficulty in ambulation.
    D. dependence on others for care.
    E. seizures.
    F. other_____

    _____

16. Self-esteem disturbance related to:
17. Sensory/perceptual alterations related to:
    A. changes in sensorium.
    B. dizziness.
    C. other_____

    _____

18. Potential impaired skin integrity related to:
    A. skin breakdown.
    B. poor mobility.
    C. pruritus.
    D. other_____

    _____

19. Altered renal tissue perfusion related to:
    A. hypovolemia.
    B. altered metabolism.
    C. other_____

    _____

20. Sleep pattern disturbance related to:
    A. headaches.
    B. back pain.

    C. chills.

    D. anuria.

    E. shortness of breath.

    F. dyspnea.

    G. chest pain.

    H. hemorrhage.

    I. vomiting.

    J. polyuria.

    K. nocturia.

    L. orthopnea.

    M. seizures.

    N. other _____

    _____

21. Powerlessness related to:

    A. advance of disease.

    B. changes in sensorium.

    C. other_____

    _____

22. Altered patterns of urinary elimination related to:

    A. advance of disease.

    B. poor administration of medication.

    C. poor fluid/dietary intake.

    D. lack of support in the home.

    E. other_____

    _____

23. Sexual dysfunction related to:

    A. weakness.

    B. headaches.

    C. other_____

    _____

24. Spiritual distress related to:

    A. fear of death.

    B. end stage of dying.

    C. other_____

    _____

II. SHORT-TERM GOALS

    1. Client/Family will contact M.D. about signs/symptoms of disease after 1–2 R.N. visits.

2. Client/Family will avoid all forms of psychologic stress after 1–2 R.N. visits.

3. Client will rest as ordered after 1–2 R.N. visits.

4. Client/Family will take seizure precautions after 1–2 R.N. visits.

5. Client/Family will assist with breathing exercises/respiratory therapy as ordered after 1–2 R.N./R.T. visits.

6. Client/Family will administer medication as ordered after 1–2–3 R.N. visits.

7. Client/Family will immediately notify M.D. of adverse effects or change in condition after 1–2 R.N. visits.

8. Client will be placed in a warm, well-ventilated room, free from drafts, after 1–2 R.N. visits.

9. Client will consume fluids/diet prescribed after 1–2 R.N. visits.

10. Client/Family will obtain a daily weight after 1–2 R.N. visits.

11. Client/Family will chart intake and output after 1–2–3 R.N. visits.

12. Client/Family will obtain urinary samples as ordered after 1–2 R.N. visits.

13. Client/Family will seek laboratory testing as ordered after 1–2 R.N. visits.

14. Client/Family will follow prescribed skin care measures after 1–2 R.N. visits.

15. Client will participate in exercise as ordered after 1–2 R.N. visits.

16. Client/Family will use proper oral hygiene/personal hygiene measures daily after 1 R.N. visit.

17. Client/Family will record vital signs every 4 hours as ordered after 1–2–3 R.N. visits.

18. Client/Family will employ adequate hand-washing techniques after 1 R.N. visit.

19. Client/Family will follow M.D. instructions for possible epistaxis after 1–2 R.N. visits.

20. Client/Family will keep routine M.D. appointments after 1–2 R.N. visits.

III. LONG-TERM GOALS

1. Improved kidney functioning will be achieved in 1–2 weeks.

2. Independent activities of daily living will be resumed in 1–2 weeks.

3. Optimal level of health will be achieved in 2–3 weeks.

4. All stages of dying will be worked through.

IV. OUTCOME CRITERIA

1. Vital signs are normal.
2. Weight remains appropriate.
3. Intake and output remain normal.
4. Vision is clear and normal.
5. Appetite is normal.
6. Client consumes nutritious meals.
7. Urine is clear, yellow, and sufficient in quantity.
8. Specific gravity is normal.
9. Laboratory test results are normal.
10. Cardiovascular system functions normally.
11. Neuromuscular system functions normally.
12. Skin is healthy and intact.
13. Chest is clear; breathing is normal.
14. Circulatory system functions normally.
15. Renal system functions normally.
16. Client is ambulatory.
17. Client states he/she feels better.

V. NURSING INTERVENTION/TREATMENT

1. R.N. will contact hospital discharge planner about rehabilitation goals for client at home.
2. R.N. will instruct client/family/H.H.A. on:
   A. proper hand-washing technique.
   B. fluid intake (usually restricted to 1200 cc or less per day)/diet (usually low in protein) as ordered.
   C. exercise/rest as ordered.
   D. strict recording of intake and output.
   E. daily recording of weight.
   F. avoidance of overexertion and overexposure to cold or to people with infections.
   G. monitoring and recording of vital signs. If possible, R.N. will teach blood pressure monitoring to family member.
   H. laboratory testing/collection of urinary samples.
   I. skin care.
   J. medication administration/adverse reactions.
   K. immediate notification of M.D. in adverse reactions or change in condition.

    L. turning/repositioning every 2 hours.

    M. oral hygiene/personal hygiene.

    N. breathing exercises/respiratory therapy and care of equipment.

    O. avoidance of stress.

    P. quiet, restful environment, free from drafts.

    Q. diversional activities.

    R. M.D. appointments or arrangements for M.D. to visit home.

3. R.N. will provide M.D. with follow-up reports and discharge summary when case closes.

4. R.N. will notify client/family/H.H.A./significant others when case will close.

5. If death is imminent, R.N. will provide psychologic support/ support of clergy in final states; will follow pronouncement-of-death procedures; will assist with funeral arrangements if necessary.

Gonorrhea
Care Plan

I. NURSING DIAGNOSIS

1. Knowledge deficit related to:
   A. acquisition/prevention of sexually transmitted disease.
   B. signs/symptoms of sexually transmitted disease.
   C. medication administration/adverse reactions.
   D. laboratory testing for sexually transmitted disease.
   E. other _____

2. Low abdominal pain/Back pain/Labial pain/Joint pain related to:
   A. acquisition of sexually transmitted disease.
   B. other _____

3. Anxiety related to acquisition/transmittal of sexually transmitted disease.

4. Potential for injury (sterility/gonorrheal arthritis/blindness/endocarditis) related to:
   A. poor administration of medication.
   B. refusal to seek medical assistance.
   C. other _____

5. Ineffective individual/family coping related to sexually transmitted disease.

6. Sexual dysfunction related to:
   A. dysuria.

B. discharge.

C. low abdominal pain.

D. back pain.

E. edema/pain in labia.

F. abscess formation.

G. infection.

H. other _____

_____

7. Noncompliance with therapy related to:

A. shame.

B. embarrassment.

C. guilt.

D. denial.

E. other _____

_____

8. Self-esteem disturbance related to:

A. acquisition/transmittal of sexually transmitted disease.

B. adultery/promiscuity.

C. other _____

_____

II. SHORT-TERM GOALS

1. Client/Spouse/Family/Contacts will seek immediate testing/ treatment after 1 R.N. visit.

2. Client/Spouse/Family/Contacts will take prescribed medication after 1 R.N. visit.

3. Client/Spouse/Family/Contacts will return for follow-up injections/ laboratory testing after 1–2 R.N. visits.

4. Client/Spouse/Family/Contacts will abstain from sexual intercourse until medical clearance is obtained after 1–2 R.N. visits.

5. Client/Spouse/Family/Contacts will wash hands thoroughly after toileting after 1–2 R.N. visits.

6. Client/Spouse/Family/Contacts will take precautions to protect eyes after 1 R.N. visit.

III. LONG-TERM GOALS

1. Control/Palliation of communicable disease will be achieved in 1–2 weeks.

2. Delivery of healthy infant will occur with normal visual response at term.

IV. OUTCOME CRITERIA

1. Pain is relieved.
2. Discharge has subsided.
3. Anus is normal and healthy.
4. Urine elimination is normal.
5. Laboratory test results are normal.
6. Vision is normal.
7. Cardiovascular system functions normally.
8. Menses are normal.
9. Vital signs are normal.
10. Client/Spouse/Family/Contacts state they feel better.

V. NURSING INTERVENTION/TREATMENT

1. The R.N. will arrange for M.D. appointment for testing/treatment of all exposed sources.
2. R.N. will instruct all infected/suspected-as-infected people on:
   A. immediate smear, culture, and sensitivity of cervix, larynx, urethra, and anus.
   B. good hand-washing technique/good personal hygiene/protection of eyes from infection.
   C. assessment of allergies.
   D. medication administration—oral or IM (aqueous procaine penicillin/probenecid/ampicillin/amoxicillin/tetracycline/ erythromycin/spectinomycin)/adverse reactions.
   E. immediate notification of M.D. of adverse reactions.
   F. follow-up M.D. appointments/prenatal visits.
   G. sexual abstinence.
3. R.N. will provide M.D. with follow-up reports and discharge summary when case closes.
4. R.N. will notify client/spouse/family/contacts/significant others when case will close.

Hemodialysis Care Plan

I. NURSING DIAGNOSIS

1. Anxiety related to:
   A. operation of hemodialysis machine.
   B. cost of hemodialysis/supplies.
   C. malfunctioning of dialysis machine.
   D. hemorrhage.
   E. other_____

   _____

2. Impaired adjustment related to:
   A. change in lifestyle to accommodate dialysis.
   B. dependence on others for care.
   C. other_____

   _____

3. Potential activity intolerance related to:
   A. weakness/fatigue.
   B. lethargy.
   C. sleep disturbances.
   D. other_____

   _____

4. Ineffective individual/family coping related to:
   A. anger.
   B. depression.
   C. change in employment status.

    D. fear of rejection by significant others.

    E. lack of support in the home.

    F. other_____

_____

5. Fear related to:

    A. possible hemorrhage.

    B. possible infection.

    C. possible loss of employment.

    D. possible death.

    E. other_____

_____

6. Noncompliance with therapy related to:

    A. denial.

    B. lack of understanding.

    C. learning disability.

    D. depression.

    E. isolation.

    F. other_____

_____

7. Self-esteem disturbance related to:

    A. dependence on others for care.

    B. possible loss of employment status.

    C. overdemands of family members.

    D. rejection by significant others.

    E. overprotection by significant others.

    F. other_____

_____

8. Powerlessness related to:

    A. kidney failure.

    B. dependence on life support kidney machine.

    C. other_____

_____

9. Altered patterns of urinary elimination: anuria/oliguria related to:

    A. hemodialysis.

    B. fluid overload.

    C. dehydration.

    D. other_____

_____

10. Potential for infection related to:
  A. poor personal hygiene.
  B. poor hand-washing technique.
  C. poor dressing technique.
  D. venous/arterial infiltration.
  E. other_____

11. Potential for injury related to:
  A. inappropriate medication administration.
  B. poor skin care.
  C. poor injection technique.
  D. poor dressing technique.
  E. poor fluid/dietary habits.
  F. overconsumption of alcohol.
  G. poor scheduling of hemodialysis.
  H. poor shunt care.
  I. venous/arterial infiltration.
  J. other_____

12. Altered nutrition: less than body requirements related to:
  A. fluid restriction.
  B. caloric restriction.
  C. sodium restriction.
  D. potassium restriction.
  E. calcium restriction.
  F. phosphorus restriction.
  G. edema.
  H. other_____

13. Altered renal tissue perfusion related to:
  A. excess fluid removal during dialysis.
  B. dry weight above normal.
  C. hypotonic dialysate.
  D. overheated dialysate.
  E. copper in the dialysate.
  F. nitrates in the dialysate.
  G. chloramines in the dialysate.
  H. formaldehyde in the dialysate.

    I. venous/arterial infiltration.

    J. spasm of fistula.

    K. kinks or clamps in venous/arterial line.

    L. other_____

_____

14. Constipation/Diarrhea related to:

    A. iron preparation administration.

    B. excessive administration of laxatives.

    C. fluids/diet.

    D. emotional stress.

    E. other_____

_____

15. Knowledge deficit related to:

    A. disease process and signs/symptoms of complications.

    B. daily recording of vital signs, blood pressure, weight, and edema.

    C. medication administration/adverse reactions.

    D. immediate notification of M.D./dialysis unit of adverse reactions.

    E. fluids/diet/vitamin administration/aluminum hydroxide (i.e., Dialume) recipes.

    F. intake and output.

    G. shunt, fistula, and graft care.

    H. complications of shunt, fistula, and graft problems.

    I. dialysis machine—setup and prime.

    J. initiation and termination of dialysis.

    K. Heparin administration.

    L. blood sampling and hematocrits.

    M. fluid maintenance and administration of normal saline prime.

    N. water treatment and reverse osmosis/dialyzer reuse.

    O. machine service and maintenance.

    P. ordering supplies and storage.

    Q. record keeping.

    R. emergency phone numbers.

    S. exercise/rest.

    T. employment/vocational counseling/college.

    U. financial assistance.

    V. support groups/education programs/resources.

    W. counseling.

    X. recreation.

    Y. home care van delivery of supplies.

    Z. travel programs.

II. SHORT-TERM GOALS

1. Client/Family will verbalize fears, anxieties, and concerns after 1–2–3 R.N. visits.
2. Client/Family will administer prescribed medication after 1–2–3 R.N. visits.
3. Client/Family will notify M.D. immediately of adverse effects of medication or signs/symptoms of complications after 1–2–3–4 R.N. visits.
4. Client/Family will strictly record intake and output after 1–2 R.N. visits.
5. Client/Family will administer prescribed fluids/diet after 1–2–3 R.N. visits.
6. Client/Family will limit sodium, potassium, calcium, phosphorus, and protein in diet as ordered after 1–2–3 R.N. visits.
7. Client/Family will obtain teaching materials for hemodialysis after 1–2–3–4 R.N. visits.
8. Client/Family will take and record daily weights, vital signs, blood pressure, and edema before hemodialysis after 1–2–3 R.N. visits.
9. Client/Family will exercise/rest as ordered after 1–2–3 R.N. visits.
10. Client/Family will obtain and properly store hemodialysis equipment and supplies after 1–2–3 R.N. visits.
11. Client/Family will use an area within a reasonable distance of a water outlet and drain after 1–2–3 R.N. visits.
12. Client/Family will use a sink with a drain capacity of 8 gallons per hour after 1–2–3 R.N. visits.
13. Client/Family will provide a plumber and/or electrical contractor to fulfill home water and electrical requirements after 1–2–3 R.N. visits.
14. Client/Family will pass hemodialysis requirements and testing before home care is established prior to hospital discharge.
15. Client/Family will state 5 complications of end-stage renal disease after 1–2–3–4 R.N. visits.
16. Client/Family will state 10 complications of hemodialysis treatment after 1–2–3–4 R.N. visits.
17. Client/Family will state function of prescribed hemodialysis machine after 4–5–6 R.N. visists.

18. Client/Family will identify and correctly utilize arterial and venous blood lines after 4–5–6 R.N. visits.
19. Client/Family will calculate and use basic formulas for fluid removal after 6–7–8 R.N. visits.
20. Client/Family will set up and prime machine correctly after 6–7–8 R.N. visits.
21. Client/Family will utilize cannulations correctly after 6–7–8 R.N. visits.
22. Client/Family will initiate dialysis correctly after 6–7–8 R.N. visits.
23. Client/Family will terminate dialysis correctly after 6–7–8 R.N. visits.
24. Client/Family will be able to troubleshoot complications after 8–9–10 R.N. visits.
25. Client/Family will collect specimens as ordered after 8–9–10 R.N. visits.
26. Client/Family will be able to disinfect and store dialysis equipment and supplies after 8–9–10 R.N. visits.
27. Client/Family will keep important phone numbers within easy reach after 1–2–3 R.N. visits.
28. Client/Family will seek laboratory testing/M.D. appointments as ordered after 1–2–3 R.N. visits.

III. LONG-TERM GOALS

1. Regulation of the fluid balance of the body will occur in 1–4 weeks.
2. Removal of toxic substances and metabolic wastes from the body will occur in 1–4 weeks.
3. Independent activities of daily living will be resumed in 1–2 weeks.
4. Optimal level of health will be achieved in 3–4 weeks.

IV. OUTCOME CRITERIA

1. Vital signs are normal.
2. Blood pressure is normal.
3. Laboratory test results are normal.
4. Shunt/Fistula/Graft functions appropriately.
5. Hemodialysis is utilized appropriately.
6. Client troubleshoots impending complications.
7. Intake and output are within normal limits.

8. Appetite is normal.

9. Increased tolerance of different foods is normal.

10. Body weight is normal.

11. Exercise tolerance is normal.

12. Libido is normal.

13. Hair growth is normal.

14. Normal puberty is achieved.

15. Liver function tests are normal.

16. Diabetes is controlled.

17. Heart/Chest sounds are normal.

18. Chest x-ray film/EKG are normal.

19. Bone growth is normal.

20. Mobility is normal.

21. Client is alert, sociable, and cooperative.

22. Client states he/she feels better.

V. NURSING INTERVENTIONS/TREATMENT

1. R.N. will contact hospital discharge planner for written instructions for hemodialysis.

2. R.N. will contact client/family to ensure proper supplies are present prior to home visit. R.N. will assess client/family level of understanding to estimate length of time needed for each training session.

3. R.N. will monitor vital signs, blood pressure, weight, color and turgor of mucous membranes and skin, signs of bleeding, intake and output, and diabetic complications.

4. R.N. will contact M.D. for recent laboratory testing, fluids and diet, hemodialysis instructions, medications, etc.

5. R.N. will allow client/family to verbalize all fears, anxieties, and concerns about condition and procedures.

6. R.N. will instruct client/family/H.H.A on:

   A. anatomy, physiology, and disease process/signs and symptoms.

   B. diabetic management if applicable.

   C. daily monitoring and recording of vital signs, including blood pressure, weights, and edema.

   D. medication administration (anticoagulants/iron preparations/ vitamins/pain medications/phosphate binders/cardiotonics/ sedatives/insulin/antihypertensives/tranquilizers/antibiotics/ androgen therapy/antiemetics/potassium binders/antipruritics/ calcium/diuretics/ingredients in over-the-counter medications/ adverse reactions)

E. immediate notification of M.D. of adverse reactions or change in condition.

F. daily recording of intake and output.

G. fluids/diet/aluminum hydroxide (i.e., Dialume) recipes.

H. complications of condition and hemodialysis procedure (air embolus, bleeding, arrythmias, respiratory distress, lethargy, blood leak, poor conductivity, cramps, hemolysis, hypotension, infiltration, clotting of dialyzer, power failure, water failure, increasing positive pressure, poor arterial flow, and separation of venous and arterial lines.

I. shunt/fistula/graft care/dressing care/AIDS precautions.

J. types of hemodialysis machines.

K. hemodialysis procedure—ultrafiltration and fluid removal, composition of dialysate, dialysis machine (controls, set up and prime), access, cannulation, initiation of treatment, blood sampling, and hematocrits, fluid maintenance, ultrafiltration rate meter, termination, water treatment, reverse osmosis unit, dialyzer reuse and alarms.

L. environment for dialysis (encourage client never to dialyze alone).

M. home dialysis program daily flow sheet.

N. cleaning and maintenance of dialysis unit and supplies.

O. monthly sterilization.

P. specimen collection.

Q. ordering supplies.

R. important phone numbers.

S. exercise/rest.

T. employment.

U. vocational counseling.

V. college.

W. financial assistance.

X. resources/home care van delivery of supplies.

Y. dental appointments.

Z. laboratory testing/M.D. appointments.

7. R.N. will provide M.D. with follow-up reports and discharge summary when case closes.

8. R.N. will notify client/family/H.H.A./significant others when case will close.

Hepatitis Surveillance Care Plan

I. NURSING DIAGNOSIS

1. Anxiety related to:
   A. potential transmittal of disease.
   B. unemployment.
   C. other_____

   _____

2. Knowledge deficit related to:
   A. proper hand-washing technique.
   B. prevention treatment of hepatitis.
   C. isolation technique.
   D. sterilization of dishes/disposal of dishes.
   E. medication administration/adverse reactions.
   F. drug abuse.
   G. sexual abstinence.
   H. blood donation.
   I. preparation of shellfish/cooking precautions.
   J. other_____

   _____

3. Ineffective individual/family coping related to:
   A. isolation.
   B. fatigue.
   C. irritability.
   D. unemployment.

    E. cost of medical care/poor insurance coverage.

    F. dependence on others for care.

    G. other_____

_____

4. Altered nutrition: potential for more than body requirements related to:

    A. anorexia.

    B. nausea/vomiting.

    C. abdominal pain.

    D. other_____

_____

5. Potential for injury related to:

    A. refusal to follow recommended instructions.

    B. denial.

    C. drug abuse.

    D. other_____

_____

6. Social isolation related to:

    A. prevention of transmittal of communicable disease.

    B. confinement to home.

    C. other_____

_____

7. Altered family processes related to:

    A. isolation of family member.

    B. other_____

_____

8. Impaired home maintenance management related to:

    A. dependence on others for care.

    B. increased demand for rest/limited activity.

    C. other_____

_____

9. Impaired home maintainance management related to:

    A. refusal to participate in therapy.

    B. drug abuse.

    C. other_____

_____

10. Altered parenting related to:

    A. fatigue.

    B. nausea/vomiting.

    C. activity intolerance.

    D. isolation.

    E. other_____

    _____

II. SHORT-TERM GOALS

1. Client will remain isolated at home until further notice from M.D. after 1–2–3 R.N. visits.
2. Client will maintain adequate rest periods throughout the day after 1–2–3 R.N. visits.
3. Client will drink 1–2 quarts fluid daily as ordered after 1–2–3 R.N. visits.
4. Client will consume diet with increased carbohydrates, protein, and moderate amount of fat after 1–2–3 R.N. visits.
5. Client will wash hands after voiding or defecating after 1 R.N. visit.
6. Client will advise all contacts to seek medical follow-up/ administration of gamma globulin after 1–2 R.N. visits.
7. Client will avoid alcohol intake as ordered after 1–2 R.N. visits.
8. Client will seek laboratory testing/M.D. appointments as ordered after 1–2 R.N. visits.

III. LONG-TERM GOALS

1. Independent activities of daily living will be resumed in 1–2 weeks.
2. Adequate diagnosis, testing, and treatment will reduce incidence of disease in community in 1–2 weeks.
3. Optimal level of health will be achieved in 1–2 weeks.

IV. OUTCOME CRITERIA

1. Vital signs are normal.
2. Skin color is clear and normal.
3. Sclera are white and healthy.
4. Appetite is normal.
5. Stools are normal.
6. Urine is clear, yellow, and sufficient in quantity.
7. Client states he/she feels better.
8. Client safely returns to play/school/work.

V. NURSING INTERVENTION/TREATMENT

1. R.N. will contact client to set up a time for interview for physical assessment and completion and submission of state surveillance record.

2. R.N. will instruct client/family on:

    A. home isolation/bed rest.

    B. monitoring and recording of vital signs.

    C. fluid intake/diet high in carbohydrates and protein, but with moderate amount of fat, as ordered by M.D.

    D. sterilization and disposal of dishes.

    E. disinfection of bathroom.

    F. proper hand-washing technique/personal hygiene.

    G. disposal of tissues into bag.

    H. garbage disposal into community.

    I. laboratory testing/M.D. appointments.

3. R.N. will instruct client to avoid blood donation.

4. R.N. will provide gamma globulin inoculation to contacts as ordered by M.D.

5. R.N. will provide M.D. with follow-up reports and discharge summary when case closes.

6. R.N. will notify client when he/she may return to play/school/ employment.

7. R.N. will notify client/family/significant others when case will close.

Herniorrhaphy
Care Plan

I. NURSING DIAGNOSIS

1. Knowledge deficit related to:
   A. breathing exercises.
   B. dressing care.
   C. ambulation.
   D. medication administration/adverse reactions.
   E. restricted weight lifting/strenuous exercise.
   G. other _____

2. Potential fluid volume deficit related to:
   A. vomiting.
   B. poor fluid intake.
   C. other _____

3. Anxiety related to:
   A. impending femoral/umbilical/incisional/internal pain.
   B. immobility.
   C. straining at stool.
   D. other _____

4. Self-care deficit: feeding/bathing/grooming/dressing/toileting related to:
   A. limited mobility.
   B. secondary infection.

C. other _____

_____

5. Impaired home maintenance management related to limited mobility.
6. Pain related to:
   A. poor skin healing.
   B. difficulty in ambulation.
   C. straining at stool.
   D. other _____

   _____

7. Noncompliance with therapy related to:
   A. confusion.
   B. poor mobility.
   C. other _____

   _____

8. Altered nutrition: potential for more than body requirements related to:
   A. wound healing.
   B. poor intake.
   C. other _____

   _____

9. Altered parenting related to restricted mobility.
10. Potential for injury related to:
    A. excessive coughing.
    B. straining at stool.
    C. excessive strenuous exercise/heavy lifting.
    D. other _____

    _____

11. Ineffective breathing patterns related to:
    A. poor demonstration of breathing exercises.
    B. incisional pain.
    C. other _____

    _____

12. Sexual dysfunction related to:
    A. healing of surgical site.
    B. secondary infection.
    C. other _____

    _____

13. Potential impaired skin integrity related to:
    A. healing of surgical site.
    B. secondary wound infection.
    C. other _____

    _____

14. Sleep pattern disturbance related to femoral/umbilical/incisional/internal pain.

II. SHORT-TERM GOALS

1. Client/Family will verbalize fears, anxieties, and concerns after 1–2 R.N. visits.
2. Client/Family will properly change dressings as ordered after 1–2 R.N. visits.
3. Client will consume fluids/diet as ordered after 1–2 R.N. visits.
4. Client will take medication as prescribed after 1–2 R.N. visits.
5. Client/Family will notify M.D. of adverse effects or impending secondary infections after 1–2 R.N. visits.
6. Client will perform exercises as ordered after 1–2 R.N. visits.
7. Client will avoid excessive coughing/smoking after 1–2 R.N. visits.
8. Client will avoid excessive lifting or strenuous exercise after 1–2 R.N. visits.
9. Client will avoid straining at stool after 1 R.N. visit.
10. Client will participate in diversional activities after 1–2 R.N. visits.

III. LONG-TERM GOALS

1. Independent activities of daily living will be resumed in 1 week.
2. Optimal level of health will be achieved in 1–2 weeks.

IV. OUTCOME CRITERIA

1. Vital signs are normal.
2. Skin is healthy and intact.
3. Normal ambulation is achieved.
4. Appetite is normal.
5. Bowel/Bladder functions normally.
6. Client consumes nutritious meals.
7. Client states he/she feels better.
8. Client can return to work.

V. NURSING INTERVENTION/TREATMENT

1. R.N. will instruct client/family/H.H.A. on:
   A. proper hand-washing technique.
   B. aseptic dressing technique.
   C. fluid intake/dietary regimen as ordered.
   D. medication administration/adverse reactions.
   E. immediate notification of M.D. of adverse reactions or signs/symptoms of impending infection.
   F. bowel/bladder regimen.
   G. avoidance/limitation of smoking and coughing.
   H. limited excessive weight lifting/strenuous exercise.
   I. prescribed ambulation/exercise.
   J. diversional activities.
2. R.N. will provide M.D. with follow-up reports and discharge summary when case closes.
3. R.N. will notify client/family/H.H.A./significant others when case will close.

Hip Fracture
Care Plan

I. NURSING DIAGNOSIS

   1. Anxiety related to:
      A. pain.
      B. possible injury or accidents.
      C. poor mobility.
      D. other _____

      _____

   2. Impaired physical mobility related to:
      A. pain.
      B. infection.
      C. limited motion.
      D. other _____

      _____

   3. Activity intolerance related to:
      A. pain.
      B. limited motion.
      C. weakness/fatigue.
      D. other _____

      _____

   4. Ineffective individual/family coping related to:
      A. irritability.
      B. cost of medical care/poor insurance coverage.
      C. dependence on others for care.
      D. other _____

      _____

5. Impaired home maintenance management related to:
   A. poor mobility.
   B. dependence on others for care.
   C. other _____

6. Sleep pattern disturbance related to:
   A. pain.
   B. confusion.
   C. other _____

7. Self-care deficit: feeding/bathing/grooming/dressing/toileting related to:
   A. pain.
   B. confusion.
   C. dependence on others for care.
   D. other _____

8. Altered patterns of urinary elimination related to:
   A. assistance needed for toileting.
   B. poor mobility.
   C. incontinence.
   D. other _____

9. Potential for injury related to:
   A. confusion.
   B. poor mobility.
   C. poor vision.
   D. dizziness.
   E. unsteadiness of gait.
   F. other _____

10. Altered nutrition: potential for more than body requirements related to:
    A. dependence on others for care.
    B. anorexia.
    C. confusion.
    D. other _____

11. Knowledge deficit related to:
    A. turning/repositioning.
    B. exercise.
    C. medication administration/adverse reaction.
    D. dressing care.
    E. other _____

    _____

12. Pain related to:
    A. poor exercise tolerance.
    B. limited movement.
    C. other _____

    _____

II. SHORT-TERM GOALS

1. Client/Family will verbalize fears, anxieties, and concerns after 1–2–3 R.N. visits.
2. Client/Family will administer medication as ordered after 1–2–3 R.N. visits.
3. Client/Family will immediately notify M.D. of adverse reactions or change in condition after 1–2 R.N. visits.
4. Client/Family will apply ace bandages/antiembolus hose/braces as ordered after 1–2–3–4 R.N./P.T. visits.
5. Client will use cane/walker/crutches/wheelchair/bed trapeze as ordered after 1–2–3–4 R.N./P.T. visits.
6. Client/Family will perform/assist with strengthening exercises after 1–2 R.N. visits in consultation with M.D. and P.T.
7. Client/Family will prepare nutritious meals/force fluids as ordered after 1–2 R.N. visits.
8. Client will visit M.D. as ordered after 1–2 R.N. visits.

III. LONG-TERM GOALS

1. Independent activities of daily living will be resumed in 1–2 weeks.
2. Ambulation will be achieved in 1–2–3 weeks.
3. Optimal level of health will be achieved in 3–4 weeks.

IV. OUTCOME CRITERIA

1. Vital signs are normal.

2. Granulation occurs; skin is normal, healthy, and intact.

3. Union occurs.

4. Urinary functioning remains normal.

5. Chest is clear.

6. Respirations are normal.

7. Weight bearing and gait remain normal.

8. Weight is appropriate for height.

9. Laboratory test results are normal.

10. Client states he/she feels better.

V. NURSING INTERVENTION/TREATMENT

1. R.N. will instruct client/family/H.H.A. on:

   A. monitoring and recording of vital signs.

   B. medication administration/adverse reactions.

   C. immediate notification of M.D. of adverse reactions or change in condition.

   D. positioning/turning/range-of-motion exercise.

   E. skin care.

   F. application of ace bandage/antiembolus hose/braces.

   G. use of overhead bed trapeze.

   H. dressing care.

   I. signs/symptoms of infection/pneumonia/decubitus ulcers/thrombus.

   J. avoidance of elevation of knees while lying in bed, to avoid flexion contractures.

   K. additional equipment (e.g., wheelchair/walker/cane).

   L. installation of grip bars along walls/shower/tub.

   M. laboratory testing/M.D. appointments.

2. R.N. will encourage independence as much as possible.

3. R.N. will provide additional services (e.g., P.T. or M.S.W.) if ordered by M.D.

4. R.N. will provide M.D. with follow-up reports and discharge summary when case closes.

5. R.N. will notify client/family/H.H.A./significant others when case will close.

Home Parenteral Nutrition Care Plan

I. NURSING DIAGNOSIS

1. Anxiety related to:
   A. possible contamination of site.
   B. air embolus/thrombus formation.
   C. hemorrhage.
   D. septicemia.
   E. operation of TPN pump.
   F. cost of medical care/poor insurance coverage.
   G. possible death.
   H. other _____

2. Knowledge deficit related to:
   A. home health agency program criteria/consent procedures.
   B. proper hand-washing technique.
   C. dressing care.
   D. irrigation of catheter/heparinization.
   E. aseptic technique.
   F. medication administration/storage/adverse reactions.
   G. operation of TPN pump.
   H. signs/symptoms of complications.
   I. insurance coverage.
   J. laboratory testing/M.D. appointments.
   K. daily vital signs.

   L. daily weight recording.

   M. fluids/diet.

   N. urine monitoring.

   O. IV tubing changes.

   P. solution preparation/inventory/ordering of supplies.

   Q. administration of fat emulsions/adverse reactions.

   R. application of catheter screw-on caps.

   S. use of a hyperalimentation vest.

   T. destruction of needles and syringes/safe garbage disposal (usually in a coffee can with tight-fitting lid).

   U. troubleshooting (e. g., air embolism/infection/thrombosis/clotted catheter/pump malfunction/catheter fracture).

   V. performance of procedures when traveling.

   W. weaning.

   X. other _____

3. Partial/Total self-care deficit: feeding/bathing/grooming/dressing/toileting/administration of solutions related to:

   A. dependence on others for care.

   B. weakness.

   C. immobility.

   D. fear.

   E. chronic vomiting/diarrhea.

   F. little or no oral intake for more than 7 days.

   G. recent loss of 10% of premorbid weight.

   H. serum albumin levels lower than 3.5 g/100 cc.

   I. poor tolerance of long-term tube feedings.

   J. constant weight loss despite adequate oral intake.

   K. other _____

4. Potential for injury related to:

   A. poor hand-washing technique.

   B. poor aseptic technique.

   C. dislodgment of catheter during sleep, play, or accidents.

   D. cracking/severing of catheter (related to improper/frequent clamping).

   E. inadequate operation of TPN pump.

   F. worn cord/worn plug/overuse of TPN pump.

   G. poor administration of medication.

    H. poor irrigation technique.

    I. other _____

    _____

5. Potential for infection related to:

    A. poor administration of medication/solutions.

    B. poor hand-washing technique.

    C. poor dressing technique.

    D. poor irrigation technique.

    E. other _____

    _____

6. Noncompliance with therapy related to:

    A. cost of medical care/poor insurance coverage.

    B. dependence on others for care.

    C. immobility.

    D. poor understanding of procedure.

    E. denial.

    F. other _____

    _____

7. Fear related to:

    A. possible hemorrhage.

    B. infection.

    C. possible air embolus.

    D. dislodgment of catheter.

    E. other _____

    _____

8. Diarrhea/Constipation related to:

    A. adverse effects of solutions.

    B. change in medication/solution.

    C. emotional stress.

    D. other _____

    _____

9. Impaired home maintenance management related to:

    A. dependence on others for care.

    B. excessive health care needs.

    C. other _____

    _____

10. Potential impaired skin integrity related to:

    A. infection.

B. tape allergy.

C. adverse reactions to medication.

D. leakage of solution.

E. other _____

_____

II. SHORT-TERM GOALS

1. Client/Family will obtain all supplies before R.N. visits home on initial evaluation.
2. Client/Family will cleanse working area (e.g., tabletop, bedside table) with soap and water after 1 R.N. visit.
3. Client/Family will wash hands as ordered after 1 R.N. visit.
4. Client/Family will prepare heparin syringe for catheter irrigation after 1–2 R.N. visits (amount of heparin will vary from client to client according to M.D.'s orders).
5. Client/Family will change heparin lock plug daily, using sterile technique, after 1–2–3 R.N. visits.
6. Client/Family will sterilize heparin caps, using alcohol solution, after 1–2 R.N. visits.

or

Client/Family will use disposable heparin caps daily after 1–2–3 R.N. visits.

7. Client/Family will tape injection-cap end of catheter after 1–2–3 R.N. visits.
8. Client/Family will wrap tape around line before clamping after 1–2–3 R.N. visits.
9. Client/Family will clamp catheter over taped area of catheter when not in use after 1–2–3 R.N. visits.
10. Client/Family will irrigate catheter with heparin/heparinized saline 3–5–10 cc as ordered after 1–2–3 R.N. visits.
11. Client/Family will fill tuberculin syringe with heparin as ordered to prepare for catheter irrigation in case of clotting after 1–2–3 R.N. visits.
12. Client/Family will inject heparin and recap line for 1 hour after 1–2–3 R.N. visits.
13. Client/Family will repeat irrigation of line if still blocked, as ordered by M.D., after 1–2–3 R.N. visits.
14. Client/Family will contact M.D. about difficulty or malfunctioning of catheter or abnormal signs/symptoms of infection after 1 R.N. visit.

15. Client/Family will change dressings over insertion and exit sites, using sterile technique, after 1–2–3 R.N. visits.

16. Client/Family will remove old dressing, apply gloves, and check for signs/symptoms of infection after 1 R.N. visit.

17. Client/Family will cleanse skin in rotating pattern, moving in an outward direction 3 inches from the exit site, using alcohol swab stick, after 1–2–3 R.N. visits.

18. Client/Family will repeat circular cleansing with 2 additional alcohol swab sticks after 1–2–3 R.N. visits.

19. Client/Family will swab site with providone-iodine, using circular motion, and dispose of swab after 1–2–3 R.N. visits.

20. Client/Family will repeat swab of site with providone-iodine, using circular motion, after 1–2–3 R.N. visits.

21. Client/Family will apply antibacterial ointment (e.g., iodophor ointment) to site after 1–2–3 R.N. visits.

22. Client/Family will apply a clean 2-inch × 2-inch gauze pad over exit site and secure with tape after 1–2–3 R.N. visits.

23. Client/Family will apply benzoin to skin around gauze in a frame-like manner, wait until it becomes tacky, remove gloves, and apply tape, completely covering gauze, after 1–2–3 R.N. visits.

24. Client/Family will loop catheter and tape to dressing with cap pointing upward after 1–2–3 R.N. visits.

25. Client/Family will change dressings 3 times weekly after 1–2–3 R.N. visits.

26. Client will shower with the use of a waterproof dressing after consulting with M.D. after 2–3 R.N. visits. (If dressing becomes wet or soiled, it must be changed immediately.)

27. Client/Family will keep a daily log of dates, intake and output (both oral and parenteral), volume infused, temperature, weight, dressing changes, urine fraction testing, and drainage after 1–2–3 R.N. visits.

28. Client/Family will obtain prescribed laboratory testing (CBC with differential, electrolytes weekly/biweekly/monthly) after 1–2 R.N. visits.

29. Client/Family will use infusion pump correctly after 1–2–3 R.N. visits.

30. Client/Family will correctly administer sterile hyperalimentation solutions on time after 1–2–3 R.N. visits.

31. Client/Family will assist in mixing of solutions as ordered after 6–8 R.N. visits.

32. Client/Family will perform regular fractional urine testing to observe for glycosuria after 1–2–3 R.N. visits.

33. Client/Family will use emergency phone numbers for contacting people who can provide instructions (e.g., M.D./pharmacist/R.N.) after 1 R.N. visit.
34. Client will keep regular M.D. appointments after 1–2 R.N. visits.
35. Client/Family will administer fat emulsion through a separate peripheral IV line, through the central catheter by means of a Y connector set or as an additive to the hyperalimentation solution as ordered after 1–2–3–4 R.N. visits.
36. Client will safely perform procedures when traveling after 6–8 R.N. visits.

III. LONG-TERM GOALS

1. Adequate nutritional status will be restored in 3–4 weeks.
2. Independent activities of daily living will be resumed in 1–2 weeks.
3. Optimal level of health will be achieved within 3–4 weeks.

IV. OUTCOME CRITERIA

1. Vital signs are normal.
2. Wound heals appropriately; skin is granulated.
3. Signs/Symptoms of infection are controlled.
4. Client/Family understand and agree on home therapy plan.
5. Client/Family are able to perform procedures for home therapy.
6. Client/Family has appropriate home environment for therapy.
7. Reimbursement for supplies/medications/skilled nursing visits/laboratory testing is obtained.
8. Serum glucose and urine fractional test results are normal.
9. Weight is appropriate for height.
10. Intake and output are normal.
11. Laboratory test results are within normal limits.
12. Normal socialization occurs.
13. Client is alert and cooperative.
14. Client states he/she feels better.
15. Client returns to school/work/play.

V. NURSING INTERVENTION/TREATMENT

1. Before admission, R.N. will meet with hospital discharge planner/parenteral nurse specialist/M.D./client, if possible, to elicit

instructions to be given to client upon returning home/to community.

2. R.N. will visit client's home before client's discharge from hospital to determine suitability of environment for parenteral nutrition therapy.

3. R.N. will arrange with hospital discharge planner to have supplies available in the home before visit.

4. R.N. will instruct client/family/H.H.A. on:

A. terminology/equipment from hospital.

B. proper hand-washing technique.

C. medication administration/adverse reactions/expiration dates/ safe needle and syringe disposal.

D. storage/inspection of medications (e.g., checking solutions for leaks, floating particles, precipitation of ingredients/discarding of solutions).

E. administration and rate of hyperalimentation solutions/sterile mixing of solutions at home if approved by M.D./administration of fat emulsions via separate peripheral IV line, central catheter by means of a Y connector set or as an additive to hyperalimentation solution/avoidance of use of a filter with fat emulsions.

F. aseptic technique for dressing changes.

G. dressing kits/depilatories for removal of excess hair around catheter.

H. administration of heparin (should be done directly after feeding if fully infused, unless otherwise specified in orders).

I. irrigation of catheter with tuberculin syringe.

J. clamping of catheter with jaw spring clamp/screw-on cap.

K. sterilization/sterile application of heparin caps to catheter (caps may also be disposable).

L. diet/fluids/tube feedings during weaning process.

M. daily rest/exercise.

N. signs/symptoms of infection/circulatory overload/dehydration/ shock/dislodgment of catheter/leaking/neck vein distension/arm or shoulder pain/purulent drainage/behavioral changes/water intoxication/electrolyte imbalances/pneumothorax/hemorrhage/ sepsis.

O. signs/symptoms of adverse reactions to intralipid infusion (chills, fever, shivering, vomiting, shortness of breath, and chest pain).

P. signs/symptoms of air embolism (coughing, shortness of breath, chest pain).

Q. signs/symptoms of hyperglycemia (polyuria, polydipsia, polyphagia, fatigue, nausea, vomiting, positive urine sugar and acetone).

R. signs/symptoms of hypoglycemia (hunger, shakiness, nervousness, cold sweats, faintness, rapid heart rate). If client becomes hypoglycemic, he/she should take sugar/hard candy/ fruit juice as ordered by M.D.

S. importance of client/family turning off infusion immediately and reporting to M.D. immediately if any signs/symptoms of complications develop.

T. safe operation and care of infusion pump: Client should avoid using water or soaking feet while connected to pump and also avoid using other electrical equipment while connected to pump.

U. personal hygiene/oral care/laboratory testing/M.D. appointments.
daily log: monitoring and recording of weight, urine fraction test results for sugar and acetone, vital signs, intake and output, wound drainage/urine specific gravity every 4–6 hours or as ordered/recording date, time, formula code, bottle/bag number, total volume of solution, dates for changing extension sets and tubing.

V. socialization/diversional activity.

W. keeping emergency listing of medical personnel near phone at all times.

X. scheduling of delivery service of all medical equipment to client's home (usually every 2 weeks or monthly); client should be able to communicate with supplier at all times.

Y. blood culture/sensitivity prior to removal of catheter/weaning.

Z. use of a hyperalimentation vest/travel arrangements.

AA. employment.

5. R.N. will provide M.D. with follow-up reports and discharge summary when case closes.

6. R.N. will provide client/family with information on additional services (e.g., medical social services/psychotherapy/career counseling/clubs/educational opportunities/organizations).

7. R.N. will notify client/family/H.H.A./significant others when case will close.

8. R.N. will provide client/family with additional resources for financial aid.

Hospice
Care Plan

I. NURSING DIAGNOSIS

1. Ineffective individual/family coping related to:
   A. the dying process.
   B. financial demands.
   C. altered levels of consciousness.
   D. hallucinations/delusions.
   E. chronic pain.
   F. other _____
   _____

2. Impaired home maintenance management related to:
   A. terminal stage of illness.
   B. excessive demands of the sick.
   C. cost of medical care.
   D. other _____
   _____

3. Anticipatory grieving of family related to impending death.
4. Knowledge deficit related to:
   A. terminal stage.
   B. medication administration/adverse reactions.
   C. pain management.
   D. operation of TENS machine.
   E. increasing dependency.
   F. family grief.
   G. the withdrawal from food and fluids.

H. altered levels of consciousness.

I. IV therapy/hyperalimentation/tube feedings.

J. home care services/hospice.

K. biohazards of antineoplastics/sources of exposure/hand washing/drug preparation, administration and disposal guidelines for contaminated waste.

L. last rites/actual death event.

M. funeral arrangements/cremation/burial.

N. financial aid/reading of a will.

O. consent for organ donation.

P. other _____

_____

5. Spiritual distress related to terminal stage.

6. Sensory/Perceptual alterations related to:

A. disease process.

B. analgesia/sedation.

C. other _____

_____

7. Altered nutrition: potential for more than body requirements related to:

A. anorexia.

B. dysphagia.

C. dependence on others for feeding/meal preparation.

D. diarrhea/constipation.

E. nausea/vomiting.

F. other _____

_____

8. Constipation/Fecal impaction/Diarrhea/Bowel incontinence related to:

A. poor fluid/dietary intake.

B. adverse reactions to medication.

C. dependence on others for care.

D. nausea/vomiting.

E. lack of exercise.

F. confusion.

G. other _____

_____

9. Ineffective breathing pattern related to:

A. semicomatose/comatose state.

    B. pain.

    C. gross abdominal enlargement.

    D. rales/rhonchi.

    E. other _____

    _____

10. Pain related to:

    A. advance of disease process.

    B. poor positioning/poor exercise tolerance.

    C. inadequate medication administration.

    D. other _____

    _____

11. Potential impaired skin integrity related to:

    A. poor medication administration (IM/IV).

    B. advance of disease process.

    C. poor positioning/turning.

    D. other _____

    _____

12. Impaired physical mobility related to:

    A. semicomatose/comatose state.

    B. paralysis.

    C. pain.

    D. infection.

    E. other _____

    _____

13. Self-care deficit: feeding/bathing/grooming/dressing/toileting related to:

    A. paralysis.

    B. infection.

    C. semicomatose/comatose state.

    D. weakness.

    E. activity intolerance.

    F. dependence on others for care.

    G. lack of support in the home.

    H. other _____

    _____

14. Self-esteem disturbance related to:

    A. unemployment/job insecurity.

    B. weakness/fatigue.

C. activity intolerance.

D. dependence on others for care.

E. other _____

_____

15. Altered family processes related to:

    A. excessive demands of the sick.

    B. lack of support in the home.

    C. grieving.

    D. other _____

    _____

16. Social isolation related to:

    A. anger.

    B. activity intolerance.

    C. grieving.

    D. increased need for sleep/rest.

    E. other _____

    _____

17. Anxiety related to:

    A. fear of dying.

    B. advance of disease process.

    C. home maintenance management.

    D. survival of spouse/children/significant others.

    E. medical costs.

    F. homemaker costs.

    G. other _____

    _____

II. SHORT-TERM GOALS

1. Client/Family will verbalize fears, anxieties, and concerns after 1–2–3–4 R.N. visits.

2. Client/Family will administer medication as prescribed after 1–2–3–4 R.N. visits.

3. Client/Family will immediately notify M.D. of adverse reactions or change in condition after 1–2 R.N. visits.

4. Family will turn/reposition client from side to side every 2 hours after 1–2 R.N. visits.

5. Client/Family will prepare nutritionally sound meals after 1–2–3 R.N. visits.

6. Client/Family will assist with enteral feedings/hyperalimentation as ordered after 1–2–3 R.N. visits.
7. Client/Family will assist with bowel/bladder habits after 1–2–3 R.N. visits.
8. Client/Family will use respiratory equipment in the home after 1–2–3 R.N. visits.
9. Client/Family will assist with all bathing and grooming activities after 1–2 R.N. visits.
10. Client/Family will assist with range-of-motion exercise to all extremities after 1–2 R.N. visits.

III. LONG-TERM GOALS

1. Client/Family will grieve normally in 6–12 months or thereafter.
2. Family will provide comfort in the terminal stages.
3. Family will provide for adequate burial/cremation.

IV. OUTCOME CRITERIA

1. Vital signs are normal.
2. Pain is eliminated.
3. Dying and death are accepted.
4. Financial status remains stable.
5. All stages of grief and grieving are worked through.

V. NURSING INTERVENTION/TREATMENT

1. R.N. will provide client/family/H.H.A. with phone numbers in case of emergency, especially on a 24-hour basis.
2. R.N. will instruct client/family/H.H.A. on:
   A. monitoring and recording of vital signs.
   B. specially balanced, high-calorie meals.
   C. bowel/bladder regimen.
   D. personal hygiene/skin care/laboratory testing/M.D. appointments.
   E. medication administration (e.g., analgesia/sedation)/adverse reactions.
   F. biohazards of antineoplastics/sources of exposure/hand washing/drug preparation, administration and contaminated waste disposal guidelines.
   G. pain management/operation of TENS machine.

H. increasing dependency/family grief/the dying person's withdrawal from food and fluids/altered levels of consciousness.
I. IV therapy/hyperalimentation/tube feedings.
J. home care services/hospice organizations/groups/individuals/clergy.
K. assistive devices/rehabilitation equipment (e.g., electrical hospital bed/air mattress with pump/feeding tubes with or without pump/Foley catheter/wheelchair/Hoyer lift/cane/walker/incontinence aids/padded side rails/restraints).
L. diversional activities for adults and children.
M. last rites/actual death event.

3. R.N. will allow client to function independently whenever possible; will allow client/family to verbalize fears, anxieties, and concerns at all times.
4. R.N. will provide additional personnel (P.T., social services, S.T., O.T., home attendant, housekeeper, homemaker) if necessary.
5. R.N. will provide M.D. with follow-up reports and discharge summary when case closes.
6. R.N. will provide for the return of all medical equipment after death.
7. R.N. will assist family with funeral arrangements/cremation, will assist with pronouncement of death according to state regulations.

Hypertension
Care Plan

I. NURSING DIAGNOSIS

1. Anxiety related to:
   A. hypertension.
   B. other _____

2. Knowledge deficit related to:
   A. avoidance of emotional stress.
   B. medication administration/adverse reactions.
   C. exercise/rest.
   D. meditation.
   E. weight loss.
   F. avoidance of tobacco/alcohol/addictive drugs.
   G. diet/fluids.
   H. reduction of intake of saturated fats and sodium.
   I. ingredients in over-the-counter medications (e.g., sugar/ caffeine/sodium/potassium).
   J. other _____

3. Potential for injury related to:
   A. refusal to comply with medical instructions.
   B. denial.
   C. other _____

4. Noncompliance with therapy related to:
   A. denial.

    B. confusion.

    C. other _____

_____

5. Self-care deficit: feeding/bathing/grooming/dressing/toileting related to:

    A. headaches.

    B. blurred vision.

    C. dizziness.

    D. other _____

_____

6. Altered patterns of urinary elimination related to:

    A. stress.

    B. medication administration.

    C. sodium retention.

    D. other _____

_____

7. Sensory/Perceptual alterations (visual) related to:

    A. refusal to adhere to medical advice.

    B. poor administration of medicine.

    C. excessive sodium intake.

    D. stress.

    E. other _____

_____

8. Increased cardiac output related to hypertension.

II. SHORT-TERM GOALS

1. Client/Family will verbalize fears, anxieties, and concerns after 1–2 R.N. visits.
2. Client/Family will immediately notify M.D. of adverse reactions or change in condition after 1–2 R.N. visits.
3. Client/Family will administer medication as ordered after 1–2 R.N. visits.
4. Client/Family will limit/omit sodium in diet as ordered after 1–2 R.N. visits.
5. Client will obtain eyeglasses as ordered after 1–2 R.N. visits.
6. Client will reduce weight as ordered after 1–2 R.N. visits.
7. Client will avoid/limit smoking and stimulants after 1–2 R.N. visits.
8. Client will exercise/rest as ordered after 1–2 R.N. visits.

9. Client/Family will monitor blood pressure as taught after 1–2 R.N. visits.

10. Client/Family will seek laboratory testing/M.D. appointments as ordered after 1–2 R.N. visits.

III. LONG-TERM GOALS

1. Normal peripheral vascular resistance will be achieved in 3–4 weeks.

2. Independent activities of daily living will be resumed in 1–2 weeks.

3. Optimal level of health will be achieved in 3–4 weeks.

IV. OUTCOME CRITERIA

1. Vital signs are normal.

2. Peripheral vascular resistance is normal at the arteriolar level.

3. Urinary functioning remains normal.

4. Laboratory test results are normal.

5. Vision remains normal.

6. Client states he/she feels better.

V. NURSING INTERVENTION/TREATMENT

1. R.N. will contact client/family to arrange home visit.

2. R.N. will instruct client/family/H.H.A. on:

   A. fluid intake/dietary restrictions, especially sodium.

   B. medication administration (e.g., thiazide diuretics/beta blockers/vasodilators/guanethidine monosulfate)/adverse reactions.

   C. ingredients in over-the-counter medications (e.g., sugar/caffeine/sodium/potassium).

   D. weight reduction.

   E. avoidance of smoking/stimulants.

   F. eye examinations.

   G. meditation/relaxation techniques.

   H. balanced rest, play, work, and sexual activity.

   I. laboratory testing/M.D. appointments.

   J. organizations for educational materials and additional assistance.

   K. teaching a family member how to take blood pressure.

3. R.N. will provide M.D. with follow-up reports and discharge summary when case closes.
4. R.N. will notify client/family/H.H.A./significant others when case will close.

Hyperthyroidism
Care Plan

I. NURSING DIAGNOSIS

1. Knowledge deficit related to:
   A. signs/symptoms of hyperthyroidism.
   B. medication administration/adverse reactions.
   C. other _____
   _____

2. Increased cardiac output related to:
   A. poor administration of medication (underdosing/overdosing).
   B. refusal to administer medication.
   C. excessive exercise.
   D. refusal to adhere to medical advice.
   E. refusal to accept radiation/surgery.
   F. advance of condition.
   G. other _____
   _____

3. Constipation/Diarrhea related to:
   A. poor fluid/dietary intake.
   B. anxiety.
   C. other _____
   _____

4. Impaired home maintenance management related to:
   A. advance in condition.
   B. stress.
   C. hyperexcitability/nervousness.

D. other _____

_____

5. Altered nutrition: potential for more than body requirements related to:
   A. increased metabolism.
   B. increased appetite.
   C. hyperexcitability.
   D. stress.
   E. other _____

   _____

6. Self-esteem disturbance related to:
   A. weight loss.
   B. altered body image.
   C. other _____

   _____

7. Altered parenting related to:
   A. hyperexcitability/nervousness.
   B. irritability.
   C. apprehension.
   D. anxiety.
   E. other _____

   _____

8. Noncompliance with therapy related to:
   A. denial.
   B. anxiety.
   C. other _____

   _____

9. Ineffective individual/family coping related to:
   A. hyperexcitability/nervousness.
   B. irritability.
   C. apprehension.
   D. anxiety.
   E. tremors.
   F. other _____

   _____

10. Potential for injury (accidents) related to fine tremors of the hands.
11. Sleep pattern disturbance related to:
    A. hyperexcitability.

    B. nervousness.

    C. anxiety.

    D. other _____

    _____

12. Activity intolerance related to weakness.

II. SHORT-TERM GOALS

1. Client will take prescribed medication as ordered after 1–2 R.N. visits.
2. Client/Family will report adverse reactions to M.D. after 1–2 R.N. visits.
3. Client will be cooperative and sociable after 1–2 R.N. visits.
4. Client/Family will prepare nutritionally satisfying meals after 1–2 R.N. visits.
5. Client will weigh self daily after 1–2 R.N. visits.
6. Client will exercise/rest appropriately daily after 1–2 R.N. visits.
7. Client/Family will maintain a fairly cool environment as ordered after 1–2 R.N. visits.
8. Client/Family will seek useful diversional activities after 1–2 R.N. visits.
9. Client will seek appropriate diagnostic testing after 1–2 R.N. visits.
10. Client will visit M.D. as ordered after 1–2 R.N. visits.

III. LONG-TERM GOALS

1. Normal metabolism will be achieved in 1–2 months.
2. Independent activities of daily living will be resumed in 1–2 weeks.
3. Optimal level of health will be achieved in 1–2 months.

IV. OUTCOME CRITERIA

1. Basal metabolic rate remains normal.
2. Vital signs are normal.
3. Appropriate weight is maintained.
4. Blood iodine-131 uptake remains normal.
5. Blood protein–bound iodine remains normal.
6. Appetite is appropriate.
7. Menses/Ovulation remains normal.
8. Bowel habits remain normal.

9. Normal sleep pattern is maintained.

10. Client states he/she feels better.

V. NURSING INTERVENTION/TREATMENT

1. R.N. will instruct client/family/H.H.A. on:

    A. monitoring and recording of vital signs.

    B. medication administration (antithyroid drugs)/adverse reactions.

    C. immediate notification of M.D. of adverse reactions or change in condition.

    D. daily weights.

    E. dietary requirements.

    F. maintenance of a cool environment.

    G. laboratory testing/M.D. appointments.

    H. skin care for excessive perspiration.

    I. radiation therapy.

    J. possible surgery.

    K. regular exercise/rest periods.

    L. diversional activities.

2. R.N. will provide M.D. with follow-up reports and discharge summary when case closes.

3. R.N. will notify client/family/H.H.A./significant others when case will close.

Hypothyroidism
Care Plan

I. NURSING DIAGNOSIS

1. Knowledge deficit related to:
   A. medication administration/adverse reactions.
   B. laboratory testing.
   C. skin care.
   D. exercise/rest.
   E. signs/symptoms of hypothyroidism.
   F. other_____

2. Impaired home maintenance management related to:
   A. lethargy.
   B. forgetfulness.
   C. fatigue.
   D. sleepiness.
   E. other_____

3. Altered parenting related to:
   A. lethargy.
   B. forgetfulness.
   C. fatigue.
   D. other_____

4. Sexual dysfunction related to:
   A. fatigue.

B. lethargy.

C. other_____

_____

5. Fatigue related to:
    A. poor administration of medication.
    B. refusal to follow medical advice.
    C. poor exercise tolerance.
    D. other_____

_____

6. Noncompliance with therapy related to:
    A. irritability.
    B. complacency.
    C. other_____

_____

7. Decreased cardiac output related to hypotension.
8. Body image disturbance related to:
    A. weight gain.
    B. thinning of hair/hair loss.
    C. other_____

_____

9. Altered nutrition: less than body requirements related to:
    A. lethargy.
    B. decreased metabolism.
    C. weight gain
    D. other_____

_____

10. Potential for injury related to:
    A. lethargy.
    B. forgetfulness.
    C. other_____

_____

II. SHORT-TERM GOALS

1. Client will take prescribed medication as ordered after 1–2 R.N. visits.
2. Client/Family will report adverse reactions or change in condition to M.D. after 1–2 R.N. visits.
3. Client will visit M.D. as order after 1–2 R.N. visits.

4. Client will seek appropriate diagnostic testing after 1–2 R.N. visits.
5. Client will be alert and responsible after 1–2 R.N. visits.
6. Client will exercise/rest appropriately daily after 1–2 R.N. visits.
7. Client/Family will maintain a warm environment as ordered after 1–2 R.N. visits.
8. Client/Family will prepare nutritionally sound meals after 1–2 R.N. visits.
9. Client/Family will seek useful diversional activities after 1–2 R.N. visits.
10. Client will weigh self daily after 1 R.N. visit.
11. Client will resume normal sexual activity after 1–2 R.N. visits.
12. Client will seek active employment after 1–2 R.N. visits.

III. LONG-TERM GOALS

1. Normal metabolism will be achieved in 1–2 months.
2. Independent activities of daily living will be resumed in 1–2 weeks.
3. Optimal level of health will be achieved in 1–2 months.

IV. OUTCOME CRITERIA

1. Basal metabolic rate remains normal.
2. Vital signs are normal.
3. Appropriate weight is maintained.
4. Menses/Ovulation is normal.
5. Hair and scalp remain healthy and intact.
6. Skin integrity remains normal.
7. Client is alert, responsible, and sociable.
8. Sensitivity to cold is eliminated.
9. Normal sleep pattern is maintained.
10. Client states he/she feels better.

V. NURSING INTERVENTION/TREATMENT

1. R.N. will instruct client/family/H.H.A. on:
   A. monitoring and recording of vital signs.
   B. skin care.
   C. daily recording of weight.
   D. regular exercise/rest.

  E. medication administration/adverse reactions.
  F. immediate notification of M.D. of adverse reactions or change in condition.
  G. maintenance of a warm environment.
  H. laboratory testing/M.D. appointments.
  I. diversional activities.
2. R.N. will provide M.D. with follow-up reports and discharge summary when case closes.
3. R.N. will notify client/family/H.H.A./significant others when case will close.

Immunizations
and Tuberculosis Testing
Care Plan

I. NURSING DIAGNOSIS

1. Anxiety related to:
   A. pain.
   B. adverse reactions to immunization.
   C. tuberculosis testing.
   D. other _____

2. Potential for injury related to:
   A. poor powers of healing/absorption.
   B. irritability/excessive movement during needle insertion.
   C. contamination of needle.
   D. other _____

3. Knowledge deficit related to:
   A. administration of immunizations/TB testing.
   B. adverse reactions.
   C. administration of antipyretics.
   D. follow-up visit.
   E. additional laboratory testing.
   F. immunizations for symptomatic/asymptomatic children with HIV infections.
   G. immunizations for children residing in the household of a patient with AIDS.

H. other _____
_____

4. Noncompliance with therapy related to:
   A. refusal to accept immunizations/TB testing.
   B. language barrier.
   C. unreliable parental supports.
   D. other _____
   _____

5. Sleep pattern disturbance related to:
   A. discomfort/pain at injection site.
   B. other _____
   _____

II. SHORT-TERM GOALS

1. Parent/Guardian will verbalize all fears, concerns, and anxieties after 1–2–3–4 R.N. visits.
2. Parent/Guardian will read literature on immunization/TB testing after 1–2 R.N. visits.
3. Parent/Guardian will sign written consent before immunizations/TB testing (in clinic).
4. Parent/Guardian will visit M.D./health center for administration of immunizations/TB testing for child/children after 1–2 R.N. visits.
5. Parent/Guardian will administer medication as prescribed for elevated temperature, irritability, or minor skin irritation after each clinic/M.D./health center visit.
6. Parent/Guardian will follow FDA guidelines for immunizations for symptomatic/asymptomatic children with HIV infections after 1–2–3–4 R.N. visits.

III. LONG-TERM GOALS

1. Sufficient immunity to a wide variety of diseases will be established for preschoolers and school-aged children.
2. Viruses will not be transmitted to immunosuppressed family members.

IV. OUTCOME CRITERIA

1. Parent/Guardian seeks immunizations/TB testing.

2. Children's vital signs remain normal after administration of immunizations/TB testing.
3. Communicable disease is prevented.

V. NURSING INTERVENTION/TREATMENT

1. R.N. will explain purpose of immunizations and assist client with choice of facility (private M.D./clinic/health center).
2. R.N. will provide parent/guardian with literature about purpose of immunizations/TB testing.
3. R.N. will arrange community education programs on immunization and TB testing in clinics, health centers, housing projects, day care centers, and schools, using filmstrips, audiocassettes, movies, records, slide presentations, handouts, and guest speakers.
4. R.N. will address immunizations for US children with HIV infections. The complete recommendations were published in *MMWR*, Sept. 26, 1986. The following is a summary of the recommendations for oral polio vaccine (OPV), Inactivated polio vaccine (IPV), and vaccines for measles, mumps, and rubella (MMR), Bacille bilié de Calmette-Guérin (BCG), diphtheria, pertussis and tetanus (DPT), *Haemophilus influenzae* type B (Hib), influenza, and pneumococcus:

Children with symptomatic HIV infections: OPV, MMR, BCG, and other live vaccines should *not be given* to children and young adults who are immunosuppressed because of HIV infection. These persons should receive IPV and should be excused for medical reasons from regulations requiring measles, rubella, and/or mumps immunization. *DPT, IPV, Hib:* The potential benefits of immunization outweigh the theoretical concern that stimulation of the immune system by immunization with inactivated vaccines might cause deterioration in immune function. Such effects have not been noted thus far among children with AIDS or other immunosuppressed persons. Immunization with DPT, IPV, and Hib vaccines *is recommended*, although immunization may be less effective than in immunocompetent children. *Flu, pneumococcal vaccines:* As with other conditions producing immunosuppression, annual immunization with inactivated influenza vaccine is recommended for children over 6 months of age, and one-time administration of pneumococcal vaccine is recommended for children over 2 years of age. *Immune globulins:* As with other immunosuppressed patients, children with clinical manifestations of HIV infection may be at increased risk for serious complications of infectious diseases such as measles and varicella;

therefore, following significant exposure to these diseases, they should receive passive immunization with immune globulin measles or varicella zoster immune globulin (varicella).

Children with previously diagnosed asymptomatic HIV infection: MMR: Pending further data, it is recommended that these children be vaccinated with MMR and followed for possible adverse reactions and for the occurrence of vaccine-preventable diseases, since immunization may be less effective than for other children. *OPV:* Available data suggest that OPV can be administered without adverse consequences to HIV-infected children who do not have overt clinical manifestations of immunosuppression. However, since family members may be immunocompromised because of HIV infection, it may be prudent to use IPV routinely to immunize these children. *DPT, Hib:* Immunization with DPT and Hib vaccines in accordance with ACIP recommendations is recommended.

Children residing in a household of a patient with AIDS: OPV: Children living with others known to be immunocompromised because of AIDS or other HIV infections should not receive OPV because they would be likely to excrete vaccine viruses that would be communicable to their immunosuppressed family members. *MMR:* MMR may be given to such a child because extensive experience has shown that live, attenuated MMR vaccine viruses are not transmitted from vaccinated persons to others.[1]

[1]*FDA Drug Bulletin,* Vol. 17, No. 2, September 1987, pp 23–24

Injection Therapy Care Plan

I. NURSING DIAGNOSIS

1. Anxiety related to:
   A. possible pain.
   B. infection.
   C. poor technique.
   D. other _____

2. Pain at injection site related to:
   A. frequent administration of injections.
   B. poor injection technique.
   C. break in aseptic technique.
   D. infection.
   E. other _____

3. Ineffective individual/family coping related to:
   A. self-administration of injections.
   B. pain.
   C. cost of medical care/poor insurance coverage.
   D. lack of assistance from significant others.
   E. fear of injury.
   F. poor technique.
   G. other _____

4. Knowledge deficit related to:
   A. aseptic technique.

B. poor comprehension/short attention span/illiteracy.
C. purchase of supplies.
D. preparation of injectable medication/storage/refrigeration.
E. proper use of syringe.
F. observation of signs/symptoms of infection.
G. rotation of injection sites.
H. blood aspiration.
I. AIDS precautions.
J. safe needle/syringe disposal.
K. intramuscular client-controlled analgesia (portable unit).
L. use of Heparin lock.
M. other _____

5. Self-care deficit: feeding/bathing/grooming/dressing/administration
of injections related to:
A. poor manual dexterity.
B. paraplegia/hemiplegia.
C. fear of handling a syringe.
D. other _____

6. Noncompliance with injection therapy related to:
A. denial.
B. refusal to administer injections.
C. pain.
D. lack of assistance from significant others.
E. cost of medical care/poor insurance coverage.
F. poor technique.
G. other _____

7. Potential for physical injury (anemia, infection, etc.) related to:
A. forgetfulness/confusion/lethargy/omission of injections.
B. refusal to administer injections.
C. poor injection technique.
D. allergic reactions (insulin lumps/fat tissue and muscle tissue
atrophy/erythema/infection/local abcess of fat necrosis).
E. air embolus.
F. poor nutritional status.
G. emaciation.

    H. poor powers of healing.

    I. other _____

_____

  8. Altered patterns of urinary elimination related to injection therapy.

II. SHORT-TERM GOALS

1. Client/Family will obtain prescriptions for parenteral medication and syringes upon discharge from hospital.
2. Client/Family will learn aseptic technique for injection therapy and proper hand-washing technique after 1–2 R.N. visits.
3. Client/Family will dispose of needle and syringe appropriately at home after 1–2 R.N. visits.
4. Client/Family will choose appropriate injection sites after 2–3 R.N. visits.
5. Client/Family will cleanse tips of vials/open ampules correctly after 1 R.N. visit.
6. Client/Family will state 5 signs/symptoms of infection after 2–3 R.N. visits.
7. Client/Family will administer subcutaneous/intramuscular injections correctly after 1–2 R.N. visits.
8. Client/Family will rub skin with alcohol and massage after needle removal after 1–2 R.N. visits.

III. LONG-TERM GOALS

1. Medication will be administered correctly in 1–2 weeks.
2. Optimal level of health will be achieved in 1–2 weeks.

IV. OUTCOME CRITERIA

1. Anxiety is overcome.
2. Injections are administered correctly and rapidly.
3. Client/Family feel relaxed and self-confident during procedure.
4. Skin integrity remains healthy and intact.
5. Client states he/she feels better.

V. NURSING INTERVENTION/TREATMENT

1. R.N. will contact client/family at home before visiting to ensure that proper supplies are present for instruction.

2. R.N. will encourage verbalization of all fears and concerns before procedure; will provide information on purpose of injections.
3. R.N. will instruct client/family/H.H.A. on:
   A. proper hand-washing technique.
   B. preparation of medication and syringe/storage of medications.
   C. cleansing and rotation of injection sites.
   D. holding skin taut.
   E. aspiration of blood and reinjection.
   F. contraindications at particular sites (e.g., impaired circulation to legs/edematous areas/bony prominences).
   G. administration of medication, withdrawal of needle, and massage of site/adverse reactions to medication.
   H. signs/symptoms of inflammation/infection.
   I. redemonstration by client/family.
   J. recording of injections.
   K. safe needle/syringe disposal.
   L. AIDS precautions.
   M. medication memory aids for forgetful clients (e.g., posters with pasted-on medications/colored dots on vials that match dots on chart/medication envelopes prepared in advance and labeled/partitioned boxes/preset medicated alarm boxes.
   N. use of intramuscular client-controlled analgesia (portable unit).
   O. use of Heparin lock.
4. R.N. will confer with M.D. whenever laboratory testing is necessary (e.g., follow-up CBC, electrolytes).
5. R.N. will arrange for nurse, laboratory technician, or M.D. to visit client's home for laboratory testing if client is unable to travel.
6. R.N. will provide follow-up reports and discharge summary to M.D. when case closes.
7. R.N. will notify client/family/H.H.A./significant others when case will close.

Intravenous Therapy
Care Plan

I. NURSING DIAGNOSIS

1. Anxiety related to fear of pain during introduction of IV needle or medication.
2. Potential for injury related to:
   A. contamination of IV needle, supplies, or site.
   B. poor hand-washing technique.
   C. lengthy use of needle at site.
   D. infiltration.
   E. obstructed flow of medication/solution.
   F. too rapid flow of medication/solution.
   G. injury or break in skin at IV site.
   H. inadequate education/hospital discharge planning for client to go home.
   I. overuse of each IV site.
   J. hemorrhage.
   K. infiltration/vein flare/phlebitis/extravasation (e.g., swelling/ burning/soreness/blister formation/necrosis).
   L. other _____

3. Pain related to:
   A. poor positioning of IV needle.
   B. poor positioning of limb.
   C. induction of caustic medication (e.g., chemotherapeutic agents)/ extravasation.

D. other _____
_____

4. Potential for infection/scarring related to:
   A. poor positioning of IV needle.
   B. poor positioning of limb.
   C. induction of caustic medication (e.g., chemotherapeutic agents)/ extravasation.
   D. incorrect flushing of IV line.
   E. other _____
_____

5. Knowledge deficit related to:
   A. poor hand-washing technique.
   B. laboratory testing/M.D. appointments.
   C. consent for IV therapy in the home.
   D. flow of solution.
   E. operation of IV pump.
   F. medication administration/adverse reactions.
   G. supplies/storage of medications/needle/syringe disposal.
   H. complications (e.g., infiltration/vein flare/phlebitis/ extravasation [swelling/burning/soreness/blister formation/ necrosis]).
   I. dressing care.
   J. cost/financial reimbursement.
   K. implantable vascular access system/accessing port/continuous infusion/medication administration/blood drawing/needle removal/troubleshooting/refill schedules/adverse reactions/ dosage compensation for fever or changes in altitude during mountain travel or airplane flights/activities to avoid (e.g., scuba diving, prolonged sun exposure, and long, hot baths are contraindicated)/signs of toxicity (e.g., nausea, vomiting, indigestion, jaundice, sore abdomen)/chemotherapy.
   L. heparinization.
   M. recording of medications and infusions.
   N. use of portable infusion pump (Ar/Med Infusor—utilizes elastomeric energy for IV delivery/Auto Syringe Pump—is battery powered/Cormed Pump is also battery powered).
   O. other _____
_____

6. Sleep pattern disturbance related to positioning of IV needle/ portable infusion pump.

7. Impaired home maintenance management related to continuous supervision of IV therapy.
8. Impaired physical mobility related to placement of IV needle.
9. Self-care deficit: feeding/bathing/grooming/dressing related to placement of IV needle.
10. Potential impaired skin integrity related to:
    A. noncompliance of client/family in supervising IV carefully.
    B. dislodgment of caustic solution into tissues.
    C. other _____
    _____

11. Potential fluid volume excess/deficit related to:
    A. rapid induction of flow rate of IV fluid.
    B. slow induction of flow rate of IV fluid.
    C. inadequate programming of IV pump.
    D. catheter malfunction.
    E. poor understanding of administration of medications/IV fluids.
    F. pump malfunctioning.
    G. other _____
    _____

12. Altered patterns of urinary elimination related to:
    A. IV infusion rate.
    B. inadequate programming of IV pump.
    C. poor delivery of infusions.
    D. excess delivery of infusions.
    E. pump malfunctioning.
    F. poor understanding of administration of medications/IV fluids.
    G. administration of diuretics.
    H. other _____
    _____

13. Social isolation related to:
    A. confinement to home for IV fluid administration.
    B. unemployment.
    C. other _____
    _____

14. Potential activity intolerance related to:
    A. confinement to IV pump.
    B. implantable catheter restrictions.
    C. other _____
    _____

II. SHORT-TERM GOALS

1. All IV equipment will be readily available in the home after 1–2 R.N. visits.
2. Client/Family will wash hands routinely before handling supplies or IV site after 1 R.N. visit.
3. Emergency drugs will be placed in the home after 1 R.N. visit if necessary and pertinent to M.D.'s plan of care.
4. Client/Family will state signs/symptoms of infection/phlebitis/cellulitis after 1–2 R.N. visits.
5. Client/Family will keep strict intake and output after 1–2 R.N. visits.
6. Client/Family will keep infusion patent by administering bags/medications/bottles of solution on time after 1–2 R.N. visits.
7. Client/Family will notify M.D./R.N. of adverse reactions or change in condition after 1–2 R.N. visits.
8. Client/Family will attach tubing properly to IV pump after 1–2–3–4 R.N. visits.
9. Client/Family will remove IV needle properly and apply pressure to site if needle infiltrates after 1–2–3 R.N. visits.
10. Client/Family will change IV dressing site daily after 1–2–3 R.N. visits.
11. Client/Family will identify any IV solution or medication that is inappropriately cloudy or contains particles and withhold administration after 1–2–3 R.N. visits.
12. Client/Family will observe IV site, solution, and rate of flow hourly after 1–2–3 R.N. visits.
13. Client/Family will safely operate implantable vascular access system after 1–2–3–4 R.N. visits.
14. Client/Family will state signs/symptoms of complications of implantable vascular access system after 1–2–3–4 R.N. visits.
15. Client/Family will check with M.D. for adjustment orders for travel or fever after 1–2–3–4 R.N. visits.
16. Client/Family will safely dispose of needles/syringes after 1–2 R.N. visits.

III. LONG-TERM GOALS

1. Adequate hydration will be achieved within 24 hours.
2. Medication/chemotherapy will be administered correctly within 24 hours.
3. Nutritional status will be maintained within 24 hours.

4. Independent activities of daily living will be resumed in 1–2–3 weeks.
5. Optimal level of health will be achieved in 3–4 weeks.

IV. OUTCOME CRITERIA

1. Client's and family's anxiety is overcome.
2. Client and family understand and agree with plan for home care.
3. Client and family are able to perform procedures.
4. Client has veins suitable for IV therapy.
5. Client has suitable home environment for IV therapy.
6. Vital signs are normal.
7. Client remains alert, responsive, and cooperative.
8. Chest is clear; respirations are normal.
9. Intake and output are normal.
10. Appetite is normal.
11. Urinary output is yellow, clear, and sufficient in quantity.
12. Circulation functions normally.
13. Client/Family state they feel relaxed and self-confident.
14. Client states he/she feels better.

V. NURSING INTERVENTION/TREATMENT

1. R.N. will check individual community health agency's policy manual for IV standards and legal implications.
2. M.D./R.N. will obtain informed written consent for client or family before the start of IV administration in the home.
3. If possible, community health R.N. will make predischarge visit to the hospital and the client's home to assess suitability of home environment for IV therapy.
4. Client/Family must have M.D./emergency room/clinic as backup coverage for IV complications.
5. A significant other must always be in attendance in the home for IV therapy.
6. R.N. will instruct client/family/H.H.A. on:
   A. purpose of IV therapy.
   B. monitoring and recording of vital signs.
   C. proper hand-washing technique.
   D. availability of all IV equipment and observation of container and of color of solution/medication before administration; observation of expiration dates before administration. Proper

storage of solution or medication should be discussed by R.N., pharmacist, or supply company.

E. allergic reactions, early signs/symptoms of infection, infiltration, hematoma formation, phlebitis, cellulitis, and bleeding/vein flare/extravasation (swelling, burning, soreness, blister formation, and necrosis).

F. antidote administration.

G. daily IV dressing and tubing change: skin preparation with Betadine or alcohol, taping of needle with application of 2-inch × 2-inch gauze pad to needle site using nonallergic tape, application of armboard, if necessary, allowing for freedom of movement and comfort (optional). Note: In some agencies, solutions may be changed every 24 hours; tubing may be changed every 48 hours; cannula may be changed every 72 hours. Policies may vary.

H. calculations for proper drip rate.

I. changing of needle site by M.D./R.N./hospital IV team/ pharmacist every 24–72 hours.

J. removal and disposal of IV needle.

K. recording of intake and output.

L. recording of date and time of each infusion and IV medication (labeling IV bag if medication is added).

M. accidental stoppage of IV fluid/irrigation of tubing.

N. principles of gravity and air and factors affecting flow.

O. air removal from tubing.

P. signs/symptoms of fluid overload (bounding pulse, weight gain, edema, increased blood pressure, headache, shortness of breath, cough, increased respirations, shock, syncope, dyspnea).

Q. signs/symptoms of dehydration and circulatory collapse (weak pulse; decreased or concentrated urinary output; thirst; cracked, dry lips and tongue; sudden weight loss; poor skin turgor).

R. operation of IV pump and alarm system, placement and changing of bag/bottle/rate of infusion/connections of tubing/ burette.

S. operation of implantable vascular access system/signs of toxicity.

T. adjustment of therapy for implantable vascular access system for fever or travel.

U. heparinization of tubing.

V. use of portable infusion pump/complications.

W. supplies/storage/ordering replacements/needle/syringe disposal.

X. cost of procedures/supplies.

Y. diversional activities/socialization.

Z. employment.

7. For clients with difficult veins, R.N. will start a new IV in an alternative site before removing old needle; will shave site if necessary.

8. R.N. will elevate arm or limb on pillow.

9. R.N. will use steel needles (butterfly or scalp vein whenever possible; clients are less prone to infections). Plastic cannulas provide a better route for administering medications. R.N. will ensure adequate lighting before IV administration.

10. R.N. will consider location of IV; will use only superficial veins of hand or forearm if possible; will consult with M.D. before using leg veins; will use large veins for viscous solutions, large quantities of solutions, irritating medications, or hypertonic solutions.

11. R.N. will encourage client/family to maintain an adequate supply of IV materials: needles, tubing, solutions, medications, Betadine, 70% alcohol, nonallergic tape, 2-inch × 2-inch gauze pads, and syringes.

12. R.N. will allow for extensive redemonstration by client/family of medication preparation and administration of IV bag/bottle, tubing changes, dressing changes, knowledge of adverse effects, knowledge of signs/symptoms of too rapid or too slow induction.

13. R.N. will confer with M.D. whenever laboratory testing is necessary.

14. R.N. will arrange for laboratory technician or M.D. to visit client's home for testing if possible.

15. R.N. will provide M.D. with follow-up reports and discharge summary when case closes.

16. R.N. will notify client/family/H.H.A./significant others when case will close.

Laminectomy
Care Plan

I. NURSING DIAGNOSIS

1. Anxiety related to:
   A. possible paralysis.
   B. possible loss of control.
   C. performing activities of daily living.
   D. loss of employment.
   E. loss of independence.
   F. other _____

2. Pain related to:
   A. poor positioning/turning.
   B. inadequate exercise.
   C. poor fluid/dietary intake.
   D. inadequate breathing exercises.
   E. poor administration of medication.
   F. other _____

3. Ineffective breathing pattern related to:
   A. poor demonstration of breathing exercises.
   B. poor use of incentive spirometer/blow bottles/IPPB.
   C. pain.
   D. muscle spasms.
   E. other _____

4. Knowledge deficit related to:
   A. medication administration/adverse reactions.
   B. turning/repositioning.
   C. fluids/diet.
   D. types of surgical procedures (e.g., disectomy/laminectomy/ spinal fusion/total laminectomy/chemonucleolysis and microsurgical dorsal root rhizotomy/facet joint rhizotomy).
   E. rehabilitative equipment/use of supportive devices (e.g., lumbar orthosis).
   F. exercising with low-heeled shoes and walking on flat, even surfaces (avoiding bending, twisting, lifting, extending, and reaching, as well as riding in cars as ordered)/physical therapy/ occupational therapy.
   G. TENS machine.
   H. sexual abstinence/contraception.
   I. other _____

5. Impaired home maintenance management related to:
   A. impaired mobility.
   B. weakness.
   C. paralysis.
   D. other _____

6. Fear related to:
   A. paralysis.
   B. immobility.
   C. ambulation.
   D. other _____

7. Impaired physical mobility related to:
   A. pain.
   B. paralysis.
   C. secondary infection.
   D. other _____

8. Noncompliance with therapy related to:
   A. poor support in the home.
   B. pain.
   C. secondary infection.

D. other _____

_____

9. Altered nutrition: potential for more/less than body requirements related to:

A. pain.

B. anorexia.

C. immobility.

D. poor tolerance in weight bearing.

E. other _____

_____

10. Altered parenting related to:

A. pain.

B. severe muscle spasms.

C. immobility.

D. poor tolerance of weight bearing.

E. other _____

_____

11. Self-care deficit: feeding/bathing/grooming/dressing/toileting related to:

A. pain.

B. immobility.

C. secondary infection.

D. other _____

_____

12. Sexual dysfunction related to:

A. pain.

B. restricted activity as ordered by M.D.

C. other _____

_____

13. Potential impaired skin integrity related to:

A. immobility.

B. secondary infection.

C. adverse reaction to medication.

D. other _____

_____

14. Sleep pattern disturbance related to:

A. pain.

B. restlessness.

    C. dyspnea.

    D. skin breakdown.

    E. other _____

    _____

15. Altered patterns of urinary elimination related to:

    A. poor fluid intake.

    B. excessive fluid intake.

    C. paralysis.

    D. immobility.

    E. difficulty assuming a standing position.

    F. other _____

    _____

II. SHORT-TERM GOALS

1. Client/Family will verbalize fears, anxieties, and concerns after 1–2 R.N. visits.
2. Client/Family will assist with logrolling in bed after 1–2 R.N. visits.
3. Client/Family will perform range-of-motion exercise as ordered after 1–2 R.N. visits.
4. Client/Family will administer medication as ordered after 1–2–3 R.N. visits.
5. Client/Family with notify M.D. immediately of adverse reactions after 1–2 R.N. visits.
6. Client/Family will notify M.D. immediately of signs/symptoms of secondary infection after 1–2 R.N. visits.
7. Client/Family will force fluids as ordered after 1–2 R.N. visits.
8. Client will consume diet as ordered after 1–2 R.N. visits.
9. Client/Family will perform good skin care after 1–2 R.N. visits.
10. Client/Family will perform all prescribed exercises after 1–2–3 R.N./P.T. visits.
11. Client/Family will assist with tube feeding/hyperalimentation as ordered after 1–2–3–4 R.N. visits.
12. Client/Family will supervise IV therapy in the home as ordered after 1–2 R.N. visits.
13. Client will perform breathing exercises as ordered after 1–2–3 R.N. visits.
14. Client/Family will utilize rehabilitative equipment as ordered after 1–2–3 R.N. visits.

15. Client will seek laboratory testing/keep appointments with M.D. after 1–2 R.N. visits.

III. LONG-TERM GOALS

1. Independent activities of daily living will be resumed in 1–2 weeks.
2. Optimal level of health will be achieved in 2–3 weeks.

IV. OUTCOME CRITERIA

1. Vital signs are normal.
2. Ambulation is normal.
3. Bilateral hand grasps are equal and strong.
4. Pupils are equal and react well to light.
5. Skin is warm, healthy, and intact.
6. All pulses are equal and palpable.
7. Bowel/Bladder functions normally.
8. Laboratory test results are normal.
9. Appetite is normal.
10. Client consumes nutritious meals.
11. Vision is clear.
12. Weight remains normal.
13. Client is alert, oriented, and sociable.
14. Client states he/she feels better.

V. NURSING INTERVENTION/TREATMENT

1. R.N. will contact hospital discharge planner for plans for home care and rehabilitation goals.
2. R.N. will instruct client/family/H.H.A. on:
   A. fluid intake/diet as ordered.
   B. enteral feedings/hyperalimentation.
   C. IV administration if ordered.
   D. bowel/bladder regimen.
   E. sexual abstinence/contraception.
   F. types of surgical procedures (e.g., disectomy/laminectomy/ spinal fusion/total laminectomy/chemonucleolysis/ microsurgical dorsal root rhizotomy/facet joint rhizotomy).
   G. prescribed turning/exercising with low-heeled shoes and walking on flat, even surfaces (avoiding bending, twisting,

lifting, extending, reaching, and riding in cars as ordered by M.D.)/physical therapy/occupational therapy.

H. TENS machine.

I. use of rehabilitative equipment in the home (e.g., commode/ wheelchair/hospital bed/supportive devices/lumbar orthosis/ long-handled brush for shower use/tub rail/raised toilet seat).

J. diversional activities/socialization.

K. skin care.

L. catheter care.

M. laboratory testing/M.D. appointments.

N. medication administration/adverse reactions.

O. immediate notification of M.D. of adverse reactions/change in condition.

P. clubs, organizations, societies for additional assistance.

3. R.N. will arrange for additional services if ordered (e.g., medical social services, vocational rehabilitation, H.H.A., home attendant, homemaker, housekeeper.

4. R.N. will provide M.D. with follow-up reports and discharge summary when case closes.

5. R.N. will notify client/family/H.H.A./significant others when case will close.

Laparoscopy
Care Plan

I. NURSING DIAGNOSIS

1. Anxiety related to:
   A. potential discomfort following procedure.
   B. postoperative diagnosis.
   C. cost of medical care/poor insurance coverage.
   D. other _____

2. Activity intolerance related to:
   A. abdominal pain.
   B. weakness/fatigue.
   C. headache.
   D. dizziness.
   E. infection.
   F. other _____

3. Constipation related to:
   A. inadequate fluids/diet.
   B. poor exercise tolerance.
   C. abdominal pain.
   D. other _____

4. Ineffective breathing pattern related to:
   A. incisional pain.
   B. abdominal pain.
   C. extreme fatigue.

    D. poor position in bed.

    E. shoulder pain.

    F. other _____

    _____

5. Pain related to:

    A. abdominal incision.

    B. poor position in bed.

    C. constipation.

    D. flatulence.

    E. shoulder pain.

    F. other _____

    _____

6. Altered family process related to:

    A. limited mobility.

    B. weakness/fatigue.

    C. dependence on others for care.

    D. other _____

    _____

7. Fear related to:

    A. postoperative results.

    B. possible sterility.

    C. possible endometriosis.

    D. other _____

    _____

8. Potential fluid volume deficit related to:

    A. nausea.

    B. vomiting.

    C. weakness/fatigue.

    D. hemorrhage.

    E. other _____

    _____

9. Impaired home maintenance management related to:

    A. abdominal pain.

    B. weakness/fatigue.

    C. dependence on others for care.

    D. nausea.

    E. other _____

    _____

10. Knowledge deficit related to:
    A. medication administration/adverse reactions.
    B. dressing care.
    C. breathing exercises.
    D. exercise/rest.
    E. poor coordination (postoperative).
    F. restricted weight lifting.
    G. fluids/diet.
    H. coitus.
    I. douching.
    J. use of tampons.
    K. bowel regularity.
    L. warm baths/showers.
    M. elimination of diagnostic dye in urine.
    N. postoperative shoulder pain.
    O. sore throat after airway removal.
    P. laboratory testing.
    Q. M.D. appointments.
    R. other _____

11. Impaired physical mobility related to:
    A. abdominal pain.
    B. shoulder pain.
    C. infection.
    D. incisional pain.
    E. other _____

12. Altered nutrition: potential for more than body requirements related to:
    A. nausea.
    B. vomiting.
    C. weakness/fatigue.
    D. other _____

13. Altered oral mucous membrane related to:
    A. sore throat after airway removal.
    B. decreased fluid intake.
    C. other _____

14. Sexual dysfunction related to:
    A. abdominal pain.
    B. incisional pain.
    C. other _____

15. Sleep pattern disturbance related to:
    A. abdominal pain.
    B. incisional pain.
    C. shoulder pain.
    D. other _____

16. Altered patterns of urinary elimination related to:
    A. decreased fluid intake.
    B. vomiting.
    C. abdominal pain.
    D. incisional pain.
    E. other _____

II. SHORT-TERM GOALS

1. Client/Spouse/Family will verbalize fears, anxieties, and concerns after 1 R.N. visit.
2. Client/Spouse/Family will properly change dressings as ordered after 1 R.N. visit.
3. Client will take medication as prescribed after 1–2 R.N. visits.
4. Client/Spouse/Family will notify M.D. of adverse effects or impending secondary infections after 1–2 R.N. visits.
5. Client will rest as ordered after 1 R.N. visit.
6. Client will avoid excessive lifting or strenuous exercise after 1–2 R.N. visits.
7. Client will avoid straining at stool after 1 R.N. visit.
8. Client will take fluids/diet as ordered after 1 R.N. visit.
9. Client will seek laboratory testing as ordered after 1 R.N. visit.
10. Client will visit M.D. as ordered after 1 R.N. visit.

III. LONG-TERM GOALS

1. Independent activities of daily living will be resumed in 1 week.
2. Optimal level of health will be achieved in 1–2 weeks.

IV. OUTCOME CRITERIA

1. Vital signs are normal.
2. Skin is healthy and intact.
3. Appetite is normal.
4. Normal ambulation is achieved.
5. Bowel/Bladder functions normally.
6. Ovaries function normally.
7. Fallopian tubes are patent.
8. Uterus functions normally.
9. Client states she feels better.
10. Client returns to work.

V. NURSING INTERVENTION/TREATMENT

1. R.N. will instruct client/family on:
   A. proper hand-washing technique.
   B. aseptic dressing technique.
   C. fluids/diet as ordered.
   D. medication administration/adverse reactions.
   E. immediate notification of M.D. of adverse reactions or signs/symptoms of impending infection.
   F. bowel/bladder regimen.
   G. limited weight lifting/strenuous exercise.
   H. prescribed ambulation/exercise.
   I. coitus.
   J. douching.
   K. use of tampons.
   L. elimination of diagnostic dye in urine.
   M. postoperative shoulder pain.
   N. warm baths/shower.
   O. sore throat after airway removal.
   P. laboratory testing.
   Q. M.D. appointments.
2. R.N. will provide M.D. with follow-up reports and discharge summary when case closes.
3. R.N. will notify client when case will close.

Laparotomy
Care Plan

I. NURSING DIAGNOSIS

1. Knowledge deficit related to:
   A. skin care/bathing.
   B. dressing care.
   C. possible insertion of urinary catheter.
   D. breathing exercises.
   E. ambulation.
   F. medication administration/adverse reactions.
   G. restricted weight lifting.
   H. exercise/rest.
   I. secondary wound infection.
   J. bowel regimen.
   K. cost of medical care/insurance coverage.
   L. other _____
   _____

2. Activity intolerance related to:
   A. weakness/fatigue.
   B. pain.
   C. pressure at surgical site.
   D. tightness at suture line.
   E. postoperative restrictions.
   F. other _____
   _____

3. Ineffective airway clearance related to:
   A. poor demonstration of breathing exercises.
   B. difficulty with expectoration.
   C. other _____

4. Anxiety related to:
   A. postoperative pain.
   B. immobility.
   C. cost of medical care/poor insurance coverage.
   D. hemorrhage.
   E. possible death.
   F. possible infection.
   G. dependence on others for care.
   H. possible infiltration of IV needle.
   I. other _____

5. Constipation related to:
   A. pain at surgical site.
   B. discomfort of bearing down on abdominal muscles.
   C. decreased mobility.
   D. poor fluid/dietary intake.
   E. other _____

6. Ineffective breathing pattern related to:
   A. poor demonstration of breathing exercises.
   B. incisional pain.
   C. noncompliance with therapy.
   D. poor positioning.
   E. other _____

7. Pain related to:
   A. abdominal distension.
   B. poor mobility.
   C. client's reluctance to request pain medication when necessary.
   D. constipation.
   E. infection.
   F. other _____

8. Ineffective individual coping related to:
   A. confinement in hospital.
   B. confinement in home.
   C. dependence on others for care/management of household chores.
   D. excessive pain.
   E. secondary infection.
   F. cost of medical care/poor insurance coverage.
   G. other _____

9. Diversional activity deficit related to:
   A. pain.
   B. immobility.
   C. fatigue.
   D. other _____

10. Fear related to:
    A. lack of support in the home.
    B. secondary infection.
    C. possible death.
    D. other _____

11. Potential fluid volume deficit related to:
    A. dysphagia following airway removal.
    B. poor intake.
    C. IV infiltration.
    D. vomiting.
    E. other _____

12. Altered health maintenance related to:
    A. noncompliance with therapy.
    B. cost of medical care/poor insurance coverage.
    C. other _____

13. Impaired home maintenance management related to:
    A. decreased ambulation.
    B. medical restrictions.

    C. dependence on others for care.

    D. lack of support in the home.

    E. other _____

_____

14. Potential for injury related to:

    A. excessive ambulation.

    B. straining upon lifting.

    C. straining at stool.

    D. poor dressing technique.

    E. other _____

_____

15. Impaired physical mobility related to:

    A. incisional pain.

    B. distension.

    C. insertion of urinary catheter.

    D. weakness/fatigue.

    E. loss of muscle tone in upper and lower extremities.

    F. other _____

_____

16. Noncompliance with therapy related to:

    A. cost of medical care/poor insurance coverage.

    B. poor understanding of procedures.

    C. grieving.

    D. denial.

    E. other _____

_____

17. Altered nutrition: more than body requirements related to:

    A. anorexia.

    B. nausea.

    C. vomiting.

    D. other _____

_____

18. Altered oral mucous membrane related to:

    A. fluid/dietary restriction.

    B. mouth breathing.

    C. other _____

_____

19. Self-care deficit: feeding/bathing/dressing/grooming/toileting related to:
    A. poor mobility/ambulation.
    B. sedation.
    C. noncompliance.
    D. other _____

20. Self-esteem disturbance related to:
    A. permanent scarring of skin.
    B. dependence on others for care.
    C. inability to work.
    D. other _____

21. Sexual dysfunction related to:
    A. medical restrictions during convalescence.
    B. abdominal pain.
    C. delayed healing of surgical site.
    D. other _____

22. Impaired skin integrity related to:
    A. upper midline incision.
    B. upper right rectus incision.
    C. transverse incision in upper abdomen.
    D. gridiron, or McBurney's incision on right.
    E. lower right rectus incision.
    F. lower midline incision.
    G. Pfannenstiel's incision.
    H. left gridiron incision.
    I. subcostal incision.
    J. discomfort of silk/wire/retention sutures.
    K. discomfort from removal of silk/wire/retention sutures.
    L. secondary infection.
    M. other _____

23. Sleep pattern disturbance related to:
    A. abdominal pain.
    B. distension.

     C. difficulty turning/repositioning.

     D. other _____

     _____

24. Social isolation related to:

     A. confinement to hospital.

     B. confinement to home.

     C. other _____

     _____

25. Altered patterns of urinary elimination related to:

     A. poor fluid/dietary intake.

     B. secondary infection.

     C. contamination at urinary catheter site.

     D. other _____

     _____

II. SHORT-TERM GOALS

1. Client/Family will verbalize fears, anxieties, and concerns after 1–2 R.N. visits.
2. Client/Family will wash hands properly before and after dressing changes after 1–2 R.N. visits.
3. Client/Family will change abdominal dressings properly after 1–2 R.N. visits.
4. Client will perform breathing exercises after 1–2 R.N. visits.
5. Client will take medication as prescribed after 1–2 R.N. visits.
6. Client/Family will notify M.D. of adverse effects of medication or impending secondary infections after 1–2 R.N. visits.
7. Client will perform exercises as ordered after 1–2 R.N. visits.
8. Client will wear abdominal binder/antiembolus hose as ordered after 1–2 R.N. visits.
9. Client will use assistive devices (e.g., cane/quad cane/walker/wheelchair/arm braces/leg braces) as ordered after 1–2 R.N. visits.
10. Client will consume fluids/diet as ordered after 1–2 R.N. visits.
11. Client will avoid excessive coughing/smoking after 1–2 R.N. visits.
12. Client will avoid excessive lifting or strenuous exercise after 1–2 R.N. visits.
13. Client will avoid straining at stool after 1–2 R.N. visits.
14. Client will participate in diversional activities after 1–2 R.N. visits.

III. LONG-TERM GOALS

1. Independent activities of daily living will be resumed in 1–2 weeks.
2. Optimum level of health will be achieved in 4–6 weeks.

IV. OUTCOME CRITERIA

1. Vital signs are normal.
2. Skin is healthy and intact.
3. Normal ambulation is achieved.
4. Appetite is normal.
5. Bowel/Bladder functions normally.
6. Chest is clear.
7. Client consumes nutritious meals.
8. Client states he/she feels better.
9. Mental outlook is healthy.
10. Client returns to work.

V. NURSING INTERVENTION/TREATMENT

1. R.N. will instruct client/family/H.H.A. on:
   A. cost of medical care/insurance coverage.
   B. proper hand-washing technique.
   C. aseptic dressing technique.
   D. fluid intake/dietary regimen as ordered.
   E. medication administration/adverse reactions.
   F. immediate notification of M.D. of adverse reactions or signs/symptoms of impending infection.
   G. bowel/bladder regimen.
   H. avoidance/limitation of smoking and coughing.
   I. limited weight lifting/strenuous exercise.
   J. prescribed ambulation/exercise.
   K. use of assistive devices (e.g., cane/quad cane/walker/wheelchair/arm brace(s)/leg brace(s).
   L. use of abdominal binder/antiembolus hose.
   M. breathing exercises.
   N. urinary catheter care.
   O. sexual activity.
   P. laboratory testing/M.D. appointments.
   Q. diversional activities.

2. R.N. will provide M.D. with follow-up reports and discharge summary when case closes.

3. R.N. will notify client/family/H.H.A./significant others when case will close.

Lead Poisoning
Care Plan

I. NURSING DIAGNOSIS

1. Knowledge deficit related to:
    A. prevention/treatment of lead poisoning.
    B. medication administration/adverse reactions.
    C. repair of ceilings/walls/other.
    D. fluid/dietary needs.
    E. other _____

    _____

2. Anxiety related to:
    A. seizures.
    B. hospitalization for lead intoxication.
    C. other _____

    _____

3. Potential for injury related to:
    A. seizures.
    B. poor parental supervision in the home.
    C. parental neglect.
    D. other _____

    _____

4. Abdominal pain related to:
    A. lead ingestion.
    B. other _____

    _____

5. Potential fluid volume deficit related to:
    A. vomiting.

B. poor fluid/dietary intake.

C. other _____

_____

6. Altered thought processes related to elevated erythrocyte protoporphyrin levels.

7. Constipation related to: elevated erythrocyte protoporphyrin levels.

8. Unilateral neglect related to elevated erythrocyte protoporphyrin levels.

9. Altered health maintenance related to:

A. repeated ingestion of lead.

B. adult essential hypertension (related to childhood lead poisoning).

C. adult gout (related to childhood lead poisoning).

D. adult renal dysfunction (related to childhood lead poisoning).

E. other _____

_____

10. Ineffective individual/family coping related to:

A. seizures.

B. coma.

C. mental retardation.

D. learning disabilities.

E. other _____

_____

II. SHORT-TERM GOALS

1. Parent will isolate child/children in lead-free rooms after 1–2 R.N. visits.

2. All responsible adults will be encouraged to supervise children at all times in a lead-free environment after 1–2 visits.

3. Parents/Landlord will repair/scrape ceilings and apply lead-free paint after 1–2 R.N./sanitary inspector visits.

4. Sanitary inspection will reveal lead content in doors, frames, window sills and frames, walls, handrails, spindles, stair treads, and any other chewable surface below 4-foot level after 1 visit.

5. Parents will allow for lead screening of other siblings after 1–2 R.N. visits.

6. Parents/Landlord will remove any cracked, chipped, blistered, peeling, flaking paint from surfaces child/children have access to after 1–2 R.N. visits.

7. R.N./Sanitary inspector will submit reports to state health department after 1 visit.

8. R.N./Sanitary inspector will revisit home to check child's/ children's health status and repair of home environment after 2–3 visits.

9. Parents will prevent child/children from chewing, sucking, inhaling, or ingesting painted surfaces, putty, painted toys, collapsible tubes, batteries, jewelry, rubber articles, talcum powders, canned foods, ointments, linoleum, dirt and dust, gasoline, insecticides, varnish, auto exhaust after 1–2 R.N. visits.

10. Adults will avoid close contact with home battery manufacturing, artist's paints, ceramic and pottery glazing at home, burning of color comics or magazine section of Sunday paper in grill after 1–2 R.N. visits.

11. Parent will administer prescribed medication (chelator drugs) as ordered to child/children after 1–2 R.N. visits.

12. Parent will immediately notify M.D. of any adverse reactions to medications or change in condition after 1–2 R.N. visits.

13. Parent will have children under age 3 tested every 6 months for lead level after 1–2 R.N. visits.

14. Parents/Landlord will wear a face mask when removing and sanding old paint after 1–2 R.N. visits.

15. Parents/Landlord will use a wet mop after cleaning up debris after 1–2 R.N. visits.

16. Family will avoid eating in any room where construction is taking place after 1–2 R.N. visits.

17. Family will keep dishes, utensils, glasswear protected from dirt and dust during construction after 1–2 R.N. visits.

III. LONG-TERM GOALS

1. Home environment will be free from lead-containing surfaces in 2–3 months.

2. Optimal level of health will be achieved in 1–2 months.

3. Prevention in community will occur after health fair/lead programs/outreach.

IV. OUTCOME CRITERIA

1. Vital signs remain normal.

2. Central nervous system functions normally.

3. Gums remain red and healthy.

4. Appetite remains adequate.

5. Bowel activity remains normal and regular.

6. GI system functions normally.

7. Blood lead level remains normal.

8. Erythrocyte protoporphyrin level is normal.

9. Hemoglobin and hematocrit levels remain normal.

10. IQ develops normally.

11. Urine study results remain normal.

12. X-ray study results are normal.

13. Cerebrospinal fluid study results are normal.

14. Home environment is free from lead-containing surfaces.

15. Child/Children are alert, sociable, and playful.

16. Developmental progress remains normal.

17. Child/Children show interest in school.

18. Parents carefully supervise child/children in the home environment.

V. NURSING INTERVENTION/TREATMENT

1. R.N./Sanitary inspector will evaluate home environment for sources of lead.

2. R.N. will screen for and counsel and educate family on lead poisoning; will also test other contact sources (playmates, friends).

3. Parents/Landlord will make arrangements to correct lead-containing sources in the home environment by removing loose paint/plaster/caulking compound/linoleum.

4. R.N. will instruct family/H.H.A. on:

   A. definition of lead poisoning and its adverse effects.

   B. sources of lead in home (e.g., painted surfaces, plaster chips, putty, varnish, painted toys, soft metal toys, collapsible tubes, batteries, jewelry, insecticides, fungicides, herbicides, neighborhood toys, dirt and dust, gasoline, talcum powders, ointments, canned goods, ceramic and pottery glazing in the home, cosmetics, gift wrapping, glazed earthenware and dinnerware, color newsprints).

   C. lead testing (blood and urine testing, x-ray testing).

   D. prescribed medication, especially chelator drugs/adverse reactions.

   E. fluid intake/dietary needs.

   F. occupations that involve lead exposure.

G. behavioral changes.

H. highly polluted environments.

5. R.N./Sanitary inspector will forward periodic reports to state department of health.

6. Additional consultation will be sought if necessary and ordered (e.g., with M.S.W. or child abuse and neglect organizations).

7. R.N. will provide M.D. with progress reports and discharge summary when case closes.

8. R.N. will notify family/H.H.A./significant others when case will close.

Lupus Erythematosus
Care Plan

I. NURSING DIAGNOSIS

1. Ineffective thermoregulation related to:
   A. advance of disease.
   B. refusal to accept medical assistance.
   C. poor administration of medication.
   D. other _____

2. Impaired skin integrity related to:
   A. skin rash (with butterfly distribution) involving face.
   B. telangiectasis of vessels of nail beds.
   C. scalp lesions.
   D. hair loss.
   E. skin atrophy, scarring, and pigmentary changes.
   F. discoid lesions involving other body parts.
   G. overexposure to sun.
   H. other _____

3. Ineffective breathing pattern related to:
   A. poor positioning in bed.
   B. exercise intolerance.
   C. other _____

4. Ineffective individual/family coping related to:
   A. dependence on others for care.
   B. cost of medical care/poor insurance coverage.

    C. permanent hair loss.

    D. atrophy, scarring, and pigmentary changes in skin.

    E. other _____

    _____

5. Diversional activity deficit related to:

    A. weakness/fatigue.

    B. restriction of activity/contact sports/heavy lifting.

    C. immobility.

    D. avoidance of exposure to sunlight.

    E. other _____

    _____

6. Fear related to:

    A. socialization.

    B. reproduction.

    C. advance of disease.

    D. skin disfigurement.

    E. baldness.

    F. remission/exacerbation.

    G. death.

    H. other _____

    _____

7. Anticipatory grieving related to:

    A. advance of disease.

    B. baldness.

    C. facial skin disfigurement.

    D. rejection by significant others.

    E. impending death.

    F. other _____

    _____

8. Impaired home maintenance management related to:

    A. weakness.

    B. immobility.

    C. dependence on others for care.

    D. poor income.

    E. other _____

    _____

9. Potential for injury related to:

    A. denial.

    B. refusal to follow medical advice.

C. overexertion.

D. exposure to sunlight.

E. poor understanding of medication administration/adverse reactions.

F. other _____

_____

10. Knowledge deficit related to:

    A. disease process.

    B. medication administration/adverse reactions.

    C. exercise/rest.

    D. laboratory testing/M.D. appointments.

    E. sun exposure.

    F. other _____

    _____

11. Impaired physical mobility related to:

    A. weakness.

    B. restriction of ambulation/activity.

    C. other _____

    _____

12. Noncompliance with therapy related to:

    A. denial.

    B. weakness/fatigue.

    C. fear.

    D. anger.

    E. embarrassment.

    F. grieving.

    G. dependence on others for care.

    H. other _____

    _____

13. Altered nutrition: potential for more than body requirements related to:

    A. refusal to follow dietary instructions.

    B. anorexia.

    C. other _____

    _____

14. Altered parenting related to:

    A. weakness.

    B. exacerbation.

    C. restricted activity.

    D. irritability.

    E. other _____

    _____

15. Self-care deficit: feeding/bathing/grooming/dressing/toileting related to:

    A. weakness.

    B. restricted activity.

    C. other _____

    _____

16. Self-esteem disturbance related to:

    A. dependence on others for care.

    B. baldness.

    C. atrophy, scarring, and pigmentary changes of skin.

    D. other _____

    _____

17. Sexual dysfunction related to:

    A. irritability.

    B. weakness.

    C. general malaise.

    D. embarrassment about condition.

    E. rejection by significant others.

    F. other _____

    _____

18. Sleep pattern disturbance related to:

    A. pain.

    B. low-grade fever.

    C. frequent toileting needs.

    D. restlessness.

    E. fear of death.

    F. other _____

    _____

19. Altered patterns of urinary elimination related to:

    A. poor fluid/dietary intake.

    B. dependence on others for care.

    C. poor administration of medication.

    D. other _____

    _____

20. Potential for violence related to:

    A. anger.

B. disturbance in self-concept.

C. rejection by significant others.

D. other _____

_____

II. SHORT-TERM GOALS

1. Client/Family will verbalize fears, anxieties, or concerns after 1–2–3–4 R.N. visits.
2. Client/Family will apply cool tap-water sponge for low-grade fever after 1–2 R.N. visits.
3. Client/Family will avoid excessive clothing or blankets to decrease body temperature after 1–2 R.N. visits.
4. Client will avoid exposure to sunlight after 1–2 R.N. visits.
5. Client/Family will administer medication as ordered after 1–2–3 R.N. visits.
6. Client/Family will immediately inform M.D. of adverse effects of medication or change in condition after 1–2 R.N. visits.
7. Client will avoid excessive activity/heavy lifting as ordered after 1–2 R.N. visits.
8. Client will exercise/rest as ordered after 1–2 R.N. visits.
9. Client/Family will record intake and output after 1–2–3 R.N. visits.
10. Client will consume fluids/diet as ordered after 1–2 R.N. visits.
11. Client/Family will practice good skin care as ordered after 1–2–3 R.N. visits.
12. Client/Family will seek appropriate laboratory testing/M.D. appointments as ordered after 1–2–3 R.N. visits.

III. LONG-TERM GOALS

1. Control and long-term remission will be achieved in 1–2 months.
2. Independent activities of daily living will be resumed in 1–2 weeks.
3. Optimal level of health will be achieved in 1–2 months.
4. All stages of dying will be worked through.

IV. OUTCOME CRITERIA

1. Vital signs are normal.
2. Skin remains healthy and intact.
3. Musculoskeletal system functions normally.
4. Cardiovascular system functions normally.

5. Renal system functions normally.

6. Intake and output are within normal limits.

7. Laboratory test results are normal.

8. Appetite is normal.

9. Fluid/dietary consumption are appropriate.

10. Chest is clear.

11. Client is sociable, cooperative, and in good spirits.

12. Client states he/she feels better.

V. NURSING INTERVENTION/TREATMENT

1. R.N. will consult with hospital discharge planner/M.D. about treatment and rehabilitation goals.

2. R.N. will instruct client/family/H.H.A. on:
   A. disease process and general treatment.
   B. monitoring and recording of vital signs. If possible, R.N. will instruct a family member in blood pressure monitoring.
   C. medication (salicylates/antimalarials/steroid hormones) administration/adverse reactions.
   D. immediate notification of M.D. of adverse effects or change in condition.
   E. intake and output.
   F. daily recording of weight.
   G. fluid intake/dietary regimen as ordered.
   H. exercise/rest as ordered.
   I. catheter care.
   J. avoidance of stress/overexertion/heavy lifting/sun exposure.
   K. laboratory testing/M.D. appointments.
   L. use of hairpiece/wig.
   M. diversional activities.
   N. insurance coverage. Chronic nature of this disease may make medical costs extensive.

3. R.N. will assign additional personnel to case (e.g., M.S.W., psychiatrist, H.H.A., home attendant, homemaker, housekeeper) if ordered.

4. R.N. will provide M.D. with follow-up reports and discharge summary when case closes.

5. R.N. will notify client/family/H.H.A./significant others when case will close.

Malnutrition
Care Plan

I. NURSING DIAGNOSIS

1. Knowledge deficit related to:
   A. proper nutritional habits.
   B. adequate meal preparation.
   C. vitamin supplementation.
   D. dental care.
   E. adequate bowel habits.
   F. medication administration/adverse reactions.
   G. other _____
   _____

2. Altered nutrition: potential for more/less than body requirements related to:
   A. poor understanding of adequate nutrition.
   B. fad diets.
   C. overconsumption of fast foods.
   D. anorexia.
   E. poor income.
   F. poor dietary habits.
   G. poor administration of vitamin therapy (overdosing/underdosing).
   H. dependence on others for care.
   I. alcohol abuse.
   J. food allergy.
   K. other _____
   _____

3. Actual/Potential fluid volume deficit related to:
   A. oliguria.
   B. marasmus.
   C. inadequate water supply.
   D. poor fluid/dietary intake.
   E. diarrhea.
   F. other _____

4. Constipation/Diarrhea related to:
   A. malnutrition.
   B. lack of roughage/fiber in diet.
   C. other _____

5. Altered patterns of urinary elimination related to:
   A. poor fluid intake.
   B. infection.
   C. poor administration of medicine.
   D. other _____

6. Potential impaired skin integrity related to:
   A. alteration in nutritional habits.
   B. vitamin deficiency.
   C. food allergy.
   D. other _____

7. Impaired home maintenance management related to:
   A. weakness.
   B. dependence on others for care.
   C. marasmus.
   D. infection.
   E. other _____

8. Ineffective breathing pattern related to:
   A. malnutrition.
   B. weakness.
   C. anemia.
   D. dyspnea.
   E. other _____

9. Decreased cardiac output related to:
   A. malnutrition.
   B. electrolyte imbalance.
   C. stress.
   D. obesity.
   E. other _____

   _____

10. Potential for infection related to:
    A. poor fluid/dietary intake.
    B. lack of knowledge of adequate nutrition.
    C. inadequate dental care.
    D. other _____

    _____

11. Ineffective individual/family coping related to:
    A. apathy.
    B. irritability.
    C. overwhelming family responsibilities.
    D. other _____

    _____

12. Impaired physical mobility related to weakness.
13. Noncompliance with therapy related to:
    A. denial.
    B. poor meal preparation.
    C. other _____

    _____

14. Potential for injury related to:
    A. malnutrition.
    B. fluid and electrolyte imbalance.
    C. poor fluid/dietary intake.
    D. refusal to comply with nutritional instructions.
    E. other _____

    _____

II. SHORT-TERM GOALS

1. Client/Family will verbalize questions after 1–2–3 R.N. visits.
2. Client will take adequate fluids/diet as ordered after 1–2 R.N. visits.

3. Client/Family will strictly record intake and output after 1–2 R.N. visits.
4. Client/Family will record weight daily after 1–2 R.N. visits.
5. Client will avoid junk foods and foods with low nutritional content after 1–2 R.N. visits.
6. Client will avoid foods that cause food allergy after 1–2 R.N. visits.
7. Client/Family will administer enteral feedings as ordered after 1–2–3 R.N. visits.
8. Client/Family will administer hyperalimentation as ordered after 1–2–3–4 R.N. visits.
9. Client will take vitamin/mineral therapy as ordered after 1–2 R.N. visits.
10. Client will take prescribed medication after 1–2–3 R.N. visits.
11. Client/Family will immediately report adverse reactions or signs/symptoms of complications to M.D. after 1–2–3 R.N. visits.
12. Client/Family will store food properly after 1–2–3 R.N. visits.
13. Client will reduce weight/gain weight as ordered after 1–2–3–4 R.N. visits.
14. Client will rest/exercise as ordered after 1–2–3 R.N. visits.
15. Client will visit dentist routinely every 6 months after 1–2 R.N. visits.

III. LONG-TERM GOALS

1. Adequate nutritional habits will be established in 1–2 weeks.
2. Independent activities of daily living will be resumed in 2–4 weeks.
3. Optimal level of health will be achieved in 2–4 weeks.

IV. OUTCOME CRITERIA

1. Vital signs remain normal.
2. Laboratory results are normal.
3. Growth and development are normal.
4. Weight remains normal.
5. Hair is shiny and healthy.
6. Skin/Mucous membrane remains healthy and intact.
7. Eyes are alert, shiny, and healthy.
8. Vision is clear.
9. GI system functions normally.
10. Client states he/she feels better.

V. NURSING INTERVENTION/TREATMENT

1. R.N. will assess physical status and nutritional habits of client/family.
2. R.N. will instruct client/family/H.H.A. on:
   A. monitoring and recording of vital signs.
   B. daily recording of weight.
   C. medication/vitamin/mineral administration/adverse reactions.
   D. immediate notification of M.D. of adverse reactions or signs/symptoms of advance of condition.
   E. laboratory testing/M.D. appointments.
   F. weight gain/weight-reduction plans.
   G. skin care.
   H. exercise/rest as ordered.
   I. bowel/bladder regimen.
   J. GI disturbances/allergies/postoperative requirements.
   K. enteral feedings/hyperalimentation.
   L. fluid intake as ordered.
   M. individualized diet.
   N. four food groups.
   O. meal planning.
   P. consumer buying.
   Q. food storage.
   R. use of food stamps.
   S. seminars, courses, clubs, organizations pertaining to ethnic food preparation.
3. R.N. will provide M.D. with follow-up reports and discharge summary when case closes.
4. R.N. will notify client/family/H.H.A./significant others when case will close.

Mastectomy
Care Plan

I. NURSING DIAGNOSIS

1. Knowledge deficit related to:
   A. medication administration/adverse reactions.
   B. dressing care.
   C. proper hand-washing technique.
   D. individualized prosthesis.
   E. exercise program/rest.
   F. proper fit of clothing.
   G. low-dose mammography.
   H. surgical procedures (e.g., lumpectomy/simple mastectomy/ modified radical mastectomy/radical mastectomy).
   I. chemotherapy.
   J. radiation/skin care.
   K. physical therapy/occupational therapy.
   L. other _____

2. Pain related to:
   A. wound granulation.
   B. infection.
   C. poor exercise tolerance.
   D. other _____

3. Ineffective individual/family coping related to:
   A. feeling of loss of femininity.
   B. fear of terminal illness.
   C. metastasis.

D. fear of loss of sexual attractiveness/desire.

E. shame.

F. rejection.

G. repulsion.

H. pain.

I. radiation administration.

J. side effects of chemotherapy.

K. grieving/loss.

L. other _____

4. Diversional activity deficit related to:

A. pain.

B. edema.

C. bulky chest dressing.

D. loss of strength in arm on affected side.

E. weakness.

F. side effects of chemotherapy/radiation.

G. other _____

5. Impaired home maintenance management related to:

A. muscle weakness.

B. toxic effects of chemotherapy/radiation.

C. other _____

6. Noncompliance with therapy related to:

A. pain.

B. denial.

C. fear.

D. anxiety.

E. other _____

7. Potential for injury related to:

A. poor administration of medications.

B. refusal to comply with exercise plan.

C. poor skin care.

D. other _____

8. Altered nutrition: potential for more than body requirements related to:
   A. dietary change.
   B. toxic effects of chemotherapy/radiation.
   C. weight reduction.
   D. other _____

   _____

9. Self-care deficit: feeding/bathing/dressing/grooming/ambulating related to:
   A. muscle weakness.
   B. pain.
   C. toxic effects of chemotherapy/radiation.
   D. other _____

   _____

10. Sexual dysfunction related to:
    A. feelings of inadequacy.
    B. shame.
    C. anxiety.
    D. lack of interest.
    E. feelings of rejection.
    F. other _____

    _____

11. Potential impaired skin integrity related to:
    A. break in aseptic dressing technique.
    B. poor hand-washing technique.
    C. skin rash.
    D. soreness linked to radiation therapy.
    E. other _____

    _____

12. Sleep pattern disturbance related to:
    A. pain.
    B. edema.
    C. discomfort of bulky chest dressing.
    D. intact sutures.
    E. other _____

    _____

II. SHORT-TERM GOALS

1. Client/Family will verbalize fears, anxieties, and concerns after 1–2–3–4 R.N. visits.
2. Client will consume appropriate fluids/diet as ordered after 1–2–3 R.N. visits.
3. Client will take prescribed medication as ordered after 1–2–3 R.N. visits.
4. Client/Family will notify M.D. of adverse reactions or change in condition after 1–2 R.N. visits.
5. Client will perform prescribed exercises as ordered after 1–2 R.N./ P.T./O.T. visits.
6. Client will obtain appropriately fitting prosthesis after 1–2 R.N. visits.
7. Client will seek diversional activities after 1–2 R.N. visits.
8. Client/Family will use gentle massage with cocoa butter on healed incision after 1–2–3 R.N. visits.
9. Client/Family will change mastectomy dressing as ordered after 1–2–3 R.N. visits.
10. Family will provide emotional support to client after 1–2 R.N. visits.
11. Client will wear elastic sleeve (from wrist to shoulder) as ordered after 1 R.N. visit.
12. Client will elevate arm as ordered after 1–2 R.N./P.T./O.T. visits.
13. Client will swing arm while walking as ordered after 1–2–3 R.N./ P.T./O.T. visits.
14. Client will wear loose, nonconstricting clothing after 1 R.N. visit.
15. Client/Family will keep surgical site, arm, and underarm as clean as possible after 1 R.N. visit.
16. Client will join mastectomy club/visit oncology clinic/request literature from professional organizations after 1–2 R.N. visits.
17. Client will seek laboratory testing/M.D. appointments as ordered after 1–2 R.N. visits.

III. LONG-TERM GOALS

1. Acceptance of condition will be achieved in 2–3 months.
2. Independent activities of daily living will be resumed in 1–2 weeks.
3. Optimal level of health will be regained in 1–2 months.

IV. OUTCOME CRITERIA

1. Vital signs are normal.
2. Laboratory test results are normal.
3. Granulation occurs; skin is healthy and intact.
4. Client is alert, cooperative, and sociable.
5. Ambulation/Mobility is normal.
6. Appetite is normal.
7. Client consumes nutritious meals.
8. Normal sleep pattern occurs.
9. Client states she feels better.
10. Client resumes employment.

V. NURSING INTERVENTION/TREATMENT

1. R.N. will visit home, assess status, and arrange for additional personnel (e.g., P.T., M.S.W., H.H.A., home attendant, homemaker, housekeeper) if necessary.
2. R.N. will instruct client/family/H.H.A. on:
   A. low-dose mammography.
   B. surgical procedures (e.g., lumpectomy/simple mastectomy/ modified radical mastectomy/radical mastectomy/radical mastectomy and lumpecotomy).
   C. chemotherapy.
   D. radiation/skin care precautions.
   E. proper hand-washing technique.
   F. aseptic dressing technique.
   G. skin care: application of cocoa butter to healed incision site if ordered by M.D.
   H. medication administration/adverse reactions.
   I. immediate notification of M.D. of adverse reactions or change in condition.
   J. personal hygiene, especially pertaining to affected arm, surgical site, and underarm.
   K. individualized prosthesis.
   L. use of elastic sleeve for edema on affected side.
   M. elevation of arm/exercises/physical therapy/occupational therapy.
   N. diversional activities/laugh therapy.
   O. wearing of loose, nonconstrictive clothing.
   P. laboratory testing/M.D. appointments.

3. R.N. will encourage client to request literature from oncology clinics, professional organizations, and clubs.
4. R.N. will provide M.D. with follow-up reports and discharge summary when case closes.
5. R.N. will notify client/family/H.H.A./significant others when case will close.

Mechanical Ventilator
Care Plan

I. NURSING DIAGNOSIS

1. Anxiety related to:
   A. mechanical failure of ventilator.
   B. possible asphyxiation while on a respirator.
   C. suctioning technique.
   D. cuffing technique.
   E. possible cross-contamination during suctioning.
   F. frequent alarm triggering.
   G. weaning.
   H. use of hand-held resuscitation bag.
   I. other _____

2. Ineffective airway clearance related to:
   A. poor suctioning technique.
   B. pulmonary congestion.
   C. ineffective use of hand-held resuscitation bag.
   D. poor/infrequent positioning/turning.
   E. inadequate/infrequent tracheostomy care.
   F. poor understanding of procedures by family members.
   G. other _____

3. Activity intolerance related to:
   A. poor respiratory status.
   B. confinement to ventilator.
   C. weakness.

D. other _____

_____

4. Ineffective breathing pattern related to:
   A. inadequate ventilator rate.
   B. inadequate oxygen concentration.
   C. inadequate tidal volume.
   D. apnea.
   E. cycle failure.
   F. rise/fall in peak airway pressure.
   G. loss of positive end-expiratory pressure (PEEP).
   H. electrical power failure.
   I. inadequate suctioning.
   J. infrequent suctioning.
   K. other _____

   _____

5. Potential altered body temperature related to:
   A. pulmonary infection.
   B. retained secretions.
   C. poor suctioning technique.
   D. chest injury.
   E. chest surgery.
   F. inadequate nutritional intake.
   G. inability to wean from respirator.
   H. lowered resistance to infection.
   I. other _____

   _____

6. Decreased cardiac output related to:
   A. retained respiratory secretions.
   B. loss of positive end-expiratory pressure (PEEP).
   C. pulmonary infection.
   D. continued elevated airway pressure (continuous positive-pressure ventilation).
   E. suctioning.
   F. other _____

   _____

7. Pain related to:
   A. immobility.
   B. restricted movement/poor positioning.

C. poor fit of tracheal tube.
D. infection.
E. subcutaneous emphysema.
F. chest injury.
G. chest surgery.
H. frequent coughing.
I. inadequate ventilator rate.
J. inappropriate use of hand-held resuscitation bag.
K. frequent tracheal dressing changes.
L. arterial blood gas sampling.
M. frequent hyperextention of neck.
N. high level of portable suctioning.
O. use of unlubricated suction catheter.
P. poor suctioning technique.
Q. swallowed air.
R. other _____

8. Bowel incontinence/Constipation/Diarrhea related to:
A. inadequate communication for expressing needs.
B. adverse reactions to medications.
C. confusion.
D. inadequate fluid/dietary intake.
E. other _____

9. Impaired verbal/physical communication related to:
A. confusion.
B. immobility.
C. paralysis of upper extremities.
D. lack of communicative devices (call bell/magic slate/hand signals/hand-held communicator with paper printout).
E. other _____

10. Ineffective family coping (compromised/disabling) related to:
A. constant need for client supervision.
B. cost of medical care/poor insurance coverage.
C. interference of household chores with client care.
D. other _____

11. Ineffective individual coping related to:
    A. social isolation.
    B. depression.
    C. dependence on others for care.
    D. rejection by significant others.
    E. other _____

12. Fear related to:
    A. lack of continuity by various caregivers.
    B. potential respiratory failure.
    C. potential death.
    D. other _____

13. Actual/Potential fluid volume deficit related to:
    A. inadequate fluid/dietary intake.
    B. vomiting.
    C. frequent suctioning.
    D. poor tolerance of oral feedings/tube feedings.
    E. diarrhea.
    F. other _____

14. Fluid volume excess related to:
    A. mechanical ventilation with humidification.
    B. electrolyte imbalances.
    C. failure to record accurate daily weights.
    D. failure to record accurate intake and output.
    E. urinary retention.
    F. hypoalbuminemia.
    G. elevation of mean airway and intrathoracic venous pressures.
    H. decreased renal perfusion.
    I. reduced lymphatic flow.
    J. other _____

15. Impaired gas exchange related to:
    A. pulmonary infection.
    B. retained pulmonary secretions/airway obstruction.
    C. infrequent suctioning.
    D. subcutaneous emphysema.

E. tracheal damage.

F. inability to wean.

G. oxygen toxicity.

H. backflow of condensation from ventilator tubing.

I. other _____

_____

16. Potential for injury related to:

    A. poor comprehension of respiratory care/operation of equipment.

    B. lack of support in the home.

    C. inadequate equipment.

    D. inadequate suctioning technique.

    E. poor use of hand-held resuscitation bag.

    F. inadequate cuffing technique.

    G. inadequate medical follow-up.

    H. inadequate chest physical therapy.

    I. disconnection from ventilator.

    J. inadequate alarm system.

    K. cycle failure.

    L. loss of positive end-expiratory pressure (PEEP).

    M. electrical power failure.

    N. fighting during suctioning.

    O. misplacement of endotracheal tube.

    P. other _____

    _____

17. Potential for infection related to:

    A. continuous ventilation with normal or low volumes.

    B. inadequate hand-washing technique.

    C. break in aseptic technique.

    D. inadequate suctioning technique.

    E. inappropriate tracheal dressing changes.

    F. inadequate fluid/dietary intake.

    G. inadequate maintenance/cleansing of respiratory equipment.

    H. other _____

    _____

18. Knowledge deficit related to:

    A. normal anatomy/physiology of respiratory system.

    B. types of mechanical-lung ventilators: controlled (machine-cycled ventilators)/assisted (client-cycled ventilators)/assist-control ventilators. There are three types of positive-pressure ventilators: volume-cycled, time-cycled, pressure-cycled.

C. types of external body ventilators (body tank ventilator/Cuirass ventilator/ventilatory belts).

D. therapy devices (Rocking devices/electrostimulator).

E. medication administration/adverse reactions.

F. signs/symptoms of complications of artificial ventilation.

G. safe operation of ventilator/malfunctioning.

H. use of hand-held resuscitation bag.

I. fluid/dietary instructions.

J. observation of client/monitoring and recording of vital signs.

K. appropriate hand-washing technique.

L. aseptic suctioning technique.

M. aseptic dressing care.

N. maintenance/cleaning/storage of medical equipment and supplies.

O. inhalation therapy.

P. bowel/bladder regimen.

Q. daily recording of intake/output.

R. cuffing technique.

S. esophageal speech techniques/communicative devices.

T. availability of emergency tracheostomy set.

U. ambulation/exercise/rest.

V. laboratory testing/M.D. appointments.

W. other _____

_____

19. Impaired physical mobility related to:

A. restriction of ventilator.

B. paralysis.

C. other _____

_____

20. Altered oral mucous membrane related to:

A. frequent suctioning.

B. frequent expectoration.

C. other _____

_____

21. Self-care deficit: feeding/bathing/hygiene/dressing/grooming/toileting related to:

A. restriction of ventilator.

    B. paralysis.

    C. other _____

          _____

22. Self-esteem disturbance related to:

    A. restriction on ventilator.

    B. loss of employment.

    C. dependence on others for care.

    D. other _____

          _____

23. Sexual dysfunction related to:

    A. restriction on ventilator.

    B. compromised respiratory status.

    C. other _____

          _____

24. Actual/Potential impaired skin integrity related to:

    A. kinked endotracheal tube.

    B. continual pulling outward and downward of tracheostomy tube.

    C. excessive movement of head and neck, causing friction on tube and cuff.

    D. excessive coughing against tube.

    E. inadequate repositioning of oral tubing.

    F. air leak around cuff.

    G. inadequate suctioning technique.

    H. inadequate dressing technique.

    I. other _____

          _____

25. Impaired swallowing related to:

    A. placement of endotracheal tube.

    B. inadequate cuffing technique.

    C. inadequate positioning of head.

    D. other _____

          _____

26. Altered cardiopulmonary tissue perfusion related to:

    A. oxygen toxicity.

    B. inadequate synchronization of client with ventilator.

    C. copious secretions.

    D. bronchospasm.

    E. infection.

    F. poor suctioning technique.

G. poor follow-up of arterial blood gas analysis.

H. mechanical overventilation.

I. inadequate administration of PEEP.

J. other _____

_____

II. SHORT-TERM GOALS

1. Client/Family will obtain all equipment/supplies before R.N. visits home on initial evaluation.

2. Client/Family will review the institution's policy concerning responsibility for the prescribed ventilator with the R.N. after 1 R.N. visit.

3. Client/Family will verbalize fears, anxieties, and concerns after 1–2–3 R.N. visits.

4. Client/Family will wash hands as ordered after 1 R.N. visit.

5. Client/Family will state the purpose for mechanical ventilation after 1–2–3–4–5 R.N. visits.

6. Client/Family will demonstrate appropriate oral/tracheal suctioning as ordered after 1–2–3–4–5 R.N. visits.

7. Client/Family will demonstrate appropriate operation of the prescribed ventilator after 1–2–3–4–5 R.N. visits.

8. Family will monitor vital signs, blood pressure, and chest auscultation as ordered after 1–2–3–4–5 R.N. visits.

9. Client/Family will state appropriate emergency phone numbers after 1–2–3 R.N. visits.

10. Client/Family will rest/exercise as ordered after 1–2–3 R.N. visits.

11. Client/Family will demonstrate appropriate use of a hand-held resuscitation bag after 1–2–3–4–5 R.N. visits.

12. Client will demonstrate use of a call bell/magic slate/hand-held communicator with paper printout after 1–2–3 R.N. visits.

13. Client/Family will record daily intake and output after 1–2–3 R.N. visits.

14. Client/Family will state signs/symptoms of mechanical ventilator complications after 1–2–3–4–5 R.N. visits.

15. Client/Family will demonstrate appropriate cuffing technique after 1–2–3–4–5 R.N. visits.

16. Client/Family will administer respiratory therapy (breathing exercises/humidification/intermittent positive-pressure breathing/inhalation therapy/chest physical therapy) as ordered after 1–2–3–4–5 R.N. visits.

17. Client/Family will change inner/outer tracheostomy cannula as ordered by M.D. after 1–2–3–4–5 R.N. visits.
18. Client/Family will have emergency tracheostomy set available at all times after 1–2–3 R.N. visits.
19. Client/Family will cleanse/sterilize tracheostomy/respiratory equipment as ordered after 1–2–3–4–5 R.N. visits.
20. Client/Family will administer prescribed medication after 1–2 R.N. visits.
21. Client/Family will immediately notify M.D. of adverse reactions or change in condition after 1–2 R.N. visits.
22. Client/Family will seek laboratory testing/M.D. appointments as ordered after 1–2 R.N. visits.
23. Client will communicate/perform esophageal speech after 4–5–6–7 R.N./S.T. visits.
24. Client/Family will perform tracheostomy dressing changes as ordered after 1–2–3 R.N. visits.
25. Client/Family will administer regular eye lubrication after 1–2–3 R.N. visits.
26. Client/Family will obtain regular sputum examinations as ordered after 1–2–3 R.N. visits.
27. Client/Family will record daily weights after 1–2–3 R.N. visits.
28. Client/Family will use Cof-Flator (portable cough machine) as ordered after 1–2–3–4–5 R.N. visits.
29. Client/Family will use portable aspirators as ordered after 1–2–3–4–5 R.N. visits.
30. Client/Family will use oxygen/liquid oxygen/oxygen concentrator as ordered after 1–2–3 R.N. visits.
31. Client/Family will apply chest shell/Cuirass shell/Pulmo-Wrap/ exsufflation belt as ordered after 1–2–3–4–5 R.N. visits.
32. Client/Family will utilize Rocking devices/electrostimulator as ordered after 1–2–3–4–5 R.N. visits.
33. Client/Family will have trouble-shooting guide available at all times after 1–2–3–4–5 R.N. visits.
34. Client will travel with equipment as ordered after 1–2–3–4–5–6 R.N. visits.
35. Client/Family will notify sales/service of respiratory equipment company when necessary after 1–2–3–4–5 R.N. visits.
36. Client will seek active employment after M.D. approval.

III. LONG-TERM GOALS

1. Mechanical ventilation will provide correct alveolar ventilation and adequate tissue oxygenation in 1–2 months.

2. Adequate respiratory functioning will be achieved in 1–2 months.
3. Spontaneous breathing will occur within 1–2–3–4–5–6 months.
4. Independent activities of daily living will be resumed in 1–2 months.
5. Communication will be achieved in 1–2 weeks.
6. Optimal level of health will be achieved within 6 months.

IV. OUTCOME CRITERIA

1. Vital signs are normal.
2. Oropharynx is clear.
3. Chest is clear bilaterally.
4. Breath sounds are normal.
5. Airway is patent.
6. Tracheostomy site is stable.
7. Skin/Mucous membrane is healthy and intact.
8. Weight is normal.
9. Swallowing is normal.
10. Appetite is normal.
11. Bowel/Bladder status is normal.
12. Intake and output are within normal limits.
13. Client is alert and sociable.
14. Ventilator functions appropriately.
15. Respiratory equipment functions without obstruction.
16. P_{O_2} and P_{CO_2} are within normal limits.
17. Laboratory test results are normal.
18. Client states he/she feels better.

V. NURSING INTERVENTION/TREATMENT

1. R.N. will contact client/family to arrange home visit and ensure all equipment/supplies are present in the home.
2. R.N. will review with the client and family upon initial evaluation the institution's policy concerning responsibility for the prescribed ventilator.
3. R.N. will obtain consent to start treatment during the initial visit.
4. R.N. will fully evaluate and observe the client and family for their capability and knowledge retention before care is initiated.
5. R.N. will conduct physical examination on initial visit and subsequent visits.

6. R.N. will instruct client/family/H.H.A./significant others on:
   A. normal anatomy/physiology of the respiratory system.
   B. close observation of the client.
   C. monitoring and recording of vital signs.
   D. appropriate hand-washing technique.
   E. aseptic suctioning/cuffing technique.
   F. aseptic tracheostomy dressing care.
   G. respiratory therapy: breathing exercises/heated and unheated humidification/intermittent positive-pressure breathing/inhalation therapy/chest physical therapy.
   H. cleaning and storage of tracheostomy equipment.
   I. availability of emergency tracheostomy set/emergency phone numbers.
   J. self-insertion of inner/outer tracheostomy cannula.
   K. medication administration/adverse reactions.
   L. signs/symptoms of infection/complications of mechanical ventilation (atelectasis/pneumothorax/subcutaneous emphysema/mediastinal emphysema/positive water balance/pulmonary edema/electrolyte imbalance/acid-base imbalances/hypoxia/hypocapnea/hypercapnea/oxygen toxicity/retrosternal pain/decreased vital capacity/sore throat/nasal congestion/cough/arrhythmias/stress ulcer/gastric rupture/GI bleeding/gastric distension/ileus/tracheal damage/decreased cardiac output/confusion/endobronchial intubation/airway obstruction/starvation/inability to wean.
   M. immediate notification of M.D. of adverse reactions or change in condition.
   N. cardiopulmonary resuscitation.
   O. types of prescribed ventilators: external body ventilators (body tank ventilator/iron lung/chest shell/Cuirass shell/ventilatory belt/Pulmo-Wrap) and lung ventilators (*controlled:* Bennett MA-1/Ohio 560; *assisted:* Bennett MA-1/Ohio 560/Portabird II; *assist-controlled:* Bennett MA-1/Bird Ventilator/iron lung/portable respirators/Engström/Emerson Volume Ventilator/Bennett PR I and PR II/Bird Mark 7).
   P. operational instructions for ventilator/trouble-shooting guide (available from respiratory equipment company or manufacturer).
   Q. use of hand-held resuscitation bag (Ambu bag).
   R. use of Rocking devices/electrostimulator/battery pack/portable aspirators/Cof-Flator/oxygen tank/liquid oxygen/oxygen concentrator.

  S. fluid/dietary intake (intake and output).

  T. gastrostomy feedings/hyperalimentation/nasogastric feedings/ oral feedings.

  U. turning/positioning/exercise/avoidance of stress and crowded areas.

  V. laboratory testing (arterial blood gases/chest x-rays/routine blood work/SMA-6/SMA-12/sputum culture and sensitivity)/ M.D. appointments.

  W. weaning from ventilator (weaning with T-piece or intermittent mandatory ventilation [IMV]).

  X. communication techniques/esophageal speech/use of writing instruments/home computer/magic slate/hand-held communicator with paper print out/call bell.

  Y. cleaning/sterilization of ventilator and all respiratory equipment.

  Z. travel/diversional activities/financial assistance/vocational counseling/employment/college.

7. R.N. will provide client/family/H.H.A./significant others with additional information/names of organizations, clubs, societies for contact with people with similar condition.

8. R.N. will assign additional personnel (e.g., M.S.W., clergy) to case if ordered.

9. R.N. will provide M.D. with follow-up reports and discharge summary when case closes.

10. R.N. will notify client/family/H.H.A./significant others when case will close.

Multiple Sclerosis Care Plan

I. NURSING DIAGNOSIS

1. Fear related to:
   A. nystagmus.
   B. blurred vision.
   C. diplopia.
   D. loss of muscle tone.
   E. advance of condition.
   F. other _____

   _____

2. Impaired physical mobility related to:
   A. ataxia.
   B. spasticity.
   C. muscular tremors.
   D. loss of muscle tone.
   E. advance of condition.
   F. other _____

   _____

3. Impaired verbal communication related to progressive loss of muscle tone.
4. Impaired home maintenance management related to generalized motor weakness.
5. Ineffective individual/family coping related to:
   A. hyperexcitability.
   B. anxiety.
   C. spastic weakness.

D. other _____
_____

6. Altered nutrition: potential for more than body requirements related to:
   A. nausea/vomiting.
   B. feeding problems/food preparation.
   C. other _____
   _____

7. Potential for injury related to:
   A. spasticity.
   B. muscular tremors.
   C. loss of control.
   D. other _____
   _____

8. Self-care deficit: feeding/bathing/dressing/grooming/ambulating related to:
   A. spasticity.
   B. muscular tremors.
   C. loss of control.
   D. other _____
   _____

9. Altered patterns of bowel/urinary elimination related to loss of abdominal reflexes.
10. Sexual dysfunction related to spasticity.
11. Anticipatory grieving related to chronic, progressive nature of illness.
12. Knowledge deficit related to:
    A. signs/symptoms of multiple sclerosis.
    B. medication administration/adverse reactions.
    C. laboratory testing/M.D. appointments.
    D. rehabilitative equipment (e.g., products from the AT&T National Special Needs Center: handsets for hearing and speech amplification/Porta Printer Plus/Portaview, Jr./emergency call systems/signaling devices/Nomad Cordless Phone/Directel/ electronic artificial larynx/Genesis Telesystem/special helpers, e.g., special coupler, larger-number decals, large-number dial overlay, operator dialer, raised faceplate).
    E. exercise/rest.
    F. fluids/diet.

G. other _____

_____

II. SHORT-TERM GOALS

1. Client will take prescribed medication after 1–2–3 R.N. visits.
2. Client will immediately notify M.D. of adverse reactions to medications or change in condition after 1–2 R.N. visits.
3. Client will take warm baths as prescribed after 1–2 R.N. visits.
4. Client will follow prescribed exercise regimen as ordered after 1–2–3–4 R.N./P.T./O.T. visits.
5. Client/Family will use warm packs and muscle relaxants if painful muscle spasms exist after 1–2–3–4 R.N./P.T./O.T. visits.
6. Client will follow prescribed bowel-training program after 1–2–3 R.N. visits.
7. Client/Family will keep commode/bedpan/urinal within easy reach after 1–2 R.N. visits.
8. Client will use incontinence aids if necessary (pads/protective pants/catheter) after 1–2 R.N. visits.
9. Client will use self-help devices (feeding devices/braces/handrails/canes/wheelchair/ramps) after 2–3–4 R.N./P.T./O.T. visits.
10. Client will wear corrective glasses after 1–2 R.N. visits.
11. Client/Family will contact organizations for information about disease after 1–2 R.N. visits.
12. Client will seek laboratory testing/M.D. appointments after 1–2 R.N. visits.

III. LONG-TERM GOALS

1. Independent activities of daily living will be resumed in 1–2 weeks.
2. Optimal level of health will be achieved in 3–4 weeks.

IV. OUTCOME CRITERIA

1. Vital signs are normal.
2. Appetite remains normal.
3. Motivation remains stable.
4. Laboratory results remain normal.
5. Joint mobility remains functional.

V. NURSING INTERVENTION/TREATMENT

1. R.N. will contact hospital/rehabilitation discharge planner about previous client education regarding nursing/S.T./P.T./O.T./M.S.W./H.H.A. for continuity in home.
2. R.N. will confer with M.S.W. about financial status/resources for payment for extensive services.
3. R.N. will instruct client/family/H.H.A. on:
   A. performing independent activities of daily living (to keep client active as long as possible).
   B. medication regimen, especially for pain and spasms/adverse reactions.
   C. promotion of rest/sleep.
   D. avoidance of excitation and stress.
   E. warm baths/packs.
   F. fluid intake and dietary regimen as ordered.
   G. avoidance of cold and dampness.
   H. mild, dry climate to encourage remission.
   I. exercise regimen as ordered by M.D. in consultation with P.T., O.T., and S.T.
   J. rehabilitative equipment (e.g., products from the AT&T National Special Needs Center: handsets for hearing and speech amplification/Porta Printer Plus/Portaview, Jr./emergency call systems/signaling devices/Nomad Cordless Phones/Directel/electronic artificial larynx/Genesis Telesystem/special helpers, e.g., special coupler, large-number decals, large-number dial overlay, operator dialer, raised faceplate).
   K. psychologic support. R.N. should answer all questions on therapy.
   L. corrective glasses.
   M. routine M.D./dental appointments.
   N. laboratory testing.
   O. socialization.
   P. organizations for additional information on multiple sclerosis.
4. R.N. will provide M.D. with follow-up reports and discharge summary when case closes.
5. R.N. will refer client to additional community resources for assistance with finances/employment/education, if necessary.
6. On admission, if possible, R.N. will notify client/family/H.H.A./significant others when case will close.

Myocardial Infarction Care Plan

I. NURSING DIAGNOSIS

1. Anxiety related to:
   A. chest pain.
   B. possible death.
   C. potential rehospitalization.
   D. potential surgery.
   E. other _____
   _____

2. Decreased cardiac output related to:
   A. poor oxygenation of heart muscle.
   B. ventricular tachycardia.
   C. ventricular fibrillation.
   D. arterial hypertension.
   E. emotional stress.
   F. other _____
   _____

3. Ineffective breathing pattern related to:
   A. dyspnea.
   B. chest pain.
   C. other _____
   _____

4. Headache/Vise-like substernal or upper abdominal pain/radiating pain to shoulders and arms, usually left arm, unrelieved by rest or nitrites related to:
   A. poor oxygenation of heart muscle.
   B. obesity.

C. emotional/physical stress.

D. other _____

_____

5. Diversional activity deficit related to:
   A. malaise.
   B. fatigue.
   C. anger.
   D. other _____

_____

6. Impaired home maintenance management related to:
   A. dyspnea on exertion.
   B. chest pain.
   C. bradycardia/tachycardia.
   D. hypertension/hypotension.
   E. vomiting.
   F. other _____

_____

7. Noncompliance with therapy related to:
   A. poor administration of medication.
   B. denial.
   C. other _____

_____

8. Sexual dysfunction related to history of severe cardiac problems.

9. Altered parenting related to cardiac disease.

10. Self-care deficit: feeding/bathing/grooming/dressing/toileting related to:
    A. dyspnea on exertion.
    B. chest pain.
    C. other _____

_____

11. Sleep pattern disturbance related to:
    A. chest pain.
    B. dyspnea.
    C. restlessness.
    D. fear of death.
    E. other _____

_____

12. Altered cardiopulmonary tissue perfusion related to:
    A. cardiac arrhythmia.

B. smoking.

C. emotional stress.

D. poor administration of medications.

E. other _____

_____

13. Potential for injury related to:

A. overexertion.

B. poor administration of medications.

C. other _____

_____

14. Self-esteem disturbance related to:

A. loss of job status.

B. dependence on others for care.

C. other _____

_____

II. SHORT-TERM GOALS

1. Client/Family will verbalize fears, anxieties, and concerns after 1–2–3–4 R.N. visits.
2. Client will take medication as ordered after 1–2–3 R.N. visits.
3. Client/Family will immediately report adverse reactions to medications/change in condition after 1–2 R.N. visits.
4. Client will limit fluid intake as ordered after 1–2 R.N. visits.
5. Client will avoid temperature extremes in fluids and weather after 1–2 R.N. visits.
6. Client/Family will limit sodium in diet as ordered after 1–2 R.N. visits.
7. Client will take potassium supplement as ordered after 1–2 R.N. visits.
8. Client will drink in moderation/eliminate alcohol according to M.D. orders after 1–2 R.N. visits.
9. Client will begin weight reduction according to M.D. orders after 1–2 R.N. visits.
10. Client will reduce/eliminate smoking after 3–4 R.N. visits.
11. Client will engage in moderate/light exercise as ordered after 1–2 R.N. visits.
12. Client will ambulate slowly after 1–2 R.N. visits.
13. Client/Family will take pulse as ordered after 1–2 R.N. visits.
14. Client will participate in diversional activities after 1–2 R.N. visits.

15. Client will seek laboratory testing/M.D. appointments as ordered after 1–2 R.N. visits.

III. LONG-TERM GOALS

1. Cardiac status will stabilize in 3–4 weeks.
2. Independent activities of daily living will be resumed in 1–2 weeks.
3. Optimal level of health will be achieved in 3–4 weeks.

IV. OUTCOME CRITERIA

1. Vital signs are normal.
2. CBC with differential remains normal.
3. Serum enzyme levels (SGOT, LDH, and CPK) are normal.
4. Chest is clear; breathing is normal.
5. Arterial blood gases are normal.
6. Venous blood gases are normal.
7. Appetite is normal.
8. Weight is appropriate.
9. Intake and output are normal.
10. Pain is relieved.
11. Peripheral pulses are normal.
12. Client is alert, oriented, and in good spirits.
13. Client assumes self-care activities.
14. Client states he/she feels better.

V. NURSING INTERVENTION/TREATMENT

1. R.N. will arrange for nursing visit in client's home.
2. R.N. will monitor and record apical and radial pulse rates, blood pressure, and laboratory testing (CBC with differential/electrolytes/ digitalis level/prothrombin time/partial thromboplastin time) as ordered by M.D.
3. R.N. will instruct client/family/H.H.A. on:
   A. disease process.
   B. apical and radial pulses.
   C. medication administration (anticoagulant therapy/nitrites/ diuretics/tranquilizers/antihypertensive/stool softeners)/adverse reactions.
   D. immediate notification of M.D. of adverse reactions.

    E. immediate notification of M.D. of any changes in present condition, onset of respiratory or localized or generalized infections.

    F. keeping emergency phone numbers at bedside or nearby. Client may also have a medical alert button to push to notify police or ambulance.

    G. laboratory testing/routine M.D. visits.

    H. prescribed exercises/stair climbing/lifting/daily rest periods.

    I. avoidance of air travel for 2–3 months, or as ordered by M.D.

    J. avoidance of temperature extremes.

    K. weight reduction as ordered.

    L. reduction in/avoidance of smoking.

    M. recording of intake and output.

    N. bed rest/chair rest.

    O. bowel regimen/avoidance of straining at stool.

    P. decreased work hours on return to work.

    Q. sexual activity.

    R. diversional activities.

4. R.N. will provide client with instructional literature/visual aids/ organizations for further assistance.

5. R.N. will assign additional personnel (e.g., M.S.W., P.T., R.T.) to case if ordered.

6. R.N. will provide M.D. with follow-up reports and discharge summary when case closes.

7. R.N. will notify client/family/H.H.A./significant others when case will close.

Nasogastric/Enteric Feeding Tube Care Plan

I. NURSING DIAGNOSIS

1. Anxiety related to:
   A. tube insertion.
   B. weight loss.
   C. malnutrition.
   D. advance of disease.
   E. other_____

2. Knowledge deficit related to:
   A. feeding preparation/preparation and measurement of tube feeding formula/feeding rate/bacterial contamination of formula/ prevention of gastrointestinal complications/passage of feeding tube.
   B. administration of tube feedings.
   C. operation of enteral pump.
   D. medication administration/adverse reactions.
   E. measurement of client with nasogastric tube prior to insertion.
   F. cost of supplies.
   G. other_____

3. Altered nutrition: potential for more/less than body requirements related to:
   A. malabsorption.
   B. diarrhea.

    C. constipation.

    D. allergic response to feedings.

    E. poor preparation of feedings.

    F. excessive weight loss/gain.

    G. other_____

    _____

4. Fluid volume deficit/excess related to:

    A. omission/delay in feeding schedule.

    B. adverse reactions to feeding.

    C. diarrhea.

    D. diuresis.

    E. excessive diaphoresis.

    F. other_____

    _____

5. Impaired swallowing related to:

    A. insertion of feeding tube.

    B. poor positioning of feeding tube.

    C. allergic response to feedings.

    D. ingestion of air into feeding tube.

    E. other_____

    _____

6. Potential for injury related to:

    A. poor passage of stylet through feeding tube.

    B. poor functioning of alarm.

    C. electrical/mechanical/battery malfunctioning of pump.

    D. aspiration.

    E. poor nutritional habits.

    F. other_____

    _____

7. Altered oral mucous membrane related to:

    A. mouth breathing.

    B. poor positioning of feeding tube.

    C. other_____

    _____

8. Ineffective airway clearance related to dislodgment of feeding tube/aspiration.

9. Impaired home maintenance management related to:

    A. overwhelming demands of caring for the sick.

    B. lack of support in the home.

    C. cost of medical care.

    D. other_____

    _____

10. Sleep pattern disturbance related to:

    A. frequent feedings.

    B. sounding of pump alarm.

    C. flatulence/distension.

    D. pain

    E. other_____

    _____

II. SHORT-TERM GOALS

1. Client/Family will verbalize all fears, anxieties, and concerns after 1–2–3–4 R.N. visits.

2. Client/Family will obtain and assemble all necessary equipment before R.N. visits.

3. Client/Family will premix/measure formula according to directions after 1–2–3 R.N. visits.

4. Client/Family will safely operate volumetric pump/enteric pump after 1–2–3 R.N. visits.

5. Client/Family will administer appropriate nose/mouth care after 1–2 R.N. visits.

6. Client/Family will state signs/symptoms of complications after 1–2–3 R.N. visits (e.g., excoriation, tracheal pressure, aspiration).

7. Client/Family will cleanse and store equipment after 1–2 R.N. visits.

8. Client will remain in sitting/semi-Fowler's position during and after feedings after 1–2–3 R.N. visits.

9. Client/Family will wash hands properly before and after feedings after 1–2 R.N. visits.

10. Client/Family will draw 10-15 cc of air into syringe after 1–2–3 R.N. visits.

11. Client/Family will insert tip of syringe into end of feeding tube after 1–2–3 R.N. visits.

12. Client/Family will open clamp on feeding tube after 1–2–3 R.N. visits.

13. Client/Family will place stethoscope over stomach area with earplugs intact after 1–2–3 R.N. visits.

14. Client/Family will inject air into feeding tube while listening with stethoscope after 1–2–3 R.N. visits.

15. Client/Family will withdraw plunger to aspirate stomach contents after 1–2–3 R.N. visits.

16. Client/Family will activate lubricant inside feeding tube by flushing with small amount of water after 1–2 R.N. visits.

17. Client/Family will insert guidewire stylet, after locking it in place behind mercury tip, after 1–2 R.N. visits (only if M.D. allows client or family to do this).

18. Client/Family will alternate nostrils after 1–2–3 R.N. visits.

19. Client will swallow small amounts of ice water/ice chips during insertion of tube after 1–2–3 R.N. visits.

20. Client/Family will remove stylet from feeding tube after insertion after 1–2–3 R.N. visits.

21. Client/Family will tape tube securely to cheek (using nonallergic tape), avoiding pressure on nares after 1–2–3 R.N. visits.

22. Client/Family will flush tubing with feeding preparation before attaching to feeding tube after 1–2–3 R.N. visits.

23. Client/Family will connect feeding tube to tubing and solution bag after 1–2–3 R.N. visits.

24. Client/Family will use syringe method/gravity drainage for feedings after 1–2–3 R.N. visits.

25. Client/Family will infuse 20-40 cc per hour and increase to 25-50 cc per hour per day after 1–2–3 R.N. visits.

26. Client/Family will measure residual stomach contents and, if greater than 100 cc, will withhold feeding for at least 2 hours, or as ordered by M.D., after 1–2–3 R.N. visits.

27. Client/Family will flush tubing with 30-50 cc water after each feeding and at regular intervals after 1–2–3 R.N. visits.

28. Client will visit M.D. as ordered after 1–2 R.N. visits.

III. LONG-TERM GOALS

1. Independent activities of daily living will be resumed in 1–2 weeks.

2. Adequate nutritional habits will be established in 1–2 weeks.

3. Normal GI functioning will resume in 1–2 weeks.

4. Optimal level of health will be achieved in 3–4 weeks.

IV. OUTCOME CRITERIA

1. Vital signs are normal.

2. Client absorbs feedings.

3. Hydration is accomplished.

4. Electrolyte balance is normal.

5. GI tract functions normally.

6. Chest remains clear.

7. Respirations are normal.

8. Weight is appropriate for height.

9. Skin remains healthy and intact.

10. Intake and output are normal.

11. Laboratory test results are normal.

12. Client states he/she feels better.

V. NURSING INTERVENTION/TREATMENT

1. R.N. will contact hospital discharge planner to assess instructions given to client for tube-feeding administration at home.

2. R.N. will arrange for all equipment and solutions to be delivered to client's home the day before client's discharge from hospital.

3. R.N. will perform complete history and physical examination on admission to home care.

4. R.N. will allow client/family to verbalize all fears, anxieties, and concerns and provide assistance.

5. R.N. will determine type of feeding to be administered: gravity-drip tube-feeding method/syringe-feeding method/pump-feeding method.

6. R.N. will instruct client/family/H.H.A. on:

   A. proper hand-washing technique.

   B. monitoring and recording of vital signs.

   C. monitoring and recording of weight daily.

   D. intake and output.

   E. skin care.

   F. mouth care.

   G. preparation of a clean working area.

   H. medication administration/adverse reactions.

   I. immediate notification of M.D. of adverse reactions or change in condition.

   J. urine testing for presence of sugar and acetone.

   K. signs/symptoms of sensitivity to nutritional preparation (e.g., diarrhea, constipation, abdominal cramping, nausea, weakness, heartburn, flatulence, vomiting, belching, dehydration, fever, weight loss of more than 2 pounds in 1 week).

L. preparation and measurement of formula/feeding rate/bacterial contamination of formula/prevention of GI complications.

M. insertion of feeding tube/measurement of tube (measure from tip of earlobe to bulge of nose to top of xiphoid process and add 9 inches and mark with tape)/stylet safety.

N. positioning of client for feedings (semi- or high Fowler's position).

O. positioning of tube/aspiration of stomach contents/ administration of feedings/checking of bowel sounds.

P. irrigation of tubing, if necessary (if plain water does not work to unclog a feeding tube, an effervescent flush using 10 cc of a carbonated beverage such as Seven-Up may work).

Q. time schedule for feedings.

R. safe operation, cleansing, storage of pump and removal of tube.

S. disposal of feeding tube (if tube contains mercury, do not incinerate because of production of toxic vapor).

T. laboratory testing/M.D. appointments.

7. R.N. will allow client/family/H.H.A. to redemonstrate procedure correctly and safely before case is closed.

8. R.N. will provide client/family/H.H.A. with sources of additional literature on feedings and nutritional advice; will consult with member of the equipment company or supplier about all instructions during admission and thereafter for deliveries made to client's home.

9. R.N. will provide client/family with names of organizations or clubs for additional information.

10. R.N. will provide M.D. with follow-up reports and discharge summary when case closes.

11. R.N. will consult with insurance company about all costs of medical care.

12. R.N. will notify client/family/H.H.A./significant others when case will close.

Neurogenic Bladder Care Plan

I. NURSING DIAGNOSIS

1. Anxiety related to:
   A. incontinence.
   B. intermittent self-catheterization.
   C. other _____

2. Knowledge deficit related to:
   A. catheterization/intermittent catheterization by family.
   B. self-catheterization.
   C. application of male external collecting device.
   D. clamping of catheter.
   E. medication administration/adverse reactions.
   F. other _____

3. Potential for infection related to:
   A. catheter leakage.
   B. poor catheterization technique.
   C. other _____

4. Ineffective individual/family coping related to:
   A. catheter leakage/odor.
   B. poor urinary output.
   C. concentrated, sedimented urinary output.
   D. other _____

5. Impaired home maintenance management related to increased client demands for frequent changing of catheters/padding/linens.

6. Self-esteem disturbance related to:
   A. urinary leakage.
   B. odor.
   C. staining of clothing or bedding.
   D. other _____

7. Sleep pattern disturbance related to catheter leakage.

8. Potential impaired skin integrity related to:
   A. poor personal hygiene.
   B. poor catheterization techniques.
   C. infection.
   D. catheter leakage.
   E. other _____

9. Altered patterns of urinary elimination related to:
   A. incorrect catheter size.
   B. catheter leakage.
   C. poor intake.
   D. poor insertion technique.
   E. delay in catheterization.
   F. other _____

10. Noncompliance with therapy related to:
    A. cost of medical supplies/poor insurance coverage.
    B. confusion/disorientation.
    C. other _____

11. Altered health maintenance related to:
    A. refusal to participate in therapy.
    B. dependence on others for care.
    C. other _____

12. Self-care deficit: feeding/bathing/grooming/dressing/toileting related to:
    A. immobility.
    B. paralysis.

C. other _____

_____

II. SHORT-TERM GOALS

1. Client/Family will seek appropriate diagnostic testing/medical intervention after 1–2–3 R.N. visits.
2. Client/Family will obtain prescribed medication after 1–2–3 R.N. visits.
3. Client/Family will obtain prescribed catheterization equipment after 1–2–3 R.N. visits.
4. Client/Family will redemonstrate intermittent self-catheterization/ catheterization/application of external catheter after 1–2–3 R.N. visits.
5. Client/Family will record vital signs as ordered after 1–2 R.N. visits.
6. Client/Family will force fluids as ordered after 1–2 R.N. visits.
7. Client/Family will state signs/symptoms of adverse reactions to medication after 1–2 R.N. visits.
8. Client/Family will immediately notify M.D. of adverse reactions or change in condition after 1 R.N. visit.

III. LONG-TERM GOALS

1. Adequate bladder functioning will result in adequate urinary output in 1–2 weeks.
2. Intermittent self-catheterization/catheterization/application of external catheter will be accomplished in 1–2 weeks.
3. Optimal level of health will be achieved in 1–2 weeks.

IV. OUTCOME CRITERIA

1. Vital signs are normal.
2. Urinary output remains clear, yellow, and sufficient in quantity.
3. Skin/Mucous membrane is healthy and intact.
4. Bladder functions appropriately.
5. Intake and output remain normal.
6. Laboratory test results remain normal.
7. Urine culture and sensitivity test results remain normal.
8. Client states he/she feels better.

V. NURSING INTERVENTION/TREATMENT

1. R.N. will instruct client/family/H.H.A. on:
   A. monitoring and recording of vital signs.
   B. proper hand-washing technique.
   C. medication administration/adverse reactions.
   D. immediate notification of M.D. of adverse reactions or change in condition.
   E. prescribed amount of fluid during and between meals.
   F. restriction of fluids after 9–10 PM.
   G. daily fluid/dietary regimen.
   H. positioning of client for catheterization (lithotomy/side-lying or prone) with blanket and sterile drapes.
   I. collection and position of catheterization equipment.
   J. sterile gloving technique.
   K. cleansing site with Betadine. If client is male, penis should be held at 45° angle to insert catheter.
   L. positioning of receptacle for collection of urine.
   M. lubrication/insertion of catheter/removal of catheter.
   N. measurement of urine. If residual urine measures 200 cc or more, catheter should be left in place after consultation with M.D.
   O. cleansing and storage of catheter.
   P. monthly urine culture and sensitivity testing.
   Q. daily recording of intake and output.
   R. application of condom/Texas catheter.
   S. use of protective absorbent pads/rubber padding/adult diapers.
   T. laboratory testing/M.D. appointments.
2. R.N. will provide follow-up reports and discharge summary to M.D. when case closes.
3. R.N. will notify client/family/H.H.A./significant others when case will close.

Ommaya Reservoir for Intrathecal Chemotherapy Care Plan

I. NURSING DIAGNOSIS

1. Knowledge deficit related to the care of the Ommaya reservoir and its adverse effects.
2. Fluid volume deficit (dehydration) related to vomiting.
3. Potential impaired skin integrity related to infected site (*Staphylococcus aureus*//*Staphylococcus epidermis*).
4. Fear related to signs/symptoms of chemotherapy.
5. Altered thought processes related to medication toxicity.
6. Pain related to:

    A. toxicity of chemotherapy.

    B. leakage at catheter site.

    C. poor catheter/skin care.

    D. other _____

    _____

7. Potential for injury related to:

    A. extreme toxicity of chemotherapy.

    B. alteration in thought processes/confusion/disorientation.

    C. ataxia.

    D. seizures.

    E. other _____

    _____

8. Altered nutrition: potential for more than body requirements related to:

    A. dysphagia.

    B. nausea.

    C. vomiting.

    D. other _____

    _____

9. Potential for infection related to:

    A. poor hand-washing technique.

    B. contamination of Ommaya site.

    C. other _____

    _____

10. Altered cerebral tissue perfusion related to:

    A. introduction of chemotherapeutic agents.

    B. other _____

    _____

II. SHORT-TERM GOALS

1. Client/Family will verbalize fears, anxieties, and concerns after 1–2–3–4 R.N. visits.
2. Client will take medication as prescribed, especially analgesics, anticonvulsants, tranquilizers, after 1–2–3–4 R.N. visits.
3. Client/Family will state three adverse reactions of chemotherapy after 1–2–3–4 R.N. visits.
4. Client/Family will cleanse Ommaya site with peroxide/Betadine as ordered after 1–2 R.N. visits.
5. Client/Family will shave area around Ommaya site before introduction of each chemotherapy injection after 1–2 R.N. visits.
6. Client will maintain rest periods throughout the day after 1–2 R.N. visits.
7. Client/Family will eliminate stress factors in the environment after 1–2 R.N. visits.
8. Client/Family will avoid placing pressure on the Ommaya site, to prevent projectile vomiting, after 1 R.N. visit.
9. After chemotherapy, client/family will report adverse reactions or change in condition after 1–2 R.N. visits.
10. Client will lie flat 30 minutes after introduction of chemotherapy injection, as requested by M.D.
11. Family will inject analgesics (especially morphine) intraventricularly as ordered by M.D. after 2–3 R.N. visits.
12. Client will seek laboratory testing/M.D. appointments as ordered after 1–2 R.N. visits.

III. LONG-TERM GOALS

1. Care and comfort of the terminally ill client will be adequately provided in 1–2 weeks.
2. Independent activities of daily living will be resumed within 1–2 weeks.
3. Disease will be controlled and catheter will be removed in 3–6 months.
4. All stages of grief and grieving will be resolved in 1 year.

IV. OUTCOME CRITERIA

1. Vital signs are normal.
2. Laboratory test results are normal.
3. Skin surrounding Ommaya site remains healthy and intact.
4. Client is oriented to person, place, and time.
5. Mobility is maintained.
6. Socialization remains normal.
7. Client is alert and cooperative.
8. Weight is appropriate for height.
9. Pain is minimal/nonexistent.
10. Client states he/she feels better.

V. NURSING INTERVENTION/TREATMENT

1. R.N. will allow verbalization by client/family of fears, anxieties, and concerns and provide psychologic support.
2. R.N. will assess vital signs once weekly, once daily, twice weekly, thrice weekly, twice monthly, or monthly as necessary.
3. R.N. will provide for additional support services (e.g., M.S.W., P.T., O.T., S.P., H.H.A., home attendant, homemaker, housekeeper) as ordered by M.D.
4. R.N. will instruct client/family/H.H.A./significant others on:
   A. purpose of Ommaya reservoir.
   B. care and cleansing of Ommaya site (using peroxide or Betadine); how to check for malfunction or displacement by pumping reservoir as ordered by M.D.
   C. precautions at site (e.g., to prevent projectile vomiting, do not place any pressure on the site unless otherwise specified by M.D.)
   D. administration of medications/adverse reactions; avoidance of

using a pillow after chemotherapy injection, to permit even dispersal of drug, especially up to 30 minutes at a time. R.N. will check with M.D. regarding this procedure, and will check with M.D. if family should be taught intrathecal injection of analgesics, especially morphine.

E. shaving of the area around reservoir very cleanly before each chemotherapy injection.

F. shunts with valves, if present.

G. fluid intake/diet.

H. exercise limitations if ordered/performing activities of daily living.

I. seizure precautions.

J. socialization.

K. laboratory testing/M.D. appointments.

5. R.N. will encourage client/family to contact M.D./R.N. about additional concerns or questions.

6. R.N. will provide literature on the Ommaya reservoir to client/ family.

7. R.N. will encourage a similar client with this reservoir to visit client to provide additional support and instructions.

8. R.N. will provide a hospice program/volunteers if necessary.

9. R.N. will support family throughout dying process if necessary.

10. R.N. will provide instructions after removal of Ommaya reservoir if client's condition is acute and not terminal.

11. R.N. will provide M.D. with follow-up reports and discharge summary when case closes.

12. R.N. will notify client/family/H.H.A./significant others when case will close.

Pacemaker
Care Plan

I. NURSING DIAGNOSIS

1. Anxiety related to:
   A. preoperative/postoperative pacemaker insertion.
   B. chest pain.
   C. overexertion.
   D. adequate meal preparation/fluid restriction.
   E. learning about pulse rate.
   F. administration of medication.
   G. pacemaker check via telephone.
   H. other _____

2. Knowledge deficit related to:
   A. pulse taking.
   B. use of stethoscope.
   C. medication administration/adverse reactions.
   D. exercise as ordered.
   E. sexual activity.
   F. avoidance of certain types of electric equipment as ordered by M.D. (depending on type and frequency of pacemaker).
   G. pacemaker check via telephone or in hospital or clinic.
   H. meal preparation/fluid intake as ordered.
   I. other _____

3. Ineffective breathing pattern related to:
   A. respiratory congestion.
   B. overexertion.

   C. poor administration of medication.

   D. dyspnea.

   E. pacemaker failure.

   F. other _____

   _____

4. Headache/Vise-like substernal or upper abdominal pain/radiating pain to shoulders and arms, usually left arm, unrelieved by rest or nitrites related to:

   A. poor oxygenation of heart muscle.

   B. poor administration of medication.

   C. medication toxicity.

   D. exercise intolerance.

   E. exposure to temperature extremes.

   F. obesity.

   G. stress.

   H. other _____

   _____

5. Potential fluid volume deficit related to vomiting.

6. Self-esteem disturbance related to:

   A. inability to perform independent activities of daily living.

   B. dependence on others for care.

   C. other _____

   _____

7. Fear/Anxiety related to impending heart failure.

8. Diversional activity deficit related to:

   A. malaise.

   B. restricted activities.

   C. chest pain.

   D. weakness/fatigue.

   E. poor mobility.

   F. other _____

   _____

9. Impaired physical mobility related to:

   A. chest pain.

   B. pain on exertion.

   C. restricted activity.

   D. bed rest.

   E. other _____

   _____

10. Impaired home maintenance management related to:
    A. dyspnea on exertion.
    B. chest pain.
    C. bradycardia/tachycardia.
    D. hypertension/hypotension.
    E. vomiting.
    F. weakness/fatigue.
    G. dependence on others for care.
    H. lack of support in the home.
    I. low income.
    J. other _____

11. Noncompliance with therapy related to:
    A. denial.
    B. poor understanding of disease.
    C. other _____

12. Decreased cardiac output related to:
    A. refusal to comply with medical advice.
    B. ventricular tachycardia/fibrillation.
    C. poor comprehension of administration of medication.
    D. arterial hypertension.
    E. emotional stress.
    F. overexertion.
    G. exposure to temperature extremes.
    H. pacemaker failure.
    I. other _____

13. Altered parenting related to history of severe cardiac problems.
14. Self-care deficit: feeding/bathing/grooming/dressing/toileting
    related to:
    A. dyspnea on exertion.
    B. chest pain.
    C. restricted activity.
    D. other _____

15. Sleep pattern disturbance related to:
    A. chest pain.
    B. dyspnea.

C. restlessness.

D. fear of death.

E. other _____

_____

16. Potential for injury related to:

 A. refusal to comply with medical instructions.

 B. poor supervision in the home.

 C. overexertion.

 D. other _____

 _____

17. Sexual dysfunction related to:

 A. restricted activity.

 B. fear of rejection.

 C. other _____

 _____

II. SHORT-TERM GOALS

1. Client/Family will verbalize fears, anxieties, and concerns after 1–2–3 R.N. visits.

2. Client/Family will administer medication as ordered after 1–2–3–4 R.N. visits.

3. Client/Family will immediately notify M.D. of adverse reactions or change in condition after 1–2 R.N. visits.

4. Client will ambulate as ordered after 1–2 R.N. visits.

5. Client will engage in light/moderate exercise as ordered after 1–2 R.N. visits.

6. Client will limit fluid intake as ordered after 1–2 R.N. visits.

7. Client will avoid temperature extremes in fluids and inclement weather after 1–2 R.N. visits.

8. Client will eliminate alcohol/drink in moderation as ordered after 1–2 R.N. visits.

9. Client will reduce weight as ordered after 1–2 R.N. visits.

10. Client will eliminate/reduce smoking after 1–2 R.N. visits.

11. Client will participate in diversional activities after 1–2 R.N. visits.

12. Client/Family will state the type of pacemaker that has been inserted after 1–2 R.N. visits.

13. Client/Family will state purpose of and set rate for asynchronous (set-rate) pacemaker after 1–2 R.N. visits.

14. Client/Family will state purpose of and normal pulse range for synchronous pacemaker after 1–2 R.N. visits.
15. Client/Family will state purpose of and normal pulse range for demand pacemaker after 1–2 R.N. visits.
16. Client will avoid certain types of electrical equipment as ordered by M.D. (depending on type and frequency of pacemaker) after 1–2 R.N. visits.
17. Client will avoid using extension cords/worn electrical cords/plugs/outlets as ordered by M.D. after 1–2 R.N. visits.
18. Client/Family will perform pacemaker check from home to hospital/clinic as ordered after 1–2–3 R.N. visits.
19. Client/Family will visit hospital/clinic for pacer check as ordered after 1–2–3 R.N. visits.
20. Client/Family will take pulse as ordered after 1–2 R.N. visits.
21. Client/Family will seek battery replacement/pacemaker replacement as ordered after 1–2–3–4 R.N. visits.
22. Client/Family will seek laboratory testing/M.D. appointments as ordered after 1–2 R.N. visits.

III. LONG-TERM GOALS

1. Adequate functioning of pacemaker will be constant in 1–2 weeks.
2. Adequate cardiac status will be achieved in 1–2 weeks.
3. Activities of daily living will be resumed in 1–2 weeks.
4. Optimal level of health will be achieved in 3–4 weeks.

IV. OUTCOME CRITERIA

1. Vital signs are normal.
2. Chest is clear; breathing is normal.
3. CBC with differential remains normal.
4. Serum enzyme levels (SGOT, LDH, and CPK) are normal.
5. Appetite is normal.
6. Weight is appropriate.
7. Intake and output are normal.
8. Skin is healthy and intact.
9. Peripheral pulse rates are normal.
10. Pacemaker batteries are changed as ordered.
11. Pacemaker functions appropriately.
12. Exercise is tolerated well.

13. Client is alert, oriented, and in good spirits.

14. Client states he/she feels better.

V. NURSING INTERVENTION/TREATMENT

1. R.N. will arrange to visit client at home.

2. R.N. will monitor and record apical and radial pulse rates, blood pressure, peripheral pulse rates, and laboratory testing (CBC with differential/electrolytes/digitalis level/prothrombin time/partial thromboplastin time and sedimentation rate) as ordered by M.D.

3. R.N. will instruct client/family/H.H.A. on:

   A. disease process.

   B. taking/apical and radial/peripheral pulse rates.

   C. medication administration (anticoagulants/nitrites/diuretics/ tranquilizers/antihypertensives/stool softeners)/adverse reactions.

   D. immediate notification of M.D. of adverse reactions or change in condition.

   E. pacemaker precautions (asynchronous [set-rate]/synchronous/ demand/external pacemaker). R.N. will stress the avoidance of certain types of electrical equipment around the pacemaker (depending on type and frequency of pacemaker) as ordered by M.D. Client should avoid the use of extension cords, worn electrical cords, plugs, or outlets around pacemaker as ordered by M.D. For external pacemaker use, client should avoid touching settings, dials, and connectors and avoid close personal contact, to prevent dislodgment. R.N. will stress that client seek pacemaker change/battery change as ordered. For adverse sign/symptom of disease or pacemaker malfunctioning, immediately contact M.D. For pacer check via telephone, client will rent/purchase pacing unit for home use. Instructions for use will be kept in home for routine check. Client or significant others will follow instructions on positioning (usually at kitchen table)/application of lubricant/wristbands (electrodes)/ placement of pacing wires/placement of magnet over pacemaker site/pacer recording over phone. For pacer check in hospital, client will keep designated appointments.

   F. emergency phone numbers to be kept at bedside.

   G. exercise/stair climbing/lifting/daily rest periods as ordered.

   H. fluid intake/dietary regimen as ordered.

   I. air travel as ordered by M.D.

   J. avoidance of temperature extremes and inclement weather.

    K. weight reduction/daily recording of weight.

    L. avoidance of/reduction in smoking.

    M. recording of intake and output.

    N. chair rest/bed rest.

    O. bowel regimen/avoidance of straining at stool.

    P. decreased work hours on returning to work.

    Q. diversional activities.

    R. sexual activity.

    S. laboratory testing/M.D. appointments.

    T. financial assistance.

    U. rehabilitative housing with elevator.

    V. insurance coverage.

4. R.N. will provide client/family with instructional literature, visual aids, organizations, clubs to contact for further assistance.

5. R.N. will assign additional personnel (e.g., M.S.W., clergy) to case if ordered.

6. R.N. will provide M.D. with follow-up reports and discharge summary when case closes.

7. R.N. will notify client/family/significant others when case will close.

Parkinson's Disease Care Plan

I. NURSING DIAGNOSIS

1. Anxiety related to:
   A. the unknown.
   B. loss of physical control.
   C. impaired body image.
   D. dependence on others for care.
   E. other _____

2. Knowledge deficit related to:
   A. signs/symptoms.
   B. medication administration/adverse reactions.
   C. exercise/rest.
   D. fluid/dietary needs.
   E. physical therapy/speech therapy.
   F. other _____

3. Altered nutrition: potential for more than body requirements related to:
   A. difficulty with mastication.
   B. anorexia.
   C. dependence on others for care.
   D. other _____

4. Potential for injury related to:
   A. bone demineralization.
   B. falls/accidents.

   C. fractures.

   D. weakness/fatigue.

   E. shuffling gait.

   F. other _____

   _____

5. Impaired physical mobility related to:

   A. weakness/fatigue.

   B. fractures.

   C. confusion.

   D. rigidity of upper/lower extremities.

   E. other _____

   _____

6. Self-care deficit: feeding/bathing/grooming/dressing/toileting related to:

   A. rigidity of upper/lower extremities.

   B. confusion.

   C. tremors.

   D. dependence on others for care.

   E. poor mobility.

   F. other _____

   _____

7. Constipation/Diarrhea related to:

   A. poor fluid/dietary intake.

   B. poor medication administration.

   C. other _____

   _____

8. Impaired home maintenance management related to:

   A. dependence on others for care.

   B. poor mobility.

   C. poor ambulation.

   D. other _____

   _____

9. Powerlessness related to:

   A. tremors.

   B. accidents/falls.

   C. confusion.

   D. difficulty with speech.

   E. other _____

   _____

10. Sleep pattern disturbance related to:
    A. tremors.
    B. anxiety.
    C. other _____

    _____

II. SHORT-TERM GOALS

1. Client/Family will verbalize fears, anxieties, and concerns after 1–2–3 R.N. visits.
2. Client/Family will administer medication as ordered after 1–2–3 R.N. visits.
3. Client/Family will immediately notify M.D. of adverse reactions or change in condition after 1–2 R.N. visits.
4. Client will ingest supplemental feedings as ordered after 1–2–3 R.N. visits.
5. Client/Family will use electric warming tray during prolonged meals after 1–2 R.N. visits.
6. Client/Family will increase fluid intake after 1–2 R.N. visits.
7. Client/Family will prepare high-residue meals as ordered after 1–2 R.N. visits.
8. Client/Family will practice/assist with stretching exercises as ordered after 1–2–3–4 R.N./P.T. visits.
9. Client will take warm baths as ordered after 1–2 R.N. visits.
10. Client will walk erect, using a broad base, after 1–2–3–4 R.N./P.T. visits.
11. Client will use a raised toilet seat after 1–2 R.N. visits.
12. Client will maintain a normal daily bowel routine after 1–2–3 R.N. visits.
13. Client will weigh self daily after 1–2 R.N. visits.
14. Client/Family will seek laboratory testing/M.D. appointments as ordered after 1–2 R.N. visits.
15. Client/Family will practice/assist with fine motor exercises after 1–2–3–4 R.N./O.T. visits.
16. Client/Family will participate in diversional activities after 1–2–3 R.N. visits.

III. LONG-TERM GOALS

1. Independent activities of daily living will be resumed in 1–2 weeks.

2. Normal ambulation will be achieved in 1–2 weeks.

3. Adequate verbal communication will be achieved in 1–2 weeks.

4. Optimal level of health will remain as long as possible, given progressive nature of disease.

IV. OUTCOME CRITERIA

1. Vital signs are normal.

2. Anxiety is overcome.

3. Tremors are controlled.

4. Regular bowel/bladder elimination occurs.

5. Appetite is normal.

6. Speech is unimpaired and coherent.

7. Weight is appropriate for height.

8. Drooling subsides.

9. Gait is normal.

10. Client states he/she feels better.

V. NURSING INTERVENTION/TREATMENT

1. R.N. will allow client/family to verbalize fears, anxieties, and concerns about parkinsonism.

2. On initial home visit, R.N. will obtain concise history and perform physical examination to determine all limitations.

3. R.N. will assess home for safety precautions and remove obstacles that may impede ambulation.

4. R.N. will instruct client/family/H.H.A. on:

A. monitoring and recording of vital signs.

B. daily recording of weight/ingesting supplemental feedings if ordered.

C. mouth care/personal hygiene.

D. meal preparation, with special attention to high-residue diet for severe constipation and warming tray for prolonged meals. R.N. will assess difficulty with mastication.

E. fluid intake as ordered: 1000–2000 cc daily to offset fluid lost in drooling or inhibited intestinal secretions.

F. medication administration/adverse reactions.

G. immediate notification of M.D. of adverse reactions or change in condition.

H. normal daily bowel routine/raised toilet seat if needed.

I. safety precautions in home.

    J. laboratory testing/M.D. appointments.

5. R.N. will consult with P.T. about active, passive, and postural exercises as ordered by M.D.; will provide client with assistive devices for ambulation (e.g., cane/quad cane/walker/wheelchair/ grab bars) and contact medical equipment company; will encourage elimination of throw rugs, to prevent falls.

6. R.N. will consult with M.D. about additional services (e.g., speech therapy, occupational therapy, social services).

7. R.N. will refer client/family to organizations, clubs, societies for additional assistance.

8. R.N. will provide M.D. with follow-up reports and discharge summary when case closes.

9. R.N. will encourage client to remain as functionally independent as possible.

10. R.N. will notify client/family/H.H.A./significant others when case will close.

Pediculosis Control Care Plan

I. NURSING DIAGNOSIS

1. Knowledge deficit related to:
   A. prevention/treatment of pediculosis capitis/corporis/pubis.
   B. medication administration/adverse reactions.
   C. signs/symptoms.
   D. good personal hygiene habits.
   E. poor understanding of transmission.
   F. other _____

2. Anxiety related to:
   A. transmission of pediculosis.
   B. social isolation.
   C. other _____

3. Noncompliance with therapy related to:
   A. denial.
   B. cost of treatment.
   C. other _____

4. Potential for infection related to:
   A. intense scratching.
   B. poor personal hygiene habits.
   C. other _____

5. Self-esteem disturbance related to embarrassment of lice infestation.

6. Potential impaired skin integrity related to:
   A. pruritus.
   B. scratching.
   C. skin irritation.
   D. other ⎯⎯⎯⎯⎯⎯⎯⎯⎯⎯⎯⎯⎯⎯⎯⎯⎯
   ⎯⎯⎯⎯⎯⎯⎯⎯⎯⎯⎯⎯⎯⎯⎯⎯⎯⎯⎯⎯⎯⎯⎯

II. SHORT-TERM GOALS

1. Client/Family will purchase necessary supplies (benzyl benzoate/benzene hexachloride) before R.N. visits home.
2. Client/Family will cut/shave hair if necessary after 1–2 R.N. visits.
3. Client/Family will apply prescribed pediculicide after 1 R.N. visit.
4. Client/Family will comb hair appropriately to remove nits after 1–2 R.N. visits.
5. Client will avoid crowded areas after 1–2 R.N. visits.

III. LONG-TERM GOALS

1. Adequate personal hygiene will be maintained after 1–2 weeks.
2. Treatment of primary contacts in community will be established in 2 weeks.
3. Lice will be eradicated in 1–2 weeks.

IV. OUTCOME CRITERIA

1. Client's/Family's hair remains clean.
2. Client/Family have established good habits of personal hygiene.
3. Client's/Family's clothing, bed linen, furniture, personal care articles remain clean.

V. NURSING INTERVENTION/TREATMENT

1. As casefinder, R.N. will examine all potential contacts in community and institute treatment as ordered by M.D.
2. R.N. will instruct client/family/H.H.A. on:
   A. prevention of cross-contamination/avoidance of contacts.
   B. shampooing, combing, cutting, shaving of hair.
   C. personal hygiene measures.
   D. application of pediculicide.

    E. cleanliness of environment (e.g., clothing, bed linen, personal care items, furniture).

3. R.N. will provide M.D. with follow-up reports and discharge summary when case closes.
4. R.N. will notify day care/school when client may reattend.
5. R.N. will notify client/family/H.H.A./significant others when case will close.

Peripheral Vascular Disease Care Plan

I. NURSING DIAGNOSIS

1. Anxiety related to:
   A. numbness/tingling in lower extremities.
   B. pain.
   C. difficulty with ambulation.
   D. gangrene.
   E. fear of amputation.
   F. other _____

2. Activity intolerance related to:
   A. pain.
   B. numbness/tingling in lower extremities.
   C. other _____

3. Ineffective individual/family coping related to:
   A. dependence on others for care.
   B. unemployment.
   C. cost of medical care/poor insurance coverage.
   D. other _____

4. Noncompliance with therapy related to:
   A. denial.
   B. lack of support in the home.

C. other _____

_____

5. Self-care deficit: feeding/bathing/grooming/dressing/toileting related to:
   A. poor mobility.
   B. dependence on others for care.
   C. confusion.
   D. other _____

_____

6. Potential for injury related to:
   A. poor fit of shoes.
   B. poor dressing care.
   C. falls/accidents.
   D. lack of exercise.
   E. other _____

_____

7. Potential impaired skin integrity related to:
   A. skin breakdown.
   B. injuries.
   C. poor skin care.
   D. poor dressing care.
   E. poor footwear.
   F. other _____

_____

8. Altered peripheral tissue perfusion related to:
   A. trophic changes.
   B. poor circulation.
   C. edema.
   D. other _____

_____

9. Knowledge deficit related to:
   A. prevention/treatment of peripheral vascular disease.
   B. medication administration/adverse reactions.
   C. exercise/rest.
   D. avoidance/limitation of smoking.
   E. avoidance of emotional stress.
   F. other _____

_____

10. Impaired home maintenance management related to:
    A. poor/restricted ambulation.
    B. lack of support in the home.
    C. dependence on others for care.
    D. other _____

    _____

II. SHORT-TERM GOALS

1. Client/Family will verbalize fears, anxieties, and concerns after 1–2 R.N. visits.
2. Client/Family will administer medication as ordered after 1–2–3 R.N. visits.
3. Client/Family will notify M.D. immediately of adverse reactions or change in condition after 1–2 R.N. visits.
4. Client will limit/abstain from smoking after 1–2–3–4 R.N. visits.
5. Client will wear properly fitting footwear after 1–2 R.N. visits.
6. Client will avoid wearing constrictive clothing (e.g., girdles, belts, circular garters) after 1–2 R.N. visits.
7. Client will wear supportive stockings after 1–2 R.N. visits.
8. Client will avoid temperature extremes after 1–2 R.N. visits.
9. Client/Family will engage in active/passive range-of-motion exercises after 1–2 R.N. visits.
10. Client/Family will limit stressful events after 1–2–3 R.N. visits.
11. Client will sleep with head of bed elevated after 1–2 R.N. visits.
12. Client will take warm baths as ordered after 1–2 R.N. visits.
13. Client/Family will apply dressings as ordered after 1–2–3 R.N. visits.
14. Client/Family will seek laboratory testing/M.D. appointments as ordered after 1–2 R.N. visits.

III. LONG-TERM GOALS

1. Independent activities of daily living will be resumed in 1–2 weeks.
2. Normal circulation to all extremities will be achieved in 1–2 weeks.
3. Optimal level of health will be achieved in 3–4 weeks.

IV. OUTCOME CRITERIA

1. Vital signs are normal.
2. All peripheral pulses are equal and palpable.
3. Skin is healthy and intact.
4. Ambulation is normal.
5. Weight is appropriate for height.
6. Client states he/she feels better.

V. NURSING INTERVENTION/TREATMENT

1. R.N. will instruct client/family/H.H.A. on:
   A. medication administration/adverse reactions.
   B. immediate notification of M.D. of adverse reactions or change in condition.
   C. limited/avoidance of smoking.
   D. nonconstricting clothing/footwear.
   E. avoidance of stress/temperature extremes.
   F. prevention of infection/injury.
   G. elevation of head of bed.
   H. dressing care.
   I. active/passive exercises.
   J. personal hygiene measures.
   K. good posture/avoidance of prolonged standing/crossing of legs.
   L. laboratory testing/M.D. appointments.
   M. diet/vitamin therapy.
   N. use of footboard/bed cradle.
2. R.N. will confer with P.T. on exercise regimen if ordered by M.D.
3. R.N. will provide M.D. with follow-up reports and discharge summary when case closes.
4. R.N. will notify client/family/H.H.A./significant others when case will close.

Postcataract
Care Plan

I. NURSING DIAGNOSIS

1. Sensory/Perceptual alterations (visual) related to:
   A. eye dressings/patches after surgery.
   B. induction of eye medication.
   C. contact lens application.
   D. application of glasses (altered prescription of glasses, possibly with darkened lens).
   E. intraocular lens implant/contact lens application.
   F. other _____
   _____

2. Knowledge deficit related to:
   A. eye medication administration/proper hand washing/adverse reactions.
   B. dressing care/application of eye patch.
   C. contact lens application/care of lenses.
   D. glasses.
   E. surgical removal of cataract/laser surgery.
   F. intraocular lens implant.
   G. signs/symptoms of pain/nausea/bleeding/floaters/veils/infection.
   H. positioning/avoidance of stooping over/jerky movements/ bumping or rubbing eye/coughing/sneezing/blowing nose/ straining at stool/reading.
   I. potential for accidents.
   J. orientation to surroundings.
   K. other _____
   _____

3. Potential for injury related to:
    A. poor hand-washing technique.
    B. poor protection during sporting events.
    C. poor safety monitoring by significant others.
    D. blindness.
    E. other _____

    _____

4. Self-care deficit: feeding/bathing/grooming/dressing/toileting related to:
    A. poor visual response.
    B. confusion.
    C. blindness.
    D. other _____

    _____

5. Impaired home maintenance management related to:
    A. poor visual response.
    B. blindness.
    C. other _____

    _____

6. Impaired physical mobility related to:
    A. altered visual response.
    B. blindness.
    C. other _____

    _____

7. Potential for infection related to:
    A. indiscriminate use of eye medication.
    B. poor hand-washing technique.
    C. injuries to eye.
    D. other _____

    _____

8. Noncompliance with therapy related to:
    A. fear.
    B. denial.
    C. cost of medication/poor insurance coverage.
    D. other _____

    _____

II. SHORT-TERM GOALS

1. Client/Family will verbalize fears, anxieties, and concerns after 1–2 R.N. visits.
2. Client/Family will wash hands correctly after 1–2 R.N. visits.
3. Client/Family will instill eye medication as ordered after 1–2 R.N. visits.
4. Client/Family will demonstrate eye dressing as ordered after 1–2 R.N. visits.
5. Client/Family will administer oral medication as ordered after 1–2 R.N. visits.
6. Client/Family will immediately notify M.D. of adverse reactions or change in condition after 1–2 R.N. visits.
7. Client/Family will remove obstacles to prevent injury after 1–2 R.N. visits.
8. Client/Family will apply contact lenses as ordered after 1–2 R.N. visits.
9. Client will wear prescribed eyeglasses after 1–2 R.N. visits.
10. Client/Family will visit M.D. as ordered after 1–2 R.N. visits.

III. LONG-TERM GOALS

1. Normal vision will resume in 2–3 weeks.
2. Independent activities of daily living will be resumed in 1–2 weeks.
3. Optimal level of health will be achieved in 3–4 weeks.

IV. OUTCOME CRITERIA

1. Vital signs are normal.
2. Corneas are healed.
3. Vision is clear in both eyes.
4. Client states he/she feels better.

V. NURSING INTERVENTION/TREATMENT

1. R.N. will contact client/family before admission to ensure proper supplies are available in the home.
2. R.N. will reorient client to home surroundings if vision is poor.
3. R.N. will instruct client/family/H.H.A. on:
   A. proper hand-washing technique.
   B. medication administration/instillation/adverse reactions.

    C. avoidance/limitation of coughing, smoking, bending, moving too rapidly, stressful situations, temperature extremes.

    D. application and care of contact lenses.

    E. immediate notification of M.D. of change in condition.

    F. cleansing of eyes.

    G. glasses.

    H. M.D. appointments.

4. R.N. will encourage client to contact organizations for those with impaired sight; will provide literature for education about condition.

5. R.N. will provide M.D. with follow-up reports and discharge summary when case closes.

6. R.N. will notify client/family/H.H.A./significant others when case will close.

Postcraniotomy
Care Plan

I. NURSING DIAGNOSIS

1. Anxiety related to:
   A. aphasia.
   B. pain.
   C. poor vision/blindness.
   D. possible malignancy.
   E. headaches.
   F. seizure disorder.
   G. other _____

2. Knowledge deficit related to:
   A. frequent need for monitoring of vital signs.
   B. dressing care.
   C. exercise/rest.
   D. medication administration/adverse reactions.
   E. placement of ventriculovenous shunt.
   F. increased intracranial pressure.
   G. avoidance of stress.
   H. other _____

3. Potential for infection related to:
   A. inadequate turning/positioning in bed.
   B. inadequate fluid/dietary intake.
   C. dependence on others for care.
   D. immobility.

    E. poor administration of medication.

    F. other _____

_____

4. Impaired verbal communication related to:
    A. aphasia.
    B. other _____

_____

5. Diversional activity deficit related to:
    A. weakness/paralysis.
    B. blindness.
    C. deafness.
    D. other _____

_____

6. Ineffective individual/family coping related to:
    A. irritability.
    B. medical costs/poor insurance coverage.
    C. extensive physical care needs.
    D. other _____

_____

7. Fear related to postoperative complications.
8. Constipation/Diarrhea/Incontinence related to:
    A. dependence on others for care.
    B. paralysis.
    C. poor fluid intake.
    D. other _____

_____

9. Impaired home maintenance management related to:
    A. weakness/paralysis.
    B. lethargy.
    C. semicomatose state.
    D. comatose state.
    E. other _____

_____

10. Altered nutrition: potential for more than body requirements
    related to:
    A. anorexia.
    B. change in diet.
    C. poor food preparation.

    D. lack of assistance in home.

    E. other ⸺⸺⸺⸺⸺⸺⸺⸺⸺⸺⸺⸺⸺⸺⸺⸺⸺⸺

11. Potential for injury related to:

    A. infection.

    B. seizure disorder.

    C. poor safety monitoring by significant others.

    D. refusal to administer medication.

    E. other ⸺⸺⸺⸺⸺⸺⸺⸺⸺⸺⸺⸺⸺⸺⸺⸺⸺⸺

12. Impaired physical mobility related to:

    A. weakness/paralysis.

    B. need for assistive devices.

    C. other ⸺⸺⸺⸺⸺⸺⸺⸺⸺⸺⸺⸺⸺⸺⸺⸺⸺⸺

13. Self-care deficit: feeding/bathing/grooming/toileting related to:

    A. immobility.

    B. weakness.

    C. paralysis.

    D. blindness.

    E. other ⸺⸺⸺⸺⸺⸺⸺⸺⸺⸺⸺⸺⸺⸺⸺⸺⸺⸺

14. Self-esteem disturbance related to:

    A. alopecia.

    B. paralysis.

    C. inability to work.

    D. other ⸺⸺⸺⸺⸺⸺⸺⸺⸺⸺⸺⸺⸺⸺⸺⸺⸺⸺

15. Sensory/Perceptual alterations (visual/auditory/tactile/kinesthetic/gustatory/olfactory) related to:

    A. altered levels of consciousness.

    B. craniotomy.

    C. advance of disease process.

    D. other ⸺⸺⸺⸺⸺⸺⸺⸺⸺⸺⸺⸺⸺⸺⸺⸺⸺⸺

16. Sexual dysfunction related to:

    A. weakness.

    B. paralysis.

C. metastasis.

D. apathy.

E. other _____

_____

17. Potential impaired skin integrity related to:

A. poor positioning in bed.

B. poor skin care.

C. leakage of Texas/Foley catheter.

D. bowel/bladder incontinence.

E. falls/accidents.

F. other _____

_____

18. Sleep pattern disturbance related to:

A. restlessness.

B. fear of dying.

C. pain.

D. bowel/bladder incontinence.

E. grieving.

F. seizure disorder.

G. other _____

_____

19. Altered patterns of urinary elimination related to:

A. altered levels of consciousness.

B. inadequate fluid intake.

C. other _____

_____

20. Social isolation related to:

A. anger/hostility.

B. confinement to home.

C. paralysis.

D. other _____

_____

II. SHORT-TERM GOALS

1. Client/Family will express fears, anxieties, and concerns to R.N. after 1–2–3–4 R.N. visits.

2. Client/Family will perform appropriate skin care after 1–2–3 R.N. visits.

3. Client/Family will apply prescribed bed cradle/heel bolsters/air mattress/footboard/bed trapeze/sandbags/waterbed/braces/splints after 1–2–3 R.N. visits.
4. Client/Family will carry out good personal hygiene measures after 1–2 R.N. visits.
5. Family will position client properly in bed every 2 hours after 1–2 R.N. visits.
6. Client/Family will provide a quiet, nonstressful environment after 1–2 R.N. visits.
7. Client/Family will maintain raised side rails in bed at all times after 1–2 R.N. visits.
8. Client/Family will administer prescribed medication as ordered after 1–2–3 R.N. visits.
9. Client/Family will notify M.D. of adverse reactions or change in condition after 1–2 R.N. visits.
10. Client/Family will exercise/rest as ordered after 1–2–3–4 R.N. visits.
11. Client/Family will administer prescribed respiratory therapy after 1–2–3–4 R.N./R.T. visits.
12. Client/Family will carry out all instructions in speech therapy/ occupational therapy/physical therapy if additional personnel are assigned after 1–2 R.N./P.T./O.T./S.T. visits.
13. Client/Family will apply for financial aid after 1–2 R.N. visits.
14. Client/Family will ambulate/assist with ambulation as ordered after 1–2 R.N. visits.
15. Client/Family will monitor IV therapy in home after 1–2–3–4 R.N. visits.
16. Client/Family will report any bleeding, infiltration, or stoppage of fluid at IV site after 1–2–3–4 R.N. visits.
17. Client will consume adequate amount fluids/diet as ordered after 1–2–3–4 R.N. visits.
18. Family will keep padded tongue blade near client at all times after 1–2 R.N. visits.
19. Client/Family will participate in diversional activities after 1–2–3 R.N. visits.
20. Client/Family will visit M.D. routinely/seek further laboratory testing after 1–2 R.N. visits.
21. Client/Family will change dressings as ordered after 1–2–3–4 R.N. visits.
22. Client/Family will obtain educational materials/information on career counseling after 5–10 R.N. visits.

III. LONG-TERM GOALS

1. Independent activities of daily living will be resumed in 1–2 weeks.
2. Optimal level of health will be achieved in 3–4 weeks.

IV. OUTCOME CRITERIA

1. Client is alert, cooperative, and sociable.
2. Speech is intelligible.
3. Communication remains adequate.
4. Vision is clear.
5. Hearing is normal.
6. Independent ambulation is resumed.
7. Skin integrity remains healthy and intact.
8. Granulation occurs.
9. Vital signs remain normal.
10. Pupils are equal and react to normal light accommodation.
11. Bowel/Bladder control is normal.
12. Reflexes are normal.
13. Appetite is normal.
14. Weight is normal.
15. Chest is clear; airway is patent.
16. Client states he/she feels better.

V. NURSING INTERVENTION/TREATMENT

1. R.N. will consult with hospital discharge planner about status of client and rehabilitation goals.
2. R.N. will arrange for any medical equipment to be delivered before or on day of hospital discharge.
3. R.N. will assess family's financial and medical coverage because therapy may become quite costly.
4. R.N. will instruct client/family/H.H.A. on:
    A. daily monitoring and recording of vital signs. R.N. will instruct a family member to monitor blood pressure if possible.
    B. seizure precautions; keeping padded tongue blade within reach at all times.
    C. medication administration/adverse reactions.
    D. immediate notification of M.D. of adverse reactions or change in condition.

    E. various types of medical equipment if needed (e.g., respiratory equipment, air mattress, water bed, sheepskin, hospital bed, padded side rails, splints, bed cradle, commode, wheelchair, crutches, cane, quad cane, walker, Hoyer lift, heel bolsters, helmet).

    F. availability of emergency phone numbers.

    G. chest physical therapy/inhalation therapy/breathing exercises.

    H. IV therapy/enteral feedings/hyperalimentation.

    I. skin care.

    J. positioning/turning every 1–2 hours.

    K. exercise/rest/ambulation as ordered.

    L. bowel/bladder regimen/catheter care/enema administration.

    M. eye care.

    N. fluid intake/dietary regimen as ordered.

    O. daily recording of weight.

    P. dressing care.

    Q. diversional activities/stimulation.

    R. respirator care.

    S. urine testing.

    T. laboratory testing/M.D. appointments.

    U. psychologic/spiritual support.

5. R.N. will assign additional personnel/services (e.g., M.S.W., P.T., O.T., S.T., cancer or rehabilitation services) to case if ordered.

6. R.N. will provide M.D. with follow-up reports and discharge summary when case closes.

7. R.N. will notify client/family/H.H.A./significant others when case will close.

Postoperative Dilation and Curettage Care Plan

I. NURSING DIAGNOSIS

1. Anxiety related to:
   A. potential discomfort following procedure.
   B. results of tissue biopsy.
   C. postoperative bleeding.
   D. postoperative incapacity.
   E. cost of medical care/poor insurance coverage.
   F. other _____

2. Constipation related to:
   A. low back pain.
   B. low pelvic pain.
   C. poor fluid intake.
   D. poor dietary intake.
   E. lack of exercise.
   F. other _____

3. Altered patterns of urinary elimination related to:
   A. low back pain.
   B. low pelvic pain.
   C. other _____

4. Activity intolerance related to:
   A. internal packing.

    B. low pelvic pain.
    C. low back pain.
    D. headache.
    E. nausea.
    F. constipation.
    G. dizziness.
    H. hemorrhage.
    I. other _____

5. Fear related to:
    A. hemorrhage.
    B. other _____

6. Impaired home maintenance management related to:
    A. postoperative fatigue.
    B. headache.
    C. pain.
    D. restricted ambulation/bed rest.
    E. other _____

7. Knowledge deficit related to:
    A. medication administration/adverse reactions.
    B. postoperative vaginal drainage.
    C. internal packing.
    D. personal hygiene/perineal care.
    E. fluids/diet.
    F. exercise/rest.
    G. hemorrhage.
    H. postoperative douche.
    I. tampon insertion.
    J. coitus.
    K. other _____

8. Impaired physical mobility related to:
    A. hemorrhage.
    B. low pelvic pain.
    C. low back pain.
    D. other _____

9. Altered nutrition: potential for more than body requirements related to:
    A. nausea.
    B. fatigue.
    C. dizziness.
    D. low pelvic pain.
    E. low back pain.
    F. hemorrhage.
    G. other _____

    _____

10. Altered oral mucous membrane related to:
    A. dysphagia after airway removal.
    B. decreased fluid intake.
    C. other _____

    _____

11. Sexual dysfunction related to:
    A. internal packing.
    B. low back pain.
    C. low pelvic pain.
    D. drainage.
    E. hemorrhage.
    F. other _____

    _____

12. Sleep pattern disturbance related to:
    A. discomfort of internal packing.
    B. low back pain.
    C. low pelvic pain.
    D. hemorrhage.
    E. other _____

    _____

II. SHORT-TERM GOALS

1. Client will report any abnormal signs of drainage or hemorrhage after 1 R.N. visit.
2. Client will perform perineal care/personal hygiene as ordered after 1 R.N. visit.
3. Client will rest/exercise as ordered after 1 R.N. visit.
4. Client will refrain from douching as ordered by M.D. after 1 R.N. visit.

   5. Client will avoid use of tampons as ordered by M.D. after 1 R.N. visit.

   6. Client will refrain from coitus as ordered by M.D. after 1 R.N. visit.

   7. Client will seek laboratory testing/M.D. appointments as ordered after 1 R.N. visit.

   8. Client will take fluids/diet as ordered after 1 R.N. visit.

   9. Client will take medications as ordered after 1 R.N. visit.

  10. Client will immediately notify M.D. of reactions to medications after 1 R.N. visit.

  11. Client will administer hot water bottle/heating pad to back or abdomen as ordered after 1 R.N. visit.

  12. Client will take warm baths/showers as ordered after 1 R.N. visit.

III. LONG-TERM GOALS

   1. Activities of daily living will be resumed in 1–2 weeks.

   2. Optimal level of health will be achieved in 2–4 weeks.

IV. OUTCOME CRITERIA

   1. Vital signs are normal.

   2. Hemoglobin and hematocrit levels remain normal.

   3. Menses are normal.

   4. Cervical/Endometrial tissue is normal.

   5. Appetite remains normal.

   6. Sleep pattern remains normal.

   7. Ambulation is normal.

   8. Bowel/Bladder status is normal.

   9. Client states she feels better.

  10. Client resumes employment.

V. NURSING INTERVENTION/TREATMENT

   1. R.N. will instruct client on:

     A. fluid/dietary intake.

     B. medication administration/adverse reactions.

     C. immediate notification of M.D. of adverse reactions or change in condition.

     D. douching.

     E. use of tampons.

    F. coitus.

    G. exercise/rest.

    H. application of hot water bottle/heating pad to abdomen or lower back.

    I. warm baths/showers.

    J. perineal care.

    K. laboratory testing.

    L. M.D. appointments.

2. R.N. will provide M.D. with follow-up reports and discharge summary when case closes.

3. R.N. will notify client when case will close.

Postoperative Ear
Care Plan

I. NURSING DIAGNOSIS

1. Potential anxiety related to:
   A. hearing impairment.
   B. vertigo.
   C. infection.
   D. edema.
   E. excess cerumen.
   F. facial nerve involvement (difficulty wrinkling forehead/closing eyes/puckering lips/baring teeth).
   G. other _____
   _____

2. Knowledge deficit related to:
   A. proper hand-washing technique.
   B. aseptic dressing technique.
   C. cleansing of external ear and surrounding skin.
   D. signs/symptoms of facial nerve injury (difficulty wrinkling forehead/closing eyes/puckering lips/baring teeth).
   E. vertigo.
   F. edema.
   G. short memory/poor comprehension/short attention span.
   H. avoidance of blowing nose/inserting foreign bodies into ear.
   I. braiding/moving hair away from surgical site.
   J. medication administration/adverse reactions.
   K. other _____
   _____

3. Potential for infection related to:
   A. facial nerve injury (difficulty wrinkling forehead/closing eyes/ puckering lips/baring teeth).
   B. poor hand-washing technique.
   C. insertion of foreign body into ear.
   D. poor irrigation technique.
   E. poor administration of medication.
   F. other _____

4. Potential for injury related to:
   A. vertigo.
   B. infection.
   C. poor aseptic technique.
   D. blowing of nose.
   E. poor personal hygiene.
   F. poor secretion of cerumen.
   G. insertion of foreign bodies into ear.
   H. poor irrigation technique.
   I. other _____

5. Noncompliance with therapy related to:
   A. vertigo.
   B. immobility.
   C. refusal to carry out orders.
   D. other _____

6. Self-care deficit: feeding/bathing/grooming/dressing/toileting/ dressing care/administration of medication related to:
   A. difficult access to ear region.
   B. hemiplegia.
   C. vertigo.
   D. other _____

7. Potential impaired skin integrity related to:
   A. frequent dressing change.
   B. tape allergy.
   C. excessive drainage.
   D. poor healing powers.

E. other _____

_____

8. Sensory/Perceptual alterations (auditory) related to:
    A. vertigo.
    B. facial nerve involvement (difficulty wrinkling forehead/closing eyes/puckering lips/baring teeth).
    C. other _____

    _____

II. SHORT-TERM GOALS

1. Client/Family will verbalize fears, anxieties, and concerns after 1–2 R.N. visits.
2. Client/Family will demonstrate proper hand-washing technique after 1–2 R.N. visits.
3. Client/Family will cleanse external ear and surrounding skin as ordered after 1–2 R.N. visits.
4. Client/Family will administer medication as ordered after 1–2 R.N. visits.
5. Client/Family will immediately notify M.D. of adverse reactions or change in condition after 1 R.N. visit.
6. Client/Family will wipe (not blow) nose if necessary after 1 R.N. visit.
7. Client/Family will braid/secure hair away from ear after 1 R.N. visit.
8. Client/Family will change ear dressings using aseptic technique as ordered after 1–2 R.N. visits.
9. Client/Family will irrigate ear as ordered after 1–2 R.N. visits.
10. Client/Family will visit M.D. as ordered after 1 R.N. visit.

III. LONG-TERM GOAL

1. Normal hearing will be restored in 1–2 weeks.

IV. OUTCOME CRITERIA

1. Vital signs are normal.
2. Wound is healed.
3. Facial muscles function appropriately.
4. Eustachian tubes are patent; hearing is normal.

5. Equilibrium is normal.

6. Client states he/she feels better.

V. NURSING INTERVENTION/TREATMENT

1. R.N. will instruct client/family on:
   A. proper hand-washing technique.
   B. medication administration/adverse reactions/immediate reporting of to M.D.
   C. aseptic dressing technique.
   D. cleansing of external ear and surrounding skin/personal hygiene habits.
   E. signs/symptoms of facial nerve involvement (difficulty wrinkling forehead, closing eyes, puckering lips, baring teeth).
   F. ear irrigations (only if ordered specifically by M.D.).
   G. avoidance of blowing of nose (wiping with tissues only).
   H. avoidance of inserting foreign bodies into ear.
   I. immediate notification of M.D. of change in condition (e.g., edema, vertigo, hemorrhage, pain, infection).
   J. excessive cerumen accumulation.
   K. application of heating pad/hot water bottle.
   L. insertion of wick soaked in aluminum acetate solution (Burrow's solution).
   M. avoidance of trauma to ear.
   N. M.D. appointments.

2. R.N. will provide M.D. with follow-up reports and discharge summary when case closes.

3. R.N. will notify client/family/significant others when case will close.

Premenstrual Syndrome Care Plan

I. NURSING DIAGNOSIS

1. Knowledge deficit related to:
   A. impending signs/symptoms of premenstrual syndrome.
   B. medication administration/adverse reactions.
   C. fluid/dietary needs.
   D. infection.
   E. other _____

2. Anxiety related to:
   A. abdominal bloating.
   B. breast tenderness/pain.
   C. joint pains.
   D. menstrual cramps.
   E. suicidal feelings/attempts.
   F. other _____

3. Headache/Menstrual cramps related to:
   A. poor fluid/dietary intake.
   B. inadequate rest.
   C. inadequate exercise.
   D. poor administration of medication.
   E. infection.
   F. other _____

4. Constipation/Diarrhea related to:
   A. poor fluid/dietary intake.
   B. inadequate rest.
   C. stress.
   D. other _____

5. Potential for violence related to:
   A. suicidal tendencies/actual attempts.
   B. fatigue.
   C. tension.
   D. anxiety.
   E. irritability.
   F. other _____

6. Impaired physical mobility related to:
   A. abdominal cramping.
   B. low back pain.
   C. edematous ankles.
   D. other _____

7. Ineffective coping related to:
   A. dysmenorrhea.
   B. clumsiness.
   C. mood swings.
   D. other _____

8. Ineffective breathing pattern related to menstrual cramps.
9. Altered nutrition: less than body requirements related to uncharacteristic craving for sweets, salty foods, or alcohol.
10. Powerlessness related to:
    A. menstrual cramps.
    B. headaches (including migraines).
    C. appetite cravings (binges).
    D. hoarseness.
    E. asthma (and hayfever).
    F. panic attacks.
    G. mood swings.
    H. excessive monthly weight gain.

    I. painful joints.

    J. bloated abdomen.

    K. other _____

    _____

11. Altered parenting related to:
    A. headaches.
    B. menstrual cramps.
    C. other _____

    _____

12. Self-care deficit: feeding/bathing/grooming/dressing related to:
    A. headaches.
    B. menstrual cramps.
    C. other _____

    _____

13. Altered patterns of urinary elimination related to fluid retention.
14. Sleep pattern disturbance related to menstrual cramps.
15. Sexual dysfunction related to:
    A. irritability.
    B. low back pain.
    C. abdominal bloating.
    D. other _____

    _____

16. Activity intolerance related to:
    A. fatigue/weakness.
    B. vertigo.
    C. low back pain.
    D. other _____

    _____

17. Diversional activity deficit related to:
    A. irritability.
    B. menstrual cramps.
    C. headaches.
    D. other _____

    _____

II. SHORT-TERM GOALS

1. Client will read current literature on PMS after 1–2 R.N. visits.
2. Client will lie down and elevate feet to reduce nausea and dizziness after 1 R.N. visit.

3. Client will consume 6 small meals per day to regulate blood sugar levels and avoid depression or severe mood swings after 1–2 R.N. visits.

4. During menses client will consume meals consisting mainly of protein and complex carbohydrates (grains) after 1–2 R.N. visits.

5. Client will limit sodium intake and foods high in sodium after 1 R.N. visit.

6. Client will take tetracycline during menses as ordered to reduce acne after 1–2 R.N. visits.

7. Client will avoid emotional stress during menses to prevent cramping after 1–2 R.N. visits.

8. Client will exercise moderately during menses to prevent or reduce cramping after 1–2 R.N. visits.

9. Client will take analgesics/diuretics/birth control pills/antibiotics/antiprostaglandins after 1 R.N. visit.

10. Client will administer progesterone suppositories as ordered after 1–2 R.N. visits.

11. Client will take vitamin therapy (B_6, multivitamins with minerals, etc.) as ordered after 1 R.N. visit.

12. Client will avoid coffee, tea, cola drinks, tobacco, and chocolate, to reduce tension and anxiety and avoid painfully swollen breasts after 1–2 R.N. visits.

13. Client will administer hot water bottles/heating pad to abdomen or lower back after 1–2 R.N. visits.

14. Client will immediately notify M.D. of adverse reactions to medications or change in condition after 1 R.N. visit.

15. Client will take warm baths as ordered after 1 R.N. visit.

16. Client will consume warm fluids (warm broths, herbal teas, etc.) after 1–2 R.N. visits.

17. Client will reduce absenteeism from school/work after 1–2 R.N. visits.

18. Client will request literature from PMS groups/join women's groups after 1–2 R.N. visits.

III. LONG-TERM GOALS

1. Menstrual cycle will return to normal in 1–2 weeks.
2. Optimal level of health will be achieved in 1–2 months.
3. Activities of daily living will be resumed in 1 week.

IV. OUTCOME CRITERIA

1. Vital signs are normal.
2. Complexion remains clear.
3. Blood sugar level remains normal.
4. Prostaglandin level remains normal.
5. Appetite remains normal.
6. Progesterone level remains normal.
7. Hemoglobin and hematocrit levels remain normal.
8. Sleep pattern remains normal.
9. Exercise is tolerated well.
10. Mental status remains healthy.
11. School/work attendance remains adequate.
12. Client states she feels better.

V. NURSING INTERVENTION/TREATMENT

1. R.N. sees that client visits M.D. for complete history and physical examination and confirmation of PMS.
2. R.N. will instruct client on:
    A. definition and treatment of PMS.
    B. fluid intake/low sodium diet consisting mainly of high protein and complex carbohydrates (6 small meals, not snacks, daily).
    C. medication regimen (administration of birth control pills/ antibiotics/oral progesterone/analgesics/antiprostaglandins/ diuretics), immediate notification of M.D. of adverse reactions or change in condition.
    D. vitamin therapy (B$_6$, multivitamin with minerals) if ordered.
    E. avoidance of coffee, tea, cola drinks, tobacco, and chocolate, to reduce tension, anxiety, and painful breasts.
    F. application of hot water bottle/heating pad to abdomen or lower back.
    G. benefits of warm baths.
    H. consumption of warm fluids (broths and herbal teas).
    I. laboratory testing.
    J. routine M.D. appointments.
    K. exercise on regular basis (fast-paced walking 1–2 times for a half hour).
    L. infection control.
3. R.N. will provide toll-free number of PMS access services for information about PMS (1-800-222-4PMS); R.N. will provide a

referral list of physicians nationwide who treat the syndrome and books, pamphlets, cassettes, videotapes, slide shows, and *PMS Access Newsletter*.

4. R.N. will provide M.D. with follow-up reports and discharge summary when case closes.

5. R.N. will notify client when case will close.

Pulmonary Tuberculosis Care Plan

I. NURSING DIAGNOSIS

1. Anxiety related to:
   A. malaise.
   B. weight loss.
   C. abnormal findings of chest x-ray/sputum culture.
   D. night sweats.
   E. high fever.
   F. anorexia.
   G. loss of strength.
   H. frequent clearing of throat.
   I. hemoptysis.
   J. other _____

2. Ineffective thermoregulation related to:
   A. poor fluid/dietary intake.
   B. poor administration of medication.
   C. inadequate rest.
   D. inadequate exercise.
   E. alcoholism.
   F. other _____

3. Ineffective individual/family coping related to:
   A. irritability.
   B. denial of symptoms.
   C. frequent cough.

D. hemoptysis.
E. night sweats.
F. loss of strength.
G. intermittent elevated temperature.
H. other _____

4. Potential fluid volume deficit related to:
   A. poor fluid/dietary intake.
   B. vomiting.
   C. elevated temperature.
   D. night sweats.
   E. other _____

5. Self-care deficit: feeding/bathing/dressing/grooming related to:
   A. weakness.
   B. vomiting.
   C. abdominal pain.
   D. fever.
   E. other _____

6. Impaired home maintenance management related to:
   A. weakness.
   B. vomiting.
   C. abdominal pain.
   D. fever.
   E. dependence on others for care.
   F. other _____

7. Knowledge deficit related to:
   A. diagnosis and treatment of TB.
   B. communicability.
   C. testing/hospitalization.
   D. restriction of activity/ambulation.
   E. adequate ventilation.
   F. avoidance of crowded areas.
   G. prognosis.
   H. medication administration/adverse reactions.
   I. other _____

8. Impaired physical mobility related to:
   A. weakness.
   B. vomiting.
   C. abdominal pain.
   D. fever.
   E. other _____

   _____

9. Noncompliance with therapy related to:
   A. alcoholism/drug abuse.
   B. denial.
   C. cost of medical care/poor insurance coverage.
   D. dependence on others for care.
   E. other _____

   _____

10. Altered nutrition: potential for more than body requirements related to:
    A. vomiting/indigestion.
    B. weight loss.
    C. anorexia.
    D. weakness.
    E. poor understanding of good nutritional habits.
    F. poor understanding of adequate meal planning.
    G. learning deficit.
    H. poor understanding of consumer buying.
    I. other _____

    _____

11. Altered parenting related to:
    A. weakness.
    B. vomiting.
    C. impaired mobility.
    D. alcoholism/drug abuse.
    E. dependence on others for care.
    F. restriction of activity.
    G. child abuse/neglect.
    H. isolation.
    I. other _____

    _____

12. Potential for injury related to:
    A. lack of supervision in the home.

B. language barrier/poor understanding of treatment.

C. learning deficit.

D. other _____

13. Ineffective breathing patterns related to:

A. frequent, unproductive cough.

B. increased sputum expectoration.

C. hemoptysis.

D. dyspnea.

E. chest pain.

F. productive cough.

G. other _____

14. Sexual dysfunction related to:

A. weakness.

B. vomiting.

C. abdominal pain.

D. chest pain.

E. frequent cough.

F. fear of rejection by significant other.

G. isolation.

H. other _____

15. Sleep pattern disturbance related to:

A. vomiting.

B. abdominal pain.

C. chest pain.

D. hemoptysis.

E. frequent expectoration.

F. frequent cough.

G. other _____

16. Altered patterns of urinary elimination related to:

A. poor intake of fluids/diet.

B. alcoholism.

C. other _____

II. SHORT-TERM GOALS

1. Client/Family will verbalize fears, anxieties, and concerns after 1–2 R.N. visits.
2. Client/Family will seek adequate TB testing after 1–2 R.N. visits.
3. Client will consume nutritionally sound meals after 1–2 R.N. visits.
4. Client will avoid alcohol/addicting drugs as ordered after 1–2–3–4 R.N. visits.
5. Client will state 3 foods from each of the 4 food groups after 1–2 R.N. visits.
6. Client/Family will wash hands properly after 1–2 R.N. visits.
7. Client/Family will adequately dispose of tissues and infected articles after 1–2 R.N. visits.
8. Client/Family will provide adequate ventilation in home after 1–2 R.N. visits.
9. Client/Family will force fluids as ordered after 1–2 R.N. visits.
10. Client/Family will take vital signs as ordered after 1–2–3 R.N. visits.
11. Client/Family will apply cool tap water sponge for high fever as ordered after 1–2–3 R.N. visits.
12. Client will perform breathing exercises as ordered after 1–2–3 R.N. visits.
13. Client/Family will perform respiratory therapy as ordered after 1–2–3– R.N. visits.
14. Client will take medication as prescribed after 1–2–3 R.N. visits.
15. Client/Family will notify M.D. of adverse effects or change in condition after 1–2 R.N. visits.
16. Client/Family will seek laboratory testing/M.D. follow-up appointments as ordered after 1 R.N. visit.

III. LONG-TERM GOALS

1. Communicable disease will be controlled in 1–2 weeks.
2. Activities of daily living will be resumed in 1–2 weeks.
3. Optimal level of health will be achieved in 1–2 months.
4. Rehabilitation for alcoholism/drug abuse will occur in 1 month.

IV. OUTCOME CRITERIA

1. Vital signs are normal.
2. Appetite is normal.

3. Client consumes nutritious meals.
4. Chest is clear; breathing is normal.
5. Skin/Mucous membrane is healthy and intact.
6. Laboratory results are normal.
7. Strength is regained.
8. Weight is appropriate for height.
9. GI system functions appropriately.
10. Client states he/she feels better.

V. NURSING INTERVENTION/TREATMENT

1. R.N. will contact hospital discharge planner about treatment and rehabilitation goals.
2. R.N. will instruct client/family/H.H.A. on:
   A. diagnosis and treatment of TB.
   B. adequate TB testing/screening for all family members.
   C. monitoring and recording of vital signs.
   D. oral hygiene.
   E. proper hand-washing technique.
   F. adequate disposal of tissues and contaminated articles.
   G. proper ventilation.
   H. fluid intake/dietary regimen as ordered/meal planning.
   I. vitamin therapy.
   J. medication administration/adverse reactions.
   K. immediate notification of M.D. of adverse reactions or change in condition.
   L. breathing exercises/respiratory therapy and care of equipment.
   M. dressing care after surgery.
   N. avoidance of alcohol/addicting drugs.
   O. rest/restricted exercise as ordered.
   P. prevention of cross-contamination/avoidance of crowded or overpolluted areas.
   Q. prevention of respiratory infections (bronchitis, pneumonia).
   R. daily recording of weight.
   S. yearly physical examinations/lifetime medical supervision/ laboratory testing.
   T. diversional activities.
3. R.N. will assign additional personnel (e.g., P.T., M.S.W., R.T., home attendant, homemaker, housekeeper) to case if ordered.

4. R.N. will encourage client to seek counseling for alcoholism/drug abuse; will provide client with names of organizations and rehabilitation centers where he/she may seek additional assistance.

5. R.N. will provide M.D. with follow-up reports and discharge summary when case closes.

6. R.N. will notify client/family/H.H.A./significant others when case will close.

Renal Calculi
Care Plan

I. NURSING DIAGNOSIS

1. Knowledge deficit related to:
   A. medication administration/adverse reactions.
   B. signs/symptoms.
   C. fluids/diet.
   D. urodynamic testing/kidney and bladder x-rays/ cystourethroscopy.
   E. other _____

2. Pain/Dull ache in groin/Anterior pain radiating to testicle in men/ Anterior pain radiating to bladder in women/Tenderness in loin area related to:
   A. passage of renal calculi in urine.
   B. inadequate fluid intake.
   C. overconsumption of calcium.
   D. other _____

3. Ineffective individual/family coping related to:
   A. excruciating pain.
   B. nausea/vomiting.
   C. syncope.
   D. passage of renal calculi in urine.
   E. other _____

4. Diversional activity deficit related to:
   A. nausea/vomiting.
   B. excruciating pain.
   C. syncope.
   D. other _____
   _____

5. Fear related to:
   A. nausea/vomiting.
   B. excruciating pain.
   C. syncope.
   D. passage of renal calculi.
   E. impending surgery.
   F. other _____
   _____

6. Potential fluid volume deficit related to:
   A. polyuria.
   B. inadequate fluid intake.
   C. other _____
   _____

7. Impaired home maintenance management related to:
   A. weakness.
   B. syncope.
   C. excruciating pain.
   D. dependence on others for care.
   E. other _____
   _____

8. Potential for injury related to:
   A. polyuria.
   B. oliguria.
   C. nausea/vomiting.
   D. syncope.
   E. lack of support in the home.
   F. refusal to follow medical instructions.
   G. poor administration of medication.
   H. obstruction.
   I. other _____
   _____

9. Ineffective breathing pattern related to renal colic.

10. Impaired physical mobility related to:
    A. weakness.
    B. excruciating pain.
    C. vomiting.
    D. other _____

11. Noncompliance with therapy related to:
    A. denial.
    B. confusion.
    C. other _____

12. Altered nutrition: potential for more than body requirements related to:
    A. formation of renal calculi.
    B. vomiting.
    C. hypovolemia.
    D. electrolyte imbalance.
    E. weakness.
    F. other _____

13. Altered parenting related to:
    A. weakness.
    B. vomiting.
    C. syncope.
    D. excruciating pain.
    E. immobility.
    F. other _____

14. Self-care deficit: feeding/bathing/grooming/dressing/toileting related to:
    A. excruciating pain.
    B. syncope.
    C. weakness.
    D. other _____

15. Sexual dysfunction related to:
    A. pain.
    B. weakness.

    C. vomiting.

    D. loin tenderness.

    E. other _____

    _____

16. Sleep pattern disturbance related to:

    A. excruciating pain.

    B. nausea/vomiting.

    C. polyuria.

    D. passage of renal calculi.

    E. other _____

    _____

17. Altered patterns of urinary elimination related to:

    A. poor fluid/dietary intake.

    B. urinary obstruction.

    C. passage of renal calculi.

    D. other _____

    _____

18. Potential for violence related to excruciating pain.

II. SHORT-TERM GOALS

1. Client/Family will verbalize fears, anxieties, and concerns after 1–2 R.N. visits.

2. Client/Family will administer prescribed medication as ordered after 1–2 R.N. visits.

3. Client/Family will notify M.D. immediately of adverse effects of medication or signs/symptoms of advance of disease after 1–2 R.N. visits.

4. Client/Family will strictly record intake and output after 1–2 R.N. visits.

5. Client will take hot baths as ordered after 1 R.N. visit.

6. Client/Family will apply moist heat to flank area as ordered after 1 R.N. visit.

7. Client/Family will force fluids as ordered after 1 R.N. visit.

8. Client/Family will strain all urine through a gauze after 1 R.N. visit.

9. Client/Family will inspect sides of urinal/bedpan for clinging stones after 1–2 R.N. visits.

10. Client/Family will crush clots that are passed in urine and inspect for stones after 1–2 R.N. visits.

11. Client will consume an acid-ash diet as ordered after 1–2 R.N. visits.

12. Client/Family will state 5 foods allowed on an acid-ash diet after 1–2 R.N. visits.

13. Client/Family will limit intake of calcium and phosphorus in diet as ordered after 1–2–3 R.N. visits.

14. Client/Family will immediately notify M.D. if no urine is excreted within 36 hours.

15. Client will avoid occupations or sports that cause excessive sweating as ordered after 1–2 R.N. visits.

16. Client will seek laboratory testing/M.D. appointments as ordered after 1–2 R.N. visits.

III. LONG-TERM GOALS

1. Normal kidney functioning will be achieved in 1–2 weeks.
2. Independent activities of daily living will be resumed in 1–2 weeks.
3. Optimal level of health will be achieved in 1–2 weeks.

IV. OUTCOME CRITERIA

1. Vital signs are normal.
2. Intake and output remain normal.
3. Laboratory test results are within normal limits.
4. Urine is clear, yellow, and sufficient in quantity.
5. Appetite is normal.
6. Client consumes nutritious meals.
7. Urine specific gravity is normal.
8. Kidney, ureter, and bladder remain patent and function well.
9. Client is alert, sociable, and cooperative.
10. Client states he/she feels better.

V. NURSING INTERVENTION/TREATMENT

1. R.N. will contact hospital discharge planner about treatment and rehabilitation goals.
2. R.N. will instruct client/family/H.H.A. on:
   A. proper hand-washing technique.
   B. monitoring and recording of vital signs.
   C. keeping strict record of intake and output.

D. prescribed medication/adverse reactions.

E. urodynamic testing/kidney and bladder x-rays/cystourethroscopy.

F. immediate notification of M.D. of adverse effects or advanced signs/symptoms of disease (pyuria, hematuria, polyuria, oliguria, anuria, pyrexia).

G. forcing of fluids as ordered.

H. diet as ordered, usually acid-ash (all breads, meats and poultry, macaroni, cranberries, plums and prunes, fish and shellfish, eggs, all types of cheese, corn and lentils, all cereals and crackers).

I. observation of urine (crushing clots and inspecting sides of urinal/bedpan for calculi).

J. straining urine through gauze.

K. hot baths/moist heat to flank area.

L. limitation of calcium and phosphorus in diet as ordered.

M. daily recording of weight.

N. avoidance of occupations and sports that cause excessive sweating as ordered.

O. avoidance of dehydration.

P. administration of aluminum hydroxide gel.

Q. avoidance of infections.

R. laboratory testing/follow-up M.D. appointments.

S. diversional activity.

T. surgery if ordered.

3. R.N. will provide follow-up reports to M.D. and discharge summary when case closes.

4. R.N. will notify client/family/H.H.A./significant others when case will close.

Renal Failure
Care Plan

I. NURSING DIAGNOSIS

  1. Anxiety related to:
    A. recent weight loss.
    B. oliguria (<400 ml per 24 hours).
    C. anuria.
    D. persistent early morning nausea/vomiting/diarrhea.
    E. dry skin and oral mucous membrane.
    F. drowsiness.
    G. headache.
    H. muscle twitching.
    I. change in taste sensation.
    J. hiccoughs.
    K. easy bruising.
    L. amenorrhea.
    M. loss of libido and potency.
    N. bone pain.
    O. convulsions.
    P. other _____

  2. Activity intolerance related to:
    A. fatigue.
    B. lethargy.
    C. weakness.
    D. shortness of breath on exertion.
    E. peripheral paresthesia/hyperesthesia.

F. bone pain.

G. lower back pain.

H. feet/ankle edema.

I. other _____
_____

3. Ineffective breathing pattern related to:

A. shortness of breath on exertion.

B. pleural pain.

C. cardiac pain.

D. hiccoughs.

E. other _____
_____

4. Altered oral mucous membrane related to:

A. vomiting.

B. dehydration.

C. other _____
_____

5. Decreased cardiac output related to:

A. shortness of breath on exertion.

B. cardiac pain.

C. hypertension.

D. ejection flow murmur.

E. other _____
_____

6. Anticipatory grieving related to:

A. loss of self-esteem.

B. increased sick time at work.

C. possible loss of job security/wages.

D. fear of end-stage renal disease.

E. other _____
_____

7. Sleep pattern disturbance related to:

A. nocturia.

B. headache.

C. muscle twitching/cramps.

D. anxiety.

E. pruritus.

F. other _____
_____

8. Potential for injury related to:
   A. knowledge deficit of disease management.
   B. denial.
   C. convulsions.
   D. suicidal ideation.
   E. other _____

9. Fear related to:
   A. potential loss of control.
   B. dependence on others for care.
   C. loss of employment status.
   D. long-term disability.
   E. death.
   F. other _____

10. Knowledge deficit related to:
    A. signs/symptoms.
    B. medication administration/adverse reactions.
    C. weight control.
    D. recording of intake and output.
    E. diet/fluid requirements/aluminum hydroxide (i.e., Dialume) recipes.
    F. importance of laboratory testing/M.D. appointments.
    G. exercise/rest.
    H. employment.
    I. complicating conditions (e.g., anemia/dehydration/stomal ulcers/hypertension/diabetes/upper and lower respiratory infections)
    J. continuous ambulatory peritoneal dialysis (CAPD).
    K. continuous cycler peritoneal dialysis (CCPD).
    L. intermittent peritoneal dialysis (IPD).
    M. hemodialysis.
    N. cost of treatment/supplies.
    O. financial assistance.
    P. support groups.
    Q. other _____

11. Noncompliance with therapy related to:
    A. cost of treatment/supplies.

    B. forgetfulness.

    C. poor concentration.

    D. learning disability.

    E. lack of support in the home.

    F. denial.

    G. other _____

12. Potential altered parenting related to:

    A. fatigue.

    B. lethargy.

    C. weakness.

    D. shortness of breath on exertion.

    E. other _____

13. Altered nutrition: more/less than body requirements related to:

    A. change in taste sensation.

    B. anorexia.

    C. nausea.

    D. vomiting.

    E. anemia.

    F. fluid/dietary restrictions.

    G. sodium/potassium/protein retention.

    H. weight gain/loss.

    I. other _____

14. Altered renal tissue perfusion related to:

    A. sodium retention.

    B. edema.

    C. oliguria.

    D. anuria.

    E. dehydration.

    F. bleeding.

    G. other _____

15. Alteration in patterns of urinary elimination: frequency/oliguria/anuria/nocturia related to:

    A. fluid/dietary intake.

    B. medication administration.

C. sodium/potassium/protein retention.

D. CAPD.

E. CCPD.

F. IPD.

G. hemodialysis.

H. other _____

_____

II. SHORT-TERM GOALS

1. Client/Family will verbalize fears, anxieties, and concerns after 1–2–3 R.N. visits.

2. Client/Family will administer prescribed medication after 1–2–3 R.N. visits.

3. Client/Family will notify M.D. immediately of adverse effects of medication or change in condition after 1–2–3 R.N. visits.

4. Client/Family will demonstrate good hand-washing technique after 1–2 R.N. visits.

5. Client/Family will strictly record intake and output after 1–2 R.N. visits.

6. Client will exercise/rest as ordered after 1–2 R.N. visits.

7. Client/Family will limit intake of sodium, potassium, protein, calcium, and phosphorus as ordered after 1–2–3 R.N. visits.

8. Client/Family will test blood glucose q.d. as ordered after 1–2 R.N. visits.

9. Client/Family will test urine q.d. as ordered after 1–2 R.N. visits.

10. Client/Family will seek/perform CAPD as ordered after 1–2–3 R.N. visits.

11. Client/Family will seek/perform IPD as ordered after 1–2–3 R.N. visits.

12. Client/Family will seek/perform CCPD as ordered after 1–2–3 R.N. visits.

13. Client/Family will seek/perform hemodialysis as ordered after 1–2–3 R.N. visits.

14. Client/Family will store supplies in appropriate areas of home after 1–2–3 R.N. visits.

15. Client will avoid occupations or sports that cause injury/bleeding after 1–2–3 R.N. visits.

16. Client will seek appropriate laboratory testing/M.D. appointments as ordered after 1–2 R.N. visits.

III. LONG-TERM GOALS

1. Normal kidney functioning will be achieved in 1–2 months.
2. Kidney functioning will be controlled by CAPD, IPD, CCPD, or hemodialysis after 1–2 months.
3. Independent activities of daily living will be resumed in 1–2 weeks.
4. Optimal level of health will be achieved in 1–2 weeks.

IV. OUTCOME CRITERIA

1. Vital signs are normal.
2. Blood pressure is normal.
3. Laboratory test results are within normal limits.
4. Appetite is good.
5. Taste sensation is normal.
6. Breath is without odor.
7. Urine is clear, yellow, and sufficient in quantity.
8. Urine specific gravity is normal.
9. Client consumes nutritious meals.
10. Liver function tests are normal.
11. EKG/Heart sounds are normal.
12. Menses are normal.
13. Skin is normal color.
14. Intake and output are within normal limits.
15. Mobility is normal.
16. Kidney, ureters, and bladder remain patent and function well.
17. Chest sounds are normal.
18. Chest x-ray film is normal.
19. Client is alert, sociable, and cooperative.
20. Client states he/she feels better.

V. NURSING INTERVENTION/TREATMENT

1. R.N. will arrange to visit client's home.
2. R.N. will monitor vital signs, including jugular venous pulse when client is supine, blood pressure (assess for postural hypotension), weight (assess for recent weight loss), skin turgor, mucous membrane, eyesight, eyeball tension (should be decreased), signs/symptoms of bleeding, and intake and output.
3. R.N. will allow client/family to verbalize all fears, anxieties, and

concerns about condition and procedures to be scheduled; will assess discharge planning instructions from hospital.

4. R.N. will contact M.D. for recent laboratory testing results of urinalysis, CBC, electrolytes, etc. (Note current sodium, potassium, protein, urea, creatinine, phosphates, uric acid, magnesium, calcium, and phosphorus levels.)

5. R.N. will instruct client/family/H.H.A. on:

   A. disease process and signs/symptoms.

   B. monitoring and recording of vital signs, including blood pressure.

   C. oral hygiene.

   D. diabetic management, if applicable.

   E. measures to improve hypotension/hypertension.

   F. exercise/rest.

   G. medication administration/adverse reactions. (Note if drug is not excreted by kidneys; if excess blood level of it affects the kidneys, adds chemically to the blood urea nitrogen level, or affects electrolyte imbalance; and if client is more susceptible because of kidney failure. Note what medications may be administered during dialysis.)

   H. immediate notification of M.D. of adverse reactions or change in condition.

   I. avoidance of smoking/alcohol.

   J. avoidance of emotional stress/injuries/infection.

   K. proper hand-washing technique.

   L. daily recording of weight and notation of suborbital, facial, peripheral, and sacral edema.

   M. fluid/dietary intake (special initial restrictions may be for sodium, potassium, protein, and phosphorus). Confer with M.D. and nutritionist. Dialume recipes may be encouraged.

   N. vitamin therapy.

   O. complicating conditions (e.g., anemia/dehydration/stomal ulcers/hypertension/diabetes/upper and lower respiratory infections).

   P. weight control.

   Q. daily recording of intake and output.

   R. CAPD.

   S. IPD/CCPD.

   T. hemodialysis.

   U. laboratory testing/M.D. appointments.

      V. dental appointments.

     W. employment/vocational training/college.

      X. financial assistance.

      Y. recreation.

      Z. support groups/counseling.

6. R.N. will provide M.D. with follow-up reports and discharge summary when case closes.

7. R.N. will notify client/family/H.H.A. when case closes.

Rheumatoid Arthritis
Care Plan

I. NURSING DIAGNOSIS

1. Knowledge deficit related to:
   A. chronic, progressive nature of disease.
   B. medication regimen/adverse reactions.
   C. daily exercise.
   D. other_____
   _____

2. Anxiety related to chronic, progressive nature of disease.
3. Joint pain/stiffness/muscular spasms related to:
   A. poor immune response.
   B. chronic, progressive nature of disease.
   C. inadequate daily exercise.
   D. other_____
   _____

4. Impaired physical mobility related to:
   A. inflammation.
   B. joint pain.
   C. deformities.
   D. dislocation.
   E. other_____
   _____

5. Sleep pattern disturbance related to:
   A. poor positioning in bed.
   B. pain.
   C. inflammation.

D. dislocation.

E. deformity.

F. stiffness.

G. muscular spasms.

H. other_____

6. Self-care deficit: feeding/bathing/grooming/dressing/toileting/ administration of medication/ambulation related to:

A. deformity.

B. dislocation.

C. stiffness.

D. pain.

E. inflammation.

F. muscular spasms.

G. other_____

7. Self-esteem disturbance related to:

A. deformity.

B. dependence on others for performance of activities of daily living.

C. other_____

8. Ineffective individual/family coping related to:

A. disabling nature of disease.

B. other_____

9. Altered patterns of urinary elimination related to:

A. poor mobility.

B. immobility.

C. other_____

10. Constipation related to:

A. poor mobility.

B. immobility.

C. other_____

11. Impaired home maintenance management related to:

A. deformity.

B. dislocation.

C. pain.

D. formation of subcutaneous nodules.

E. other_____

_____

12. Potential impaired skin integrity related to thinning of skin.

II. SHORT-TERM GOALS

1. Client/Family will verbalize fears, anxieties, and concerns after 1–2–3 R.N. visits.

2. Client/Family will obtain prescribed medication as ordered after 1–2 R.N. visits.

3. Client/Family will correctly administer prescribed medication as ordered after 1–2–3 R.N. visits.

4. Client/Family will immediately report to M.D. adverse reactions to medication or change in condition after 1–2 R.N. visits.

5. Client/Family will prepare nutritionally sound meals after 1–2 R.N. visits.

6. Client/Family will follow a prescribed pattern of rest each day after 1–2 R.N. visits.

7. Client/Family will use pillows/bed cradles/bed boards/raised toilet/splints/supports/Hoyer lift when necessary after 1–2–3–4 R.N./P.T./O.T. visits.

8. Client will avoid emotional stress whenever possible after 1–2 R.N. visits.

9. Client will take a warm bath or shower on rising after 1–2 R.N. visits.

10. Client/Family will apply warm, moist compresses as ordered after 1–2 R.N. visits.

11. Client/Family will use flannel sheets/electric blanket as ordered after 1–2 R.N. visits.

12. Client/Family will perform each prescribed exercise slowly after 1–2–3 R.N./P.T./O.T. visits.

13. Client/Family will use paraffin applications as ordered after 1–2–3 R.N./P.T./O.T. visits.

14. Client/Family will seek laboratory testing/M.D. appointments as ordered after 1–2 R.N. visits.

III. LONG-TERM GOALS

1. Independent activities of daily living will be resumed in 1–2 weeks.

2. Optimal level of health will be achieved in 3–4 weeks.

IV. OUTCOME CRITERIA

1. Joints can be placed in full range of motion; muscle tone is preserved.
2. Pain is relieved.
3. Laboratory test results remain normal.
4. Ambulation remains steady.
5. Bowel/Bladder functions normally.
6. Intake and output are within normal range.
7. Vital signs remain normal.
8. Skin surface remains healthy and intact.
9. Vision remains clear.
10. Cardiac output remains strong.
11. Lungs remain clear.
12. Reflexes remain present with normal response.

V. NURSING INTERVENTION/TREATMENT

1. R.N. will provide psychologic support to client/family regarding chronic, progressive nature of disease.
2. R.N. will instruct client/family/H.H.A. on:
   A. medication regimen (salicylates/hormones/corticosteroids/methotrexate/chrysotherapy/gold injections)/adverse reactions.
   B. immediate notification of M.D. of adverse reactions or change in condition.
   C. avoidance of pain precipitation factors (e.g., emotional stress, dampness, temperature extremes).
   D. good body mechanics for transfer, ambulation, lifting, reaching.
   E. use of splints/supports/bed cradle/footboard/wheelchair/crutches/braces/corrective shoes/raised toilet/overhead trapeze/bed board/canes/sandbags/bath lift/exercise equipment.
   F. surgical correction (synovectomy/ankylosis/arthroplasty/arthrodesis/resection with prosthetic implantation).
   G. weight reduction if necessary.
   H. scheduled daily rest periods.
   I. avoidance of overactivity/prolonged sitting, walking, or standing/sudden, jerky movements.
   J. use of heat treatments (paraffin applications/warm showers or baths/contrast (hot and cold) baths/electric blanket).

K. prescribed exercise plan (muscle setting/range-of-motion activities/breathing exercises/swimming).

3. R.N. will encourage client to be as functionally independent as possible.

4. R.N. will encourage client to visit M.D. routinely for examination and laboratory testing.

5. R.N. will confer with M.D., P.T., O.T., M.S.W., if ordered, regarding all types of therapy and continued progress being made.

6. R.N. will provide M.D. with follow-up reports and discharge summary when case closes.

7. R.N. will notify client/family/H.H.A./significant others when case will close.

Rocky Mountain
Spotted Fever
Care Plan

I. NURSING DIAGNOSIS

   1. Anxiety related to:
      A. chills.
      B. severe pain in bones and muscles.
      C. headaches.
      D. profuse skin eruptions.
      E. skin necrosis.
      F. restlessness.
      G. insomnia.
      H. deafness.
      I. visual disturbances.
      J. subcutaneous hemorrhages.
      K. fever.
      L. other _____

   2. Knowledge deficit related to:
      A. Rocky Mountain spotted fever.
      B. skin care.
      C. fluid intake/dietary regimen as ordered.
      D. complications.
      E. medication administration/adverse reactions.
      F. high-risk environmental areas.
      G. other _____

3. Impaired verbal communication related to deafness.
4. Ineffective individual/family coping related to:
   A. dependence on others for care.
   B. altered levels of consciousness.
   C. cost of medical care/poor insurance coverage.
   D. other _____

   _____

5. Diversional activity deficit related to:
   A. chills.
   B. severe bone and muscle pain.
   C. skin necrosis.
   D. visual disturbances.
   E. mental confusion/delirium.
   F. coma.
   G. other _____

   _____

6. Fear related to:
   A. profuse skin eruptions.
   B. skin necrosis.
   C. subcutaneous hemorrhages.
   D. delirium.
   E. potential pneumonia.
   F. fever.
   G. secondary anemia.
   H. pigmented, scarred skin.
   I. other _____

   _____

7. Potential fluid volume deficit related to:
   A. poor intake.
   B. fever.
   C. general malaise.
   D. delirium/mental confusion.
   E. subcutaneous hemorrhages.
   F. macular rash on mucous membrane of mouth and pharynx.
   G. other _____

   _____

8. Anticipatory grieving related to:
   A. possibility of coma.

    B. possibility of death.

    C. other _____

    _____

9. Impaired home maintenance management related to:

    A. extreme fatigue.

    B. dependence on others for care.

    C. delirium.

    D. coma.

    E. increased demands posed by care of the sick at home.

    F. other _____

    _____

10. Potential for injury related to:

    A. possible skin necrosis.

    B. poor supervision in the home.

    C. delirium.

    D. deafness.

    E. visual disturbances.

    F. mental confusion.

    G. pigmented, scarred skin.

    H. other _____

    _____

11. Severe pain in bones and muscles related to:

    A. tick infestation.

    B. other _____

    _____

12. Impaired physical mobility related to:

    A. severe bone and muscle pain.

    B. weakness.

    C. delirium.

    D. mental confusion.

    E. visual disturbances.

    F. other _____

    _____

13. Noncompliance with therapy related to:

    A. lack of support in the home.

    B. denial.

    C. weakness.

    D. delirium.

    E. visual changes.

    F. deafness.

    G. mental confusion.

    H. other _____

    _____

14. Altered nutrition: potential for more than body requirements related to:

    A. poor understanding of disease.

    B. weakness.

    C. anorexia.

    D. fever.

    E. other _____

    _____

15. Altered oral mucous membrane related to tick infestation.

16. Self-care deficit: feeding/grooming/bathing/dressing/toileting related to:

    A. weakness.

    B. severe bone and muscle pain.

    C. visual changes.

    D. pneumonia.

    E. delirium.

    F. mental changes.

    G. coma.

    H. other _____

    _____

17. Self-esteem disturbance related to dependence on others for care.

18. Social isolation related to:

    A. skin necrosis.

    B. bed rest.

    C. other _____

    _____

19. Sensory/Perceptual alterations (visual) related to:

    A. mental confusion.

    B. delirium.

    C. coma.

    D. other _____

    _____

20. Sexual dysfunction related to:

    A. severe muscle and bone pain.

   B. mental confusion.

   C. delirium.

   D. coma.

   E. other _____

   _____

21. Potential impaired skin integrity related to:

   A. extensive rose-colored macular and petechial rash.

   B. skin necrosis.

   C. permanently pigmented, scarred skin.

   D. other _____

   _____

22. Sleep pattern disturbance related to:

   A. severe bone and muscle pain.

   B. restlessness.

   C. exhausting insomnia.

   D. other _____

   _____

23. Powerlessness related to:

   A. mental confusion.

   B. delirium.

   C. coma.

   D. other _____

   _____

24. Altered patterns of urinary elimination related to:

   A. poor intake.

   B. delirium.

   C. coma.

   D. other _____

   _____

II. SHORT-TERM GOALS

   1. Client/Family will verbalize fears, anxieties, and concerns after 1–2 R.N. visits.
   2. Client/Family will administer prescribed medication as ordered after 1–2 R.N. visits.
   3. Client/Family will notify M.D. of adverse effects or signs/symptoms of advance of disease after 1–2 R.N. visits.
   4. Client/Family will use appropriate skin care measures after 1–2 R.N. visits.

5. Client/Family will rest/exercise as ordered after 1–2 R.N. visits.

6. Client/Family will seek annual vaccination against Rocky Mountain spotted fever if necessary after 1 R.N. visit.

7. Client/Family will examine self/client twice daily for ticks as ordered after 1–2 R.N. visits.

8. Client/Family will apply tick repellant to clothes as ordered after 1–2 R.N. visits.

9. Client/Family will remove ticks with tweezers by pulling firmly but gently after 1–2 R.N. visits.

10. Client will consume a high-protein diet as ordered after 1 R.N. visit.

11. Client/Family will force fluids as ordered after 1–2 R.N. visits.

12. Client/Family will strictly record intake and output after 1–2 R.N. visits.

13. Client/Family will avoid emotional stress after 1–2 R.N. visits.

14. Client will be placed in a warm, restful environment after 1–2 R.N. visits.

15. Client/Family will seek correction for visual disturbances after 2–3 R.N. visits.

16. Client will seek laboratory testing/M.D. appointments as ordered after 1–2 R.N. visits.

III. LONG-TERM GOALS

1. Independent activities of daily living will be resumed in 2–4 weeks.

2. Optimal level of health will be achieved in 4 weeks.

3. Tick eradication/Vaccination will be accomplished in prevalent regions.

4. All stages of death and dying will be worked through.

IV. OUTCOME CRITERIA

1. Vital signs are normal.

2. Skin/Mucous membrane is healthy and intact.

3. Chest is clear; breathing normal.

4. Vision is clear and normal.

5. Hearing is normal.

6. Circulatory status remains normal.

7. Laboratory test results (CBC with differential) are normal.

8. Normal sleep pattern occurs.

9. Appetite is normal.

10. Client consumes nutritious meals.

11. Bowel/Bladder elimination is normal.

12. Client states he/she feels better.

V. NURSING INTERVENTION/TREATMENT

1. R.N. will assess complete history and perform physical examination on initial home visit.

2. R.N. will instruct client/family/H.H.A. on:

   A. monitoring and recording of vital signs every 4 hours.

   B. medication administration/adverse reactions.

   C. immediate notification of M.D. of adverse reactions or signs/symptoms of advance of disease.

   D. appropriate skin care measures.

   E. quiet, restful environment.

   F. forcing of fluids/consuming high-protein diet.

   G. exercise/rest as ordered.

   H. breathing exercises/respiratory therapy.

   I. changes in sensorium.

   J. bowel/bladder elimination.

   K. laboratory testing/M.D. appointments.

   L. diversional activities.

   M. immunization/annual revaccination against disease if necessary.

   N. tick examination twice daily.

   O. tick repellant application to clothes.

   P. tick removal with tweezers.

3. R.N. will report disease to local board of health.

4. R.N. will provide M.D. with follow-up reports and discharge summary when case closes.

5. R.N. will notify client/family/H.H.A./significant others when case will close.

6. If death is imminent, R.N. will provide psychologic support/ support of clergy in final stages; will follow pronouncement-of-death procedures; will assist with funeral arrangements if necessary.

Scabies
Care Plan

I. NURSING DIAGNOSIS

1. Knowledge deficit related to:
   A. prevention/treatment of scabies.
   B. medication administration/adverse reactions.
   C. signs/symptoms.
   D. good personal hygiene habits.
   E. poor understanding of transmission.
   F. other _____

2. Anxiety related to:
   A. transmission of scabies.
   B. social isolation.
   C. other _____

3. Noncompliance with therapy related to:
   A. denial.
   B. cost of treatment.
   C. other _____

4. Potential for infection related to:
   A. intense scratching.
   B. poor administration of medication.
   C. other _____

    5. Self-esteem disturbance related to embarrassment over skin lesions.
    6. Impaired skin integrity related to:
       A. intense pruritus.
       B. excoriation.
       C. burrows.
       D. papular/vesicular lesions.
       E. other _____

       _____

    7. Potential for injury related to intense scratching.
    8. Ineffective individual/family coping related to intense scratching.
    9. Impaired home maintenance management related to:
       A. intense pruritus/scratching.
       B. papular/vesicular lesions.
       C. other _____

       _____

  10. Diversional activity deficit related to:
       A. severe pruritus.
       B. embarrassment about lesions.
       C. other _____

       _____

  11. Self-care deficit: bathing/dressing/grooming related to extensive
      skin lesions in interdigital surfaces; axillary, cubital, and popliteal
      folds; inguinal region; and areola in women.
  12. Sleep pattern disturbance related to severe pruritus.
  13. Sexual dysfunction related to:
       A. intense pruritus.
       B. scabies communicability.
       C. other _____

       _____

II. SHORT-TERM GOALS

    1. Client/Family will visit M.D. routinely for treatment of scabies after
      1–2 R.N. visits.
    2. Client/Family will apply prescribed lotion/cream/ointment (lindane
      1%/benzyl benzoate/4%–5% sulfur ointment) as ordered after
      1–2 R.N. visits.
    3. Client/Family will bathe as ordered (after 8–24–48 hours) following
      application of prescribed lotion/cream/ointment after 1–2 R.N.
      visits.

4. Client/Family will dispose of padded mattress if necessary after 1–2 R.N. visits.
5. Client/Family will change clothing frequently as ordered after 1–2 R.N. visits.
6. Client/Family will launder clothing as ordered after 1–2 R.N. visits.
7. Client/Family will notify M.D. of adverse effects of medication after 1–2 R.N. visits.
8. Client/Family will seek medical clearance to return to play/school/work after 2–3 R.N. visits.

III. LONG-TERM GOALS

1. Communicable disease will be controlled in 1–2 weeks.
2. Home maintenance management will be functional in 1–2 weeks.

IV. OUTCOME CRITERIA

1. Skin integrity remains healthy and intact.
2. Sexuality remains normal.
3. Sleep pattern remains normal.
4. Good personal hygiene measures are employed.
5. Client's/Family's personal care items, clothing, furniture remain clean.
6. Client/Family returns to play/school/work.
7. Client/Family state they feel better.

V. NURSING INTERVENTION/TREATMENT

1. R.N. will make home visit to investigate all communicable sources.
2. R.N. will instruct client/family/H.H.A. on:
   A. isolation of all suspected cases.
   B. protection of primary caregiver when providing prescribed treatment: proper hand-washing techniques; disposal of apron, gown, gloves.
   C. thorough bathing/personal hygiene.
   D. disposal/disinfection of clothing, bedding, furniture if necessary.
   E. application/administration of medication/lotion/cream/ ointment; explicit instructions for bathing as ordered by M.D. (lotions/creams/ointments are usually applied thinly from the neck down and washed off thoroughly after 8, 24, or 48 hours).

    F. literature, books, pamphlets on scabies.

    G. notification of M.D. of adverse reactions to medication/creams/lotions/ointments or of secondary infections.

    H. routine M.D. appointments.

3. R.N. will provide M.D. with follow-up reports and discharge summary when case closes.

4. R.N. will notify client/family/H.H.A./significant others when case will close.

Scarlet Fever
Care Plan

I. NURSING DIAGNOSIS

1. Anxiety related to:
   A. vomiting.
   B. fever.
   C. flushed cheeks.
   D. erythematous skin rash.
   E. malaise.
   F. circumoral pallor.
   G. petechiae.
   H. strawberry tongue.
   I. sore throat.
   J. other _____

2. Ineffective thermoregulation related to:
   A. generalized bacterial infection.
   B. poor fluid/dietary intake.
   C. other _____

3. Self-care deficit: feeding/bathing/grooming/dressing/toileting related to:
   A. fever.
   B. vomiting.
   C. extreme weakness.
   D. malaise.

E. other _____

_____

4. Knowledge deficit related to:
   A. treatment of scarlet fever.
   B. medication administration/adverse reactions.
   C. tepid-sponge administration.
   D. monitoring of vital signs.
   E. other _____

   _____

5. Potential fluid volume deficit related to:
   A. vomiting.
   B. sore throat.
   C. poor fluid intake.
   D. other _____

   _____

6. Impaired home maintenance management related to:
   A. increasing demands posed by care of sick child.
   B. isolation precautions.
   C. other _____

   _____

7. Potential for injury related to:
   A. refusal to take medication.
   B. other _____

   _____

8. Ineffective breathing pattern related to:
   A. sore throat.
   B. coated tongue.
   C. congestion.
   D. other _____

   _____

9. Potential impaired skin integrity related to:
   A. petechiae.
   B. bright erythematous, finely papular generalized rash (may begin on border of lower jaw/face/base of neck/axilla/groin, then proceed to trunk and extremities).
   C. sandpaper feel of rash, with peeling.
   D. other _____

   _____

10. Altered nutrition: potential for more than body requirements related to:
    A. vomiting.
    B. malaise.
    C. poor fluid/dietary intake.
    D. other _____

_____

11. Sleep pattern disturbance related to:
    A. vomiting.
    B. malaise.
    C. sore throat.
    D. restlessness.
    E. other _____

_____

12. Social isolation related to home confinement.

II. SHORT-TERM GOALS

1. Parent will place child in a quiet, restful environment after 1 R.N. visit.
2. Child will consume fluids/diet as tolerated after 1 R.N. visit.
3. Child will rest appropriately after 1 R.N. visit.
4. Parent will take body temperature every 3–4 hours as ordered after 1 R.N. visit.
5. Parent will report disease to local board of health after 1 R.N. visit.
6. Parent will administer prescribed medication to child after 1–2 R.N. visits.
7. Parent will immediately notify M.D. of adverse reactions to medications or change in condition after 1–2 R.N. visits.
8. Child will amuse self with books, TV, radio, videogames after 1 R.N. visit.
9. Child will stay home until medical clearance is given to return to school after 1–2 R.N. visits.
10. Parent will seek laboratory testing/M.D. appointments as ordered after 1–2 R.N. visits.

III. LONG-TERM GOALS

1. Communicable disease is controlled and possible spread to community is prevented in 1 week.

2. Independent activities of daily living will be resumed in 1–2 weeks.

3. Optimal level of health achieved in 2–3 weeks.

IV. OUTCOME CRITERIA

1. Vital signs are normal.
2. Vision is clear.
3. Skin is clear, warm, healthy, and intact.
4. Appetite is normal.
5. Client consumes nutritious meals.
6. Bowel/Bladder habits are normal.
7. Skin/Mucous membrane is healthy and intact.
8. Chest is clear.
9. Child states he/she feels better.
10. Child attends school/play.

V. NURSING INTERVENTION/TREATMENT

1. Parent will contact M.D. about earliest possible signs/symptoms of disease.
2. Parent will report disease to local board of health.
3. R.N. will instruct parent on:
   A. isolation of child.
   B. monitoring and recording of vital signs.
   C. proper hand-washing technique.
   D. fluid intake/dietary regimen as ordered.
   E. bowel/bladder functioning.
   F. medication administration/adverse reactions.
   G. immediate notification of M.D. of adverse reactions or change in condition.
   H. skin care measures.
   I. diversional activities.
4. R.N. will provide M.D. with follow-up reports and discharge summary when case closes.
5. R.N. will notify client/parents when case will close and when child may return to school.

Seizure Disorder Care Plan

I. NURSING DIAGNOSIS

1. Anxiety related to:
   A. uncontrolled seizures.
   B. medication administration.
   C. loss of control during seizures.
   D. incontinence.
   E. other _____

2. Potential for injury related to:
   A. failure to administer medication on time.
   B. loss of control during seizures.
   C. other _____

3. Altered parenting related to:
   A. loss of control during seizures.
   B. other _____

4. Ineffective individual/family coping related to:
   A. uncontrolled seizures.
   B. constant fear of injury.
   C. other _____

5. Knowledge deficit related to:
   A. etiology of seizures.

    B. medication regimen/adverse reactions.

    C. safety precautions.

    D. diet/exercise/rest.

    E. other _____

    _____

6. Ineffective airway clearance related to seizures.

7. Noncompliance with medication regimen related to:

    A. refusal to take medications.

    B. denial.

    C. other _____

    _____

8. Powerlessness related to loss of control during seizures.

9. Social isolation related to:

    A. uncontrolled seizures.

    B. embarrassment.

    C. fear of injury in community.

    D. fear of rejection by significant others.

    E. other _____

    _____

10. Alterations in health maintenance related to:

    A. frequent alterations in medication regimen.

    B. poor safety precautions in home and community.

    C. refusal to comply with therapy.

    D. other _____

    _____

II. SHORT-TERM GOALS

1. Client/Family will verbalize all fears, anxieties, and concerns after 1–2–3 R.N. visits.

2. Client/Family will remove obstacles for injury whenever and wherever possible in the home environment after 1 R.N. visit.

3. Client/Family will administer medication correctly after 1–2 R.N. visits.

4. Client/Family will state adverse reactions to medications after 1–2 R.N. visits.

5. Client/Family will notify M.D. immediately of adverse reactions or any change in condition after 1–2 R.N. visits.

6. Client/Family will note precipitating factors influencing seizures after 1–2 R.N. visits.

7. Client will carry emergency medical identification after 1–2 R.N. visits.

8. Client/Family will regulate diet and fluids on a daily basis as ordered after 1–2 R.N. visits.

9. Client/Family will regulate exercise on a daily basis after 1–2 R.N. visits.

10. Client/Family will schedule daily rest periods after 1–2 R.N. visits.

11. Client will refrain from driving or operating dangerous machinery as ordered after 1–2 R.N. visits.

12. Client/Family will avoid temperature extremes after 1 R.N. visit.

13. Client will refrain from drinking excessive amounts of alcohol after 1–2–3–4 R.N. visits.

14. Client/Family will seek laboratory testing/M.D. appointments as ordered after 1–2 R.N. visits.

III. LONG-TERM GOALS

1. Independent activities of daily living will be resumed in 1–2 weeks.
2. Seizure disorder will be controlled in 1–2 weeks.
3. Optimal level of health will be achieved in 1–2 weeks.

IV. OUTCOME CRITERIA

1. Vital signs remain normal.
2. Teeth, tongue, and lips remain healthy and intact.
3. Tremors/convulsive movements are controlled.
4. Laboratory test results remain within normal limits.
5. Pain is relieved.
6. Mental status remains alert and oriented to person, place, and time.

V. NURSING INTERVENTION/TREATMENT

1. R.N. will allow client/family to verbalize fears, anxieties, and concerns about seizure disorder.
2. R.N. will instruct client/family/H.H.A. on:
   A. type of seizure disorder specific to client.
   B. monitoring and recording of vital signs.
   C. medication administration/adverse effects.

D. regulation of diet, fluids, rest, exercise; avoidance of temperature extremes, alcohol, and stress.

E. keeping padded tongue blade available at all times.

F. wearing of medical identification (e.g., ID bracelet, necklace, wallet card).

G. awareness of aura and impending seizure activity.

H. recording of characteristics of each seizure (how seizure begins, types of tremors, movements sustained, size of pupils, bowel or bladder incontinence, unconsciousness, sleep activity afterward, duration of seizure).

I. examination of teeth, tongue, gums, cheeks, head, and extremities after seizure activity.

J. laboratory testing/x-ray testing/CT scans/EEGs.

K. avoidance of driving or operating dangerous machinery as ordered by M.D.

L. routine M.D. appointments.

M. positioning of self/client during seizure.

N. career counseling.

O. hereditary characteristics as discussed with M.D.

3. R.N. will provide M.D. with follow-up reports and discharge summary when case closes.

4. R.N. will encourage client to meet with individuals or groups to assist with acceptance of condition; will refer client to organizations or foundations for educational materials.

5. R.N. will notify client/family/H.H.A./significant others when case will close.

Spinal Cord Injury Care Plan

I. NURSING DIAGNOSIS

1. Knowledge deficit related to:
   - A. fluid intake/dietary regimen as ordered.
   - B. medication administration/adverse reactions.
   - C. exercise/rest.
   - D. dressing care.
   - E. hemiplegia/diplegia/paraplegia/quadriplegia.
   - F. sexual activity.
   - G. urinary/bowel elimination.
   - H. employment/recreation.
   - I. other _____

2. Anxiety related to:
   - A. immobility.
   - B. dependence on others for care.
   - C. loss of control.
   - D. paralysis.
   - E. other _____

3. Partial/Total self-care deficit: feeding/dressing/bathing/grooming/ toileting related to:
   - A. hemiplegia/diplegia/paraplegia/quadriplegia.
   - B. weakness.
   - C. dependence on others for care.

D. other _____

_____

4. Potential for injury related to:
   A. stress/grieving.
   B. poor nutritional habits.
   C. excessive smoking.
   D. poor administration of medication.
   E. feeding problems.
   F. falls/accidents.
   G. other _____

   _____

5. Constipation/Diarrhea related to:
   A. immobility.
   B. poor fluid/dietary intake.
   C. poor administration of medication.
   D. other _____

   _____

6. Potential for infection related to:
   A. paralysis.
   B. poor fluid/dietary intake.
   C. poor personal hygiene habits.
   D. other _____

   _____

7. Potential fluid volume deficit related to:
   A. poor intake.
   B. excessive diuresis.
   C. other _____

   _____

8. Potential impaired skin integrity related to:
   A. immobility.
   B. poor personal hygiene.
   C. other _____

   _____

9. Ineffective breathing patterns related to:
   A. poor fluid intake.
   B. immobility.
   C. inappropriate use of respiratory equipment.
   D. poor breathing exercises.

E. infection.

F. other _____

_____

10. Self-esteem disturbance related to:

    A. fear of rejection by significant others.

    B. loss of muscle tone.

    C. immobility.

    D. alterations in body image.

    E. other _____

    _____

11. Sexual dysfunction related to:

    A. paralysis.

    B. anger.

    C. inadequate sexual rehabilitation.

    D. other _____

    _____

12. Sleep pattern disturbance related to:

    A. anxiety.

    B. paralysis.

    C. dependence on others for care.

    D. other _____

    _____

II. SHORT-TERM GOALS

1. Client/Family will verbalize all fears, anxieties, and concerns after 1–2–3–4 R.N. visits.

2. Through appropriate hospital discharge planning, client/family will purchase/rent prescribed medical equipment before R.N. visits.

3. Client will drink 2000-3000 cc of fluids daily after 1–2 R.N. visits.

4. Client/Family will administer medication as ordered after 1–2–3 R.N. visits.

5. Client/Family will immediately notify M.D. of adverse reactions or change in condition after 1–2 R.N. visits.

6. Client/Family will exercise/rest as ordered after 1–2 R.N. visits.

7. Client/Family will bathe self/client after 1–2 R.N. visits.

8. Client/Family will feed self/use assistive devices for feeding after 1–2 R.N./P.T./O.T. visits.

9. Client/Family will catheterize and measure urinary output after 1–2 R.N. visits.
10. Client/Family will apply crutches/cane/braces independently after 1–2–3 R.N./P.T./O.T. visits.
11. Client/Family will propel wheelchair after 1–2 R.N. visits.
12. Client/Family will apply Texas catheter as ordered after 1–2 R.N. visits.
13. Client/Family will transfer to bed/commode/chair/tub/car/ wheelchair after 5–6 R.N./P.T. visits.
14. Client/Family will assist with bowel care after 1–2 R.N. visits.
15. Client/Family will participate in sports activities as ordered after 3–4 R.N. visits.
16. Client will drive with adaptive equipment after 9–10 R.N./P.T./ O.T. visits.
17. Client/Family will seek laboratory testing/M.D. appointments as ordered after 1–2 R.N. visits.
18. Client will seek employment after 9–10 visits.

III. LONG-TERM GOALS

1. Independent activities of daily living will be resumed in 1–2 months.
2. Ambulation will be achieved in 1–2 months.
3. Optimal level of health will be achieved in 1–2 months.
4. Employment will be obtained in 1–2 months.

IV. OUTCOME CRITERIA

1. Vital signs are normal.
2. Chest is clear.
3. Bowel/Bladder functions normally.
4. Respirations are normal.
5. Sexual relations are normal.
6. Weight is appropriate for height.
7. Laboratory test results are normal.
8. Peripheral circulation is normal.
9. Mental health remains normal.
10. Client states he/she feels better.

V. NURSING INTERVENTION/TREATMENT

1. R.N. will contact client/family before admission to community

health agency to arrange for additional supplies or rehabilitation equipment if necessary.

2. R.N. will consult with M.D. if additional personnel are needed (e.g., P.T., S.T., M.S.W., H.H.A., home attendant, housekeeper, homemaker).

3. R.N. will allow client/family to verbalize fears, anxieties, and concerns and will provide psychologic support.

4. R.N. will instruct client/family/H.H.A./significant others on:

   A. monitoring and recording of vital signs.

   B. fluid intake/dietary regimen as ordered.

   C. medication administration/adverse reactions.

   D. immediate notification of M.D. of adverse reactions.

   E. skin care.

   F. exercise/rest.

   G. bowel/bladder routine.

   H. positioning/turning.

   I. respiratory therapy.

   J. rehabilitation equipment (e.g., air mattress with pump/water bed/flotation pad/electric wheelchair/chair lift/Hoyer lift/bed trapeze/transfer board/hospital bed/patient lifter/environmental controls/raised toilet seat/commode/standing frame/grab bars/ramps).

   K. self-aid devices.

   L. recording of intake and output.

   M. strengthening/weight-bearing activities/physical therapy as ordered/muscle testing/occupational therapy as ordered.

   N. transportation/potential driving ability.

   O. sexual rehabilitation.

   P. career counseling.

   Q. housing.

   R. financial assistance.

   S. dental care.

   T. laboratory testing/M.D. appointments.

   U. socialization groups, organizations, clubs.

5. R.N. will provide M.D. with follow-up reports and discharge summary when case closes.

6. R.N. will notify client/family/H.H.A./significant others when case will close.

Staphylococcus/Salmonella/ Shigella Surveillance Care Plan

I. NURSING DIAGNOSIS

   1. Anxiety related to:
- A. headache.
- B. nausea/vomiting.
- C. diarrhea.
- D. abdominal pain.
- E. fever.
- F. other _____

   2. Knowledge deficit related to:
- A. management of nausea/vomiting/diarrhea (limited fluids/ avoidance of sugar and fatty and fried foods).
- B. medication administration/adverse reactions.
- C. isolation of the sick.
- D. adequate nutrition.
- E. proper hand-washing technique.
- F. collection of stool specimens.
- G. laboratory testing/M.D. appointments.
- H. other _____

   3. Abdominal pain related to:
- A. contaminated food.
- B. contaminated water supply.

C. other _____

4. Ineffective individual/family coping related to:
    A. malaise.
    B. frequent diarrhea.
    C. abdominal pain.
    D. anorexia.
    E. nausea/vomiting.
    F. bloody stools.
    G. irritability.
    H. other _____

5. Self-care deficit: feeding/bathing/grooming/dressing/toileting
   related to:
    A. abdominal pain.
    B. nausea/vomiting.
    C. diarrhea.
    D. dependence on others for care.
    E. other _____

6. Impaired home maintenance management related to:
    A. general malaise.
    B. frequent diarrhea.
    C. excessive demands posed by caring for the sick.
    D. dependence on others for care.
    E. loss of income.
    F. other _____

7. Diarrhea/Bloody stools related to:
    A. contaminated food.
    B. contaminated water supply.
    C. other _____

8. Impaired physical mobility related to:
    A. weakness.
    B. abdominal pain.
    C. nausea/vomiting.
    D. other _____

9. Noncompliance with therapy related to:
   A. denial.
   B. language barrier.
   C. lack of assistance in the home.
   D. other _____

   _____

10. Altered nutrition: potential for more than body requirements related to:
    A. nausea/vomiting.
    B. dependence on others for care.
    C. diarrhea.
    D. weight loss.
    E. temporary dietary restrictions.
    F. bacterial contamination.
    G. other _____

    _____

11. Altered parenting related to:
    A. weakness.
    B. immobility.
    C. other _____

    _____

12. Potential fluid volume deficit related to:
    A. anorexia.
    B. nausea/vomiting.
    C. diarrhea.
    D. poor/restricted fluid/dietary intake.
    E. other _____

    _____

13. Sleep pattern disturbance related to:
    A. diarrhea.
    B. nausea/vomiting.
    C. abdominal pain.
    D. other _____

    _____

14. Activity intolerance related to:
    A. fatigue/weakness.
    B. nausea/vomiting/diarrhea.
    C. abdominal pain.

D. other _____

_____

II. SHORT-TERM GOALS

1. Client/Family will wash hands before and after defecating after 1–2 R.N. visits.
2. Client/Family will collect stool specimens from client and 1 each from family members and submit to state for laboratory testing after 1–2 R.N. visits.
3. Client/Family will prepare meals in a clean environment after 1–2 R.N. visits.
4. Client/Family will administer medication for diarrheal stools as ordered after 1–2 R.N. visits.
5. Client/Family will adequately store food to retard spoilage after 1–2 R.N. visits.
6. Client/Family will seek laboratory testing/M.D. appointments as ordered after 1–2 R.N. visits.

III. LONG-TERM GOALS

1. Infectious agent will be eradicated in 1–2 weeks.
2. Independent activities of daily living will be resumed in 1–2 weeks.
3. Optimal level of health will be achieved in 1–2 weeks.
4. Client/Family will safely reintegrate into community in 1–2 weeks.

IV. OUTCOME CRITERIA

1. Vital signs are normal.
2. Bowel elimination is normal.
3. Appetite remains normal.
4. Client consumes adequate fluids/nutritious meals.
5. Tissue turgor remains normal.
6. Client prepares meals in clean environment.
7. Proper hand washing is carried out.
8. Client states he/she feels better.

V. NURSING INTERVENTION/TREATMENT

1. R.N. will arrange appointment for home visit for interview and preparation of state surveillance record.

2. R.N. will collect 1–3 or more specimens according to local board of health/state regulations concerning period of communicability and testing.
3. R.N. will encourage client/family to visit M.D. for treatment.
4. R.N. will provide instructions in good hand-washing technique/ preparation of food in clean environment/adequate food storage/ disposal of human waste/prevention of cross-contamination/ *Staphylococcus aureus* enterotoxin (most common sources: processed meat, cream-filled or custard pastries, potato salad and milk at room temperature)/*Shigella* (food, particularly dairy products, contaminated by excreta)/*Salmonella* (undercooked poultry, fish, and pork; contaminated milk, water, ice cream, eggs, and precooked beef).
5. R.N. will consult with sanitarian about possible inspection of home or eating establishment if necessary.
6. R.N. will provide M.D. with follow-up reports and discharge summary when case closes.
7. R.N. will notify client/family/significant others when case will close.

Suprapubic Prostatectomy Care Plan

I. NURSING DIAGNOSIS

1. Knowledge deficit related to:
   A. aseptic technique.
   B. proper hand-washing technique.
   C. medication administration/adverse reactions.
   D. ambulation.
   E. catheter care.
   F. fluid/dietary needs.
   G. other _____

2. Potential for injury related to:
   A. poor dressing technique.
   B. inadequate fluid intake.
   C. other _____

3. Pain related to:
   A. wound granulation.
   B. inadequate exercise.
   C. poor fluid/dietary intake.
   D. poor administration of medication.
   E. infection.
   F. kinking of catheter.
   G. other _____

4. Potential fluid volume deficit related to:
   A. frequency of need to urinate.
   B. poor urinary output (or small stream).
   C. poor fluid/dietary intake.
   D. diuresis.
   E. obstruction of catheter.
   F. other _____
   _____

5. Impaired physical mobility related to:
   A. pain.
   B. infection.
   C. other _____
   _____

6. Noncompliance with therapy related to:
   A. confusion.
   B. denial.
   C. dependence on others for care.
   D. lack of support in home.
   E. other _____
   _____

7. Sexual dysfunction related to:
   A. pain.
   B. infection.
   C. other _____
   _____

8. Altered health maintenance related to:
   A. lack of support in the home.
   B. refusal to comply with medical treatment.
   C. other _____
   _____

9. Self-care deficit: feeding/bathing/grooming/dressing/toileting
   related to:
   A. pain.
   B. poor mobility.
   C. other _____
   _____

10. Altered patterns of urinary elimination related to:
    A. pain.
    B. poor fluid intake.

    C. infection.

    D. obstruction of catheter.

    E. other _____

_____

11. Ineffective individual/family coping related to:

    A. excessive pain.

    B. slow healing of surgical site.

    C. dependence on others for care.

    D. other _____

_____

12. Self-esteem disturbance related to:

    A. inability to perform activities of daily living.

    B. unemployment.

    C. poor prognosis.

    D. other _____

_____

II. SHORT-TERM GOALS

1. Client/Family will verbalize all fears, anxieties, and concerns after 1–2–3 R.N. visits.
2. Client/Family will record vital signs daily as ordered after 1–2 R.N. visits.
3. Client/Family will change suprapubic dressings aseptically as ordered after 1–2 R.N. visits.
4. Client/Family will apply prescribed ointments/creams to suprapubic site as ordered after 1–2 R.N. visits.
5. Client will avoid alcohol intake for approximately 1 month or as ordered after 1–2–3–4 R.N. visits.
6. Client/Family will state signs/symptoms of infection after 1–2 R.N. visits.
7. Client/Family will obtain prescribed medication after 1–2 R.N. visits.
8. Client/Family will notify M.D. of adverse reactions after 1–2 R.N. visits.
9. Client/Family will notify M.D./R.N. of increased pain, infection, or bleeding after 1–2 R.N. visits.
10. Client will consume fluids/diet as ordered after 1–2 R.N. visits.
11. Client/Family will obtain irrigation equipment for Foley catheter after 1–2 R.N. visits.

12. Client/Family will obtain extra catheter, gloves, and insertion kits to keep in home after 1–2 R.N. visits.
13. Client/Family will correctly irrigate catheter as ordered after 1–2–3 R.N. visits.
14. Client/Family will keep urinary drainage bag lower than client's bladder at all times after 1–2–3 R.N. visits.
15. Client/Family will keep accurate daily record of intake and output after 1–2–3 R.N. visits.
16. Client will perform own independent activities of daily living after 1–2 R.N. visits.
17. Client will ambulate/exercise/rest as ordered after 1–2 R.N. visits.
18. Client/Family will change urinary draining bag once monthly at home or as ordered by R.N. after 1–2 R.N. visits.
19. Client will participate in diversional activities (e.g., reading, card games, videogames, painting, computer programming) after 1–2 R.N. visits.
20. Client/Family will seek laboratory testing/M.D. appointments as ordered after 1–2 R.N. visits.

III. LONG-TERM GOALS

1. Independent activities of daily living will be resumed in 1–2 weeks.
2. GU system will function adequately in 1–2 weeks.
3. Optimal level of health will be achieved in 3–4 weeks.

IV. OUTCOME CRITERIA

1. Vital signs are normal.
2. Urine is clear, yellow, and sufficient in quantity.
3. Surgical site is well-healed; skin/mucous membrane is healthy and intact.
4. Ambulation is normal.
5. Sexual relations are normal.
6. Client states he feels better.

V. NURSING INTERVENTION/TREATMENT

1. R.N. will contact client/family to ensure that proper supplies are present before home visit.
2. R.N. will instruct client/family/H.H.A. on:
   A. monitoring and recording of vital signs.

    B. signs/symptoms of infection, hemorrhage, urinary obstruction, frequency, dribbling.

    C. medication administration/adverse reactions.

    D. immediate notification of M.D. of adverse reactions or change in condition.

    E. daily recording of intake and output.

    F. avoidance of emotional stress.

    G. exercise/rest.

    H. fluid/dietary needs: 3000 cc fluids daily as ordered by M.D.

    I. avoidance of straining at stool.

    J. exercise of perineal muscles.

    K. Foley catheter irrigation/equipment to be kept in the home.

    L. monthly change of Foley bag and catheter if necessary.

    M. aseptic dressing technique.

    N. laboratory testing/M.D. appointments.

    O. diversional activities.

4. R.N. will provide follow-up reports and discharge summary to M.D. when case closes.

5. R.N. will notify client/family/H.H.A./significant others when case will close.

Syphilis
Care Plan

I. NURSING DIAGNOSIS

1. Knowledge deficit related to:
   A. prevention and treatment of syphilis.
   B. transmission of disease.
   C. signs/symptoms.
   D. source of infection.
   E. congenital defects.
   F. state/local laboratory testing.
   G. medication administration/adverse reactions.
   H. other _____

   _____

2. Anxiety related to:
   A. source of infection.
   B. transmission of communicable disease.
   C. congenital defects.
   D. other _____

   _____

3. Headache/joint pain/bone pain related to:
   A. acquisition of sexually transmitted disease.
   B. promiscuity.
   C. poor administration of medication.
   D. refusal to seek adequate medical help.
   E. other _____

   _____

4. Noncompliance with therapy related to:
   A. shame.
   B. embarrassment.
   C. guilt.
   D. denial.
   E. other _____

5. Potential for injury/birth defects related to:
   A. procrastination/refusal of treatment.
   B. other _____

6. Altered health maintenance related to:
   A. acquisition of sexually transmitted disease.
   B. transmission of sexually transmitted disease.
   C. other _____

7. Altered nutrition: potential for more than body requirements related to weight loss.
8. Potential impaired skin integrity related to generalized infection.
9. Altered thought processes related to generalized infection.
10. Sexual dysfunction related to:
    A. lymphadenopathy.
    B. chancre formation.
    C. macular/papular skin rash.
    D. painful joints.
    E. bone pain.
    F. fever.
    G. enlargement of liver and spleen.
    H. anemia.
    I. bilateral earache.
    J. headaches.
    K. other _____

11. Self-esteem disturbance related to acquisition/transmission of communicable disease.
12. Social isolation related to acquisition/transmission of communicable disease.

II. SHORT-TERM GOALS

1. Client/Spouse/Family/Contacts will seek immediate testing/treatment after 1–2–3 R.N. visits.
2. Client/Spouse/Family/Contacts will take prescribed medication as ordered after 1–2 R.N. visits.
3. Client/Spouse/Family/Contacts will immediately notify M.D. of adverse reactions to medications or change in condition after 1–2 R.N. visits.
4. Client/Spouse/Family/Contacts will return for follow-up injections/laboratory testing as ordered after 1–2 R.N. visits.
5. Client/Spouse/Family/Contacts will abstain from sexual intercourse until medical clearance is obtained after 1–2 R.N. visits.
6. Client/Spouse/Family/Contacts will consent to hospitalization as ordered after 1–2 R.N. visits.

III. LONG-TERM GOAL

1. Control/Palliation of communicable disease will be achieved in 1–2 weeks.

IV. OUTCOME CRITERIA

1. Venereal Disease Research Laboratory (VDRL) and rapid plasma reagin (RPR) test remain at very low dilution.
2. FTA (fluorescent treponemal antibody absorption test) or MHA-TP (microhemagglutination-treponemal test) remains nonreactive.
3. Skin remains healthy and intact.
4. Client/Spouse/Family/Contacts are alert and cooperative.
5. Hemoglobin/Hematocrit levels/WBC remain normal.
6. Liver and spleen function normally.
7. Weight remains normal.
8. Vision remains clear.
9. Musculoskeletal system functions normally.
10. Client/Spouse/Family/Contacts state he/she/they feel better.

V. NURSING INTERVENTION/TREATMENT

1. R.N. will arrange for M.D. appointment for laboratory testing/treatment of all exposed sources.

2. R.N. will instruct all infected/suspected as infected people on:
   A. proper hand-washing technique/personal hygiene.
   B. immediate blood testing.
   C. assessment of allergies.
   D. medication administration—oral or IM (benzathine penicillin/ probenecid/ampicillin/tetracycline/erythromycin)/adverse reactions.
   E. immediate notification of M.D. of adverse reactions.
   F. follow-up M.D./clinic visits.
   G. sexual abstinence as ordered/use of latex condom.
3. R.N. will provide M.D. with follow-up reports and discharge summary when case closes.
4. R.N. will notify client/spouse/family/contacts when case will close.
5. R.N. will notify client/spouse/family/contacts/significant others that VDRL/RPR may remain positive throughout life.

Tracheostomy/Laryngectomy Care Plan

I. NURSING DIAGNOSIS

1. Anxiety related to:
   A. emergency/elective tracheostomy.
   B. suctioning.
   C. loss of communication.
   D. possibility of death.
   E. hyperoxygenation.
   F. other _____

2. Knowledge deficit related to:
   A. proper hand-washing technique.
   B. dressing care.
   C. suctioning technique.
   D. cleaning and storage of equipment.
   E. inhalation therapy.
   F. cuffing technique.
   G. esophageal speech techniques.
   H. portable computer-synthesized speech unit (Texas Instruments Vocaid)
   I. hand-held communicator.
   J. medication administration/adverse reactions.
   K. other _____

3. Potential for injury related to:
   A. poor fit of tracheal tube.

B. poor cuffing technique.

C. poor hand-washing technique.

D. skin breakdown.

E. poor suctioning technique.

F. refusal to suction.

G. poor dressing technique.

H. depressed immune system.

I. other _____

_____

4. Impaired verbal communication related to:

A. tracheostomy.

B. difficulty with esophageal speech techniques.

C. other _____

_____

5. Self-care deficit: feeding/bathing/grooming/dressing/performing household chores related to:

A. weakness.

B. paralysis.

C. refusal to assist with therapy.

D. dependence on others for care.

E. other _____

_____

6. Ineffective airway clearance related to:

A. retained respiratory secretions.

B. poor suctioning techniques.

C. infection.

D. edema.

E. hemorrhage.

F. poor dressing care.

G. other _____

_____

7. Noncompliance with therapy related to:

A. fear of injury.

B. fear of death.

C. cost of medical care/poor insurance coverage.

D. lack of support in the home.

E. dependence on others for care.

F. other _____

_____

8. Potential impaired skin integrity related to:
   A. infection.
   B. poor suctioning technique.
   C. other _____

   _____

9. Self-esteem disturbance related to:
   A. tracheostomy.
   B. communication deficit.
   C. unemployment.
   D. other _____

   _____

10. Ineffective breathing pattern related to:
    A. poor suctioning technique.
    B. infection.
    C. retained respiratory secretions.
    D. other _____

    _____

II. SHORT-TERM GOALS

1. Client/Family will verbalize fears, anxieties, and concerns after 1–2–3–4 R.N./R.T./S.T. visits.
2. Client/Family will obtain all medical equipment as ordered after 1–2–3 R.N./R.T./S.T. visits.
3. Client/Family will administer respiratory therapy (breathing exercises/inhalation therapy/chest physical therapy) as ordered after 1–2–3 R.N./R.T. visits.
4. Client/Family will wash hands as ordered after 1 R.N. visit.
5. Client/Family will demonstrate appropriate suctioning technique after 1–2–3 R.N./R.T. visits.
6. Client/Family will demonstrate appropriate cuffing technique after 1–2–3 R.N./R.T. visits.
7. Client/Family will change inner/outer tracheostomy cannula as ordered by M.D. after 1–2–3 R.N./R.T. visits.
8. Client/Family will keep an emergency tracheostomy set on hand at all times after 1–2 R.N./R.T. visits.
9. Client/Family will cleanse tracheostomy/respiratory equipment as ordered after 1–2 R.N./R.T. visits.
10. Client/Family will administer prescribed medication after 1–2 R.N. visits.

11. Client/Family will immediately notify M.D. of adverse reactions or change in condition after 1–2 R.N. visits.

12. Client will perform communication/esophageal speech after 1–2–3–4–5–6 R.N./S.T. visits.

13. Client will carry writing materials at all times after 1–2 R.N. visits.

14. Client/Family will seek laboratory testing/M.D. appointments as ordered after 1–2 R.N. visits.

15. Client will avoid crowded areas, infected people, lint, and dust contamination as ordered after 1–2 R.N. visits.

III. LONG-TERM GOALS

1. Adequate respiratory functioning will be achieved in 1–2 weeks.
2. Independent activities of daily living will be resumed in 1–2 weeks.
3. Communication will be achieved in 1–2 weeks.
4. Optimal level of health will be achieved in 3–4 weeks.

IV. OUTCOME CRITERIA

1. Vital signs are normal.
2. Chest is clear.
3. Breath sounds are normal.
4. Airway is patent.
5. Appetite is normal.
6. Weight is normal.
7. Laboratory test results are normal.
8. Skin/Mucous membrane is healthy and intact.
9. Client is alert and sociable.
10. Client states he/she feels better.

V. NURSING INTERVENTION/TREATMENT

1. R.N. will contact client to arrange home visit and ensure all supplies are present in home.
2. R.N. will perform physical examination on initial visit.
3. R.N. will instruct client/family/H.H.A. on:
   A. monitoring and recording of vital signs.
   B. proper hand-washing technique.
   C. dressing care/aseptic technique.
   D. suctioning techniques.

E. cuffing.

F. respiratory therapy (breathing exercises/chest physical therapy/inhalation therapy) as ordered.

G. cleaning and storage of tracheostomy equipment.

H. storage of emergency tracheostomy set.

I. self-insertion of inner/outer tracheostomy cannula.

J. medication administration/adverse reactions.

K. signs/symptoms of infection.

L. immediate notification of M.D. of adverse reactions or change in condition.

M. laboratory testing/M.D. appointments.

N. communication techniques, esophageal speech/portable computer-synthesized speech unit (Texas Instruments Vocaid/hand-held communicator/R.N. will confer with S.T.).

O. avoidance of air pollution, people with infections, overcrowded areas.

P. appropriate clothing.

4. R.N. will provide client/family with additional information/names of organizations, clubs, societies to contact about talking with people with similar condition.

5. R.N. will provide M.D. with follow-up reports and discharge summary when case closes.

6. R.N. will notify client/family/H.H.A./significant others when case will close.

Transcutaneous Electrical Nerve Stimulation (TENS) Care Plan

I. NURSING DIAGNOSIS

1. Knowledge deficit related to:
   A. pain management.
   B. operation of TENS machine.
   C. adverse reactions.
   D. other _____
   _____

2. Pain related to:
   A. poor supervision/operation of TENS machine.
   B. advance of disease process.
   C. other _____
   _____

3. Ineffective individual/family coping related to pain.
4. Diversional activity deficit related to pain.
5. Ineffective breathing pattern related to chest pain.
6. Impaired home maintenance management related to pain.
7. Impaired physical mobility related to pain.
8. Noncompliance with operation of TENS machine related to:
   A. refusal to operate TENS machine.
   B. mechanical problems.
   C. previous dissatisfaction/lack of pain relief.
   D. burns.
   E. rash.

F. other _____
_____

9. Fear related to operating TENS machine.
10. Altered parenting related to pain.
11. Self-care deficit: feeding/bathing/dressing/grooming/household chores related to pain.
12. Sexual dysfunction related to pain.
13. Potential impaired skin integrity related to:
    A. burns from TENS administration.
    B. other _____
    _____

14. Sleep pattern disturbance related to pain.
15. Potential for injury related to:
    A. poor application of electrodes.
    B. contact of electrode with metal, producing shocking sensation.
    C. burning of skin.
    D. other _____
    _____

II. SHORT-TERM GOALS

1. Client/Family will verbalize fears, anxieties, and questions about TENS machine after 1–2–3 R.N. visits.
2. Client will state location and severity of pain after 1–2 R.N. visits.
3. Client/Family will state 2 common side effects of the TENS machine after 1–2–3 R.N. visits.
4. Client will state he/she feels tingling and then numbness after 1–2 R.N. visits.
5. Client/Family will turn off TENS stimulator before bathing after 1 R.N. visit.
6. Client/Family will apply TENS before coughing, deep breathing, turning, ambulation, or physical therapy after 1–2 R.N. visits.
7. Client/Family will correctly apply electrode gel to intact, healthy skin after 1–2 R.N. visits.
8. Client/Family will correctly apply electrodes to skin after 1–2 R.N. visits.
9. Client/Family will increase current level of TENS until tingling discomfort is felt and then will turn it down slightly after 1–2 R.N. visits.
10. Client/Family will correctly replace batteries in TENS machine after 1–2 R.N. visits.

11. Client/Family will apply prescribed medication to contact dermatitis or burn site after 1–2 R.N. visits.
12. Client/Family will use TENS machine in place of medication after 1–2 R.N. visits.

III. LONG-TERM GOALS

1. Pain management will be achieved in 1–2 weeks.
2. Independent activities of daily living will be resumed in 1–2 weeks.
3. Optimal level of health will be achieved in 1–2 weeks.

IV. OUTCOME CRITERIA

1. Vital signs are normal.
2. Circulation is normal.
3. Skin is healthy and intact.
4. Pain is relieved.
5. Need for pain medication or TENS is eliminated.
6. Wound heals appropriately.
7. Ambulation occurs normally.
8. Client states he/she feels better.

V. NURSING INTERVENTION/TREATMENT

1. R.N. will consult with hospital discharge planner for arrangements to be made for TENS therapy to occur in the home.
2. R.N. will instruct client/family/H.H.A. on:
    A. purpose, operation, and care of TENS machine.
    B. potential mechanical problems.
    C. adjusting of machine for elimination of various levels of pain.
    D. elimination of additional oral/IM pain medications.
    E. potential side effects of TENS: contact dermatitis and burns.
    F. possible purchase of machine.
    G. laboratory testing/M.D. appointments.
3. R.N. will provide M.D. with follow-up reports and discharge summary when case closes.
4. R.N. will notify client/family/H.H.A./significant others when case will close.

Transurethral Resection
Care Plan

I. NURSING DIAGNOSIS

1. Knowledge deficit related to:
   A. dressing change.
   B. aseptic technique.
   C. intake and output.
   D. medication administration/adverse reactions.
   E. ambulation.
   F. other _____
      _____

2. Pain related to:
   A. wound granulation.
   B. inadequate exercise.
   C. infection.
   D. poor administration of medication.
   E. other _____
      _____

3. Potential fluid volume deficit related to:
   A. frequency of urination.
   B. poor output (or small stream).
   C. hemorrhage.
   D. obstruction of catheter.
   E. other _____
      _____

4. Impaired physical mobility related to:
   A. pain.

B. other _____

_____

5. Noncompliance with therapy related to:
   A. confusion.
   B. denial.
   C. dependence on others for care.
   D. other _____

_____

6. Altered nutrition: potential for more than body requirements related to:
   A. anorexia.
   B. lack of support in the home.
   C. other _____

_____

7. Potential for injury related to:
   A. poor fluid intake.
   B. poor catheter care.
   C. other _____

_____

8. Self-care deficit: feeding/bathing/dressing/grooming/toileting/ household chores related to:
   A. pain.
   B. lethargy.
   C. poor mobility.
   D. infection.
   E. confusion.
   F. other _____

_____

9. Sexual dysfunction related to:
   A. pain.
   B. occlusive dressing.
   C. weakness.
   D. other _____

_____

10. Altered patterns of urinary elimination related to:
   A. muscle spasms.
   B. poor fluid intake.
   C. infection.

    D. obstruction of catheter.

    E. other _____

    _____

11. Ineffective individual/family coping related to:

    A. pain.

    B. irritability.

    C. slow healing of surgical site.

    D. immobility.

    E. dependence on others for care.

    F. other _____

    _____

12. Self-esteem disturbance related to:

    A. unemployment.

    B. sexual dysfunction.

    C. other _____

    _____

II. SHORT-TERM GOALS

1. Client/Family will obtain prescribed medication after 1–2 R.N. visits.
2. Client/Family will correctly administer prescribed medication after 1–2 R.N. visits.
3. Client/Family will notify M.D. of adverse reactions or change in condition after 1–2 R.N. visits.
4. Client/Family will notify M.D./R.N. of increased pain, infection, or bleeding after 1–2 R.N. visits.
5. Client will consume fluids/diet as ordered after 1–2 R.N. visits.
6. Client/Family will obtain extra catheter, gloves, insertion kits, and bags to keep in home after 1–2 R.N. visits.
7. Client/Family will obtain irrigation equipment for Foley catheter after 1–2 R.N. visits.
8. Client/Family will correctly irrigate catheter as ordered after 1–2 R.N. visits.
9. Client/Family will keep urinary drainage bag lower than client's bladder at all times after 1–2 R.N. visits.
10. Client/Family will keep accurate daily record of intake and output after 1 R.N. visit.
11. Client will ambulate/exercise/rest as ordered after 1–2 R.N. visits.
12. Client/Family will change urinary drainage bag once monthly at home or as ordered by R.N. after 1–2 R.N. visits.

13. Client will participate in diversional activities (e.g., card games, videogames, painting) as ordered after 1–2 R.N. visits.
14. Client/Family will seek laboratory testing/M.D. appointments after 1 R.N. visit.

III. LONG-TERM GOALS

1. Adequate healing of surgical site will result in adequate urinary output in 1–2 weeks.
2. Independent activities of daily living will be resumed in 1–2 weeks.
3. Optimal level of health will be achieved in 1–2 weeks.

IV. OUTCOME CRITERIA

1. Vital signs are normal.
2. Urine is yellow, clear, and sufficient in quantity.
3. Intake and output are adequate.
4. Voiding is normal.
5. Surgical site is well-healed; granulation occurs.
6. Ambulation is normal.
7. Client states he feels better.
8. Client returns to work.

V. NURSING INTERVENTION/TREATMENT

1. R.N. will assess signs/symptoms of hemorrhage, infection, or obstruction.
2. R.N. will instruct client/family/H.H.A. on:
   A. monitoring and recording of vital signs (especially temperature).
   B. signs/symptoms of infection, hemorrhage, urinary obstruction, frequency of urination, dribbling, and pain.
   C. immediate notification of M.D./R.N. of pain, infection, bleeding, urinary obstruction, frequency of urination, or dribbling.
   D. medication administration (analgesics/antispasmodics/antibiotics)/adverse reactions.
   E. immediate notification of M.D of adverse reactions.
   F. recording of intake and output.
   G. avoidance of emotional stress.
   H. exercise/rest as ordered.
   I. avoidance of straining at stool.

    J. exercise of perineal muscles.

    K. fluid intake/dietary instructions; 3000 cc fluid daily unless otherwise ordered by M.D.

    L. Foley catheter irrigation, equipment, gloves, catheters, insertion sets to be kept in the home.

    M. performance of Foley catheter irrigations with normal saline if ordered.

    N. monthly change of urinary drainage bag and catheter.

    O. bladder training.

    P. urinalysis/urine culture and sensitivity tests if ordered.

    Q. diversional activities.

    R. blood testing.

    S. laboratory testing/M.D. appointments.

3. R.N. will provide M.D. with follow-up reports and discharge summary when case closes.

4. R.N. will notify client/family/H.H.A./significant others when case will close.

Two-Way
Foley Catheter
Care Plan

I. NURSING DIAGNOSIS

1. Anxiety related to:
   A. catheter insertion.
   B. infection.
   C. other _____
   _____

2. Knowledge deficit related to:
   A. purpose of Foley catheter.
   B. fluid intake.
   C. personal hygiene/perineal care/meatal care.
   D. types of urinary incontinence (i.e., stress incontinence/
      urge incontinence/overflow incontinence/reflex incontinence/
      functional incontinence/total incontinence)/etiology.
   E. urodynamic testing/kidney and bladder x-rays/
      cystourethroscopy.
   F. bladder training.
   G. catheterization equipment/appliances.
   H. pelvic floor exercises.
   I. biofeedback.
   J. surgery.
   K. intermittent catheterization.
   L. odor control.
   M. intake and output.

N. infection.

O. catheterization equipment.

P. medication administration/adverse reactions.

Q. removal of catheter.

R. other _____

_____

3. Altered patterns of urinary elimination related to:

A. poor fluid intake.

B. abnormal fluid retention.

C. immobility.

D. poor exercise.

E. kinking of catheter.

F. obstruction of catheter with sedimentation.

G. unauthorized removal of catheter by client or family.

H. infection.

I. poor irrigation techniques.

J. other _____

_____

4. Potential for injury related to:

A. poor catheterization technique.

B. poor hand-washing technique.

C. inadequate fluid intake.

D. skin breakdown.

E. other _____

_____

5. Ineffective individual/family coping related to:

A. catheter discomfort.

B. infection.

C. dependence on others for care.

D. other _____

_____

6. Sexual dysfunction related to:

A. catheterization.

B. other _____

_____

7. Self-care deficit: feeding/bathing/grooming/dressing/toileting related to:

A. paralysis.

    B. dependence on others for care.

    C. other _____

    _____

8. Actual/Potential impaired skin integrity related to:

    A. poor personal hygiene.

    B. catheter leakage.

    C. poor removal of catheter.

    D. other _____

    _____

9. Actual/Potential fluid volume deficit related to:

    A. poor intake.

    B. excessive diuresis.

    C. lack of support in the home.

    D. other _____

    _____

10. Social isolation related to:

    A. confinement to home.

    B. embarrassment about catheter placement.

    C. other _____

    _____

II. SHORT-TERM GOALS

1. Client/Family will verbalize fears, anxieties, and concerns after 1–2–3 R.N. visits.
2. Client/Family will administer adequate fluids as ordered after 1–2 R.N. visits.
3. Client/Family will irrigate catheter as ordered after 1–2–3 R.N. visits.
4. Client/Family will lubricate catheter after 1–2–3 R.N. visits.
5. Client/Family will practice adequate personal hygiene/perineal care after 1–2 R.N. visits.
6. Client/Family will record daily intake and output after 1–2–3 R.N. visits.
7. Client/Family will change Foley bag once monthly or prn after 1–2–3 R.N. visits.
8. Client/Family will maintain catheter equipment in home after 1–2 R.N. visits.
9. Client/Family will administer medication as ordered after 1–2 R.N. visits.

10. Client/Family will state three signs/symptoms of adverse reactions to medications after 1–2–3 R.N. visits.
11. Client/Family will immediately notify M.D. of adverse reactions or change in condition after 1–2 R.N. visits.
12. Client will seek laboratory testing/M.D. appointments after 1–2 R.N. visits.

III. LONG-TERM GOALS

1. Urinary functioning will resume in 1–2 weeks.
2. Independent activities of daily living will be resumed in 1–2 weeks.
3. Optimal level of health will be achieved in 2–4 weeks.

IV. OUTCOME CRITERIA

1. Vital signs are normal.
2. Intake and output are normal.
3. Urinary output is clear, yellow, and sufficient in quantity.
4. Weight is normal for height.
5. Skin/Mucous membrane is healthy and intact.
6. Laboratory test results are normal.
7. Appetite is normal.
8. Voiding resumes.
9. Client states he/she feels better.
10. Client returns to work.

V. NURSING INTERVENTION/TREATMENT

1. R.N. will contact client/family to arrange for home visit and assessment of general physical status.
2. R.N. will instruct client/family to assemble all equipment before home visit.
3. R.N. will instruct client/family on:
   A. types of urinary incontinence (i.e., stress incontinence/ reflex incontinence/urge incontinence/functional incontinence/ overflow incontinence/total incontinence)/etiology.
   B. urodynamic testing/kidney and bladder x-rays/ cystourethroscopy.
   C. catheterization equipment/appliances.
   D. proper hand-washing technique.

E. positioning.

F. monitoring and recording of vital signs.

G. signs/symptoms of infection.

H. skin care/personal hygiene/perineal care/meatal care.

I. assessment of color, amount, and consistency of urine/odor control.

J. milking* of tubing.

K. positioning of tubing (dependent position at all times lower than bladder).

L. fluid intake/diet as ordered.

M. intake and output.

N. daily recording of weight.

O. medication administration/adverse reactions.

P. biofeedback.

Q. surgery.

R. immediate notification of M.D. of adverse reactions or change in condition.

S. catheter irrigation/intermittent catheterization.

T. urinalysis/culture and sensitivity tests.

U. bladder training/pelvic floor exercises.

V. disinfection of urinary receptacle when emptying Foley bag.

W. exercise/rest.

X. laboratory testing/M.D. appointments.

4. R.N. will change Foley catheter as ordered by M.D.

5. R.N. will provide M.D. with follow-up reports and discharge summary when case closes.

6. R.N. will notify client/family/H.H.A./significant others when case will close.

*"Milking": assisting tubing in downward position periodically to prevent pooling of fluids.

Ulcerative Colitis Care Plan

I. NURSING DIAGNOSIS

1. Diarrhea/Bloody stools related to:
   A. psychologic stress.
   B. poor nutritional habits.
   C. other _____

   _____

2. Anxiety related to:
   A. frequent diarrhea.
   B. abdominal pain.
   C. bloody stools.
   D. weight loss.
   E. other _____

   _____

3. Potential fluid volume deficit related to diarrhea.
4. Abdominal pain/Painful rectal spasms related to:
   A. psychologic stress.
   B. poor administration of medication/vitamins.
   C. inappropriate fluid/dietary intake.
   D. refusal to comply with medical orders.
   E. other _____

   _____

5. Knowledge deficit related to:
   A. fluid/dietary intake.
   B. medication/vitamin administration.
   C. rest/exercise.

    D. nature of chronic disease.

    E. biofeedback.

    F. other _____

    _____

6. Body image disturbance related to weight loss.

II. SHORT-TERM GOALS

1. Client will consume well-balanced, bland, low-residue, high-protein diet after 1–2 R.N. visits.
2. Client/Family will administer medication as ordered after 1–2 R.N. visits.
3. Client/Family will immediately notify M.D. of adverse reactions to medications or change in condition after 1–2 R.N. visits.
4. Client will take vitamin therapy as ordered after 1 R.N. visit.
5. Client will rest periodically each day as ordered after 1 R.N. visit.
6. Client will avoid emotional stress as much as possible after 1–2 R.N. visits.
7. Client will weigh self daily after 1 R.N. visit.
8. Client will seek laboratory testing/M.D. appointments after 1–2 R.N. visits.

III. LONG-TERM GOALS

1. Independent activities of daily living will be resumed in 1–2 weeks.
2. GI functioning will remain normal as a result of proper dietary intake in 1–2 weeks.
3. Optimal level of health will be achieved in 6–8 weeks.

IV. OUTCOME CRITERIA

1. Vital signs are normal.
2. Peristalsis remains normal.
3. Mucous membrane remains healthy and intact.
4. Weight remains normal for stature.
5. Stools are formed and of normal quantity and color.
6. Laboratory test results remain normal.
7. Client states he/she feels better.

V. NURSING INTERVENTION/TREATMENT

1. R.N. will assess probable etiologic factors in severe bouts of diarrhea.
2. R.N. will encourage verbalization of fears and anxieties in everyday life; will provide psychologic support; will encourage client to seek further professional counseling, if necessary, and to join professional organizations, to learn how to deal better with chronic nature of disease.
3. R.N. will instruct client/family/H.H.A. on:
   A. monitoring and recording of vital signs.
   B. well-balanced, bland, low-residue, high-protein diet; fluid intake as ordered.
   C. recording of intake and output.
   D. recording of weight daily.
   E. medication administration (sedatives/sulfa preparations/cortisone preparations/iron replacement/anticholinergics/vitamin therapy)/adverse reactions.
   F. immediate notification of M.D. of adverse reactions or change in condition.
   G. rest/exercise/biofeedback/meditation.
   H. avoidance of temperature extremes in fluids to prevent excessive gastric motility.
   I. rectal installations of cortisone preparations.
   J. laboratory testing/collection of stool specimens.
   K. routine M.D. appointments.
4. R.N. will provide M.D. with follow-up reports and discharge summary when case closes.
5. R.N. will notify client/family/significant others/H.H.A./home attendant when case will close.

Antepartal Care Plan

I. NURSING DIAGNOSIS

1. Anxiety related to:
   A. the unknown.
   B. altered body image.
   C. mental/physical well-being of fetus.
   D. unwanted pregnancy.
   E. single parenthood.
   F. marital discord.
   G. other _____

2. Knowledge deficit related to:
   A. normal anatomy/physiology of reproductive tract.
   B. growth and development of fetus.
   C. fetal circulation.
   D. methods/locations (home or hospital) of delivery.
   E. financial decisions regarding all aspects of pregnancy.
   F. nutrition/vitamin therapy.
   G. laboratory testing.
   H. marital relations/abstinence.
   I. daily exercise/rest periods.
   J. care of breasts/bathing.
   K. morning sickness/danger signals/signs of labor.
   L. quickening.
   M. physiologic changes (skin changes/dyspnea/fatigue/urinary frequency/edema/increased pulse/diaphoresis/weight gain/mood swings).

    N. clothing/footwear.

    O. prevention of sexually transmitted diseases.

    P. nonstress test/contraction stress test/biophysical profile.

    Q. medication administration/adverse reactions.

    R. douching.

    S. avoidance of smoking/alcohol/caffeine/drug abuse.

    T. dental care.

    U. contraception/sterilization.

    V. amniocentesis/chorion villus biopsy/ultrasonography/fetal monitoring.

    W. fetoscopic tissue sampling.

    X. newborn care (formula preparation/breast-feeding/clothing/ bathing/cord care/infant stimulation techniques/rest periods/ immunizations/TB testing/clinic or M.D appointments).

    Y. follow-up M.D. appointments.

    Z. other _____

    _____

3. Body image disturbance related to:

    A. increased weight gain.

    B. excessive food intake.

    C. excessive sodium intake.

    D. inadequate exercise.

    E. other _____

    _____

4. Impaired physical mobility related to:

    A. increased weight gain.

    B. edema.

    C. other _____

    _____

5. Sleep pattern disturbance related to:

    A. urinary frequency.

    B. nausea/vomiting.

    C. other _____

    _____

6. Altered nutrition: more than body requirements related to:

    A. nausea/anorexia/vomiting.

    B. increased appetite.

    C. dyspepsia.

    D. constipation/diarrhea.

    E. fetal growth.

    F. other ————————————————————————

————————————————————————————————————

7. Constipation/Diarrhea related to:

    A. poor fluid/dietary intake.

    B. refusal to follow medical advice.

    C. other ————————————————————————

————————————————————————————————————

8. Ineffective individual/family coping related to:

    A. demands of single parenthood.

    B. inadequate support system.

    C. marital/family discord.

    D. financial instability.

    E. unwanted pregnancy.

    F. other ————————————————————————

————————————————————————————————————

9. Personal identity disturbance related to:

    A. unemployment.

    B. dependence on others for care/financial support.

    C. altered body image.

    D. other ————————————————————————

————————————————————————————————————

10. Increased cardiac output related to:

    A. increased body size/weight gain.

    B. exercise intolerance.

    C. stress.

    D. increased vital capacity.

    E. growing fetus.

    F. other ————————————————————————

————————————————————————————————————

11. Sexual dysfunction related to:

    A. fatigue.

    B. mood swings.

    C. estimated date of delivery (abstinence).

    D. other ————————————————————————

————————————————————————————————————

12. Potential impaired skin integrity related to:

    A. use of constrictive clothing.

B. poor personal hygiene.

C. other _____

_____

13. Impaired home maintenance management related to:
    A. fatigue.
    B. difficulty with ambulation.
    C. dependence on others for care.
    D. insufficient income.
    E. other _____

    _____

14. Altered family processes related to:
    A. increased financial responsibilities.
    B. need for baby-sitting/day care services.
    C. other _____

    _____

II. SHORT-TERM GOALS

1. Client will visit M.D. routinely as advised after 1–2 R.N. visits.
2. Client/Spouse/Father will verbalize all fears, anxieties, and questions after 2–3 R.N. visits.
3. Client/Spouse/Father will attend specific classes in prenatal care if desired after 1–2 R.N. visits.
4. Client will drink 1–2 qt of fluid daily if ordered after 1–2 R.N. visits.
5. Client will eat nutritionally balanced meals after 1–2 R.N. visits.
6. Client will exercise and rest routinely every day after 1–2 R.N. visits.
7. Client/Spouse/Father will read instructional literature in preparation for childbearing after 1–2 R.N. visits.
8. Client will wear a supportive brassiere after 1–2 R.N. visits.
9. Client will care for breasts after 1–2 R.N. visits.
10. Client will wear appropriate clothing/footwear after 1–2 R.N. visits.
11. Client will engage in social activities after 1–2 R.N. visits.
12. Client will avoid/limit smoking after 1–2 R.N. visits.
13. Client will abstain from alcohol intake after 1–2 R.N. visits.
14. Client will seek appropriate dental care as ordered after 1–2 R.N. visits.
15. Client will seek laboratory testing as ordered after 1–2 R.N. visits.

16. Client will apply appropriate creams/lotions/emollients to skin after 1–2 R.N. visits.
17. Client/Spouse/Father will prepare newborn environment after 8–9 R.N. visits.
18. Client will engage in marital relations after consulting with M.D. after 1–2 R.N. visits.
19. Client will undergo ultrasonography as ordered after 1–2–3 R.N. visits.
20. Client will undergo nonstress testing/oxytocin challenge testing as ordered after 1–2–3 R.N. visits.
21. Client will wear external fetal monitor as ordered after 1–2–3 R.N. visits.
22. Client/Spouse/Father will attend Lamaze classes after 1–2–3 R.N. visits.

III. LONG-TERM GOALS

1. Client will resume independent activities of daily living throughout pregnancy.
2. Marital relationship will be stable throughout pregnancy and thereafter.
3. Delivery of normal, healthy, infant will occur in 9 months.
4. Optimal level of health will be achieved by both mother and fetus in 9 months.

IV. OUTCOME CRITERIA

1. Vital signs remain normal.
2. Reproductive system functions normally.
3. Cardiovascular system functions normally.
4. GU system functions normally.
5. Endocrine system functions normally.
6. Respiratory system functions normally.
7. Mental status is normal.
8. Laboratory test results remain normal.
9. Skin/Mucous membrane is healthy and intact.
10. Prenatal classes are attended.
11. Nutritional status is normal.
12. Clinic/M.D. appointments are attended.
13. Social contact with relatives/friends is maintained.

14. Financial status is stable.
15. Infant is normal and healthy.

V. NURSING INTERVENTION/TREATMENT

1. R.N. will encourage regular checkups with M.D. throughout course of pregnancy.
2. R.N. will encourage verbalization and provide psychological support at all times.
3. R.N. will instruct client/spouse/father on:
    A. normal anatomy and physiology of reproductive tract.
    B. growth and development of fetus.
    C. fetal circulation.
    D. methods and locations (home and hospital) of delivery.
    E. monitoring and recording of vital signs if necessary.
    F. financial decisions regarding all aspects of delivery.
    G. nutrition/vitamin therapy.
    H. laboratory testing.
    I. marital relations/abstinence.
    J. daily exercise/rest periods.
    K. care of breasts/bathing.
    L. morning sickness, danger signals, signs of labor.
    M. quickening.
    N. physiologic changes (skin changes, dyspnea, fatigue, urinary frequency, edema, increased pulse, diaphoresis, weight gain, mood swings).
    O. clothing/footwear.
    P. douching.
    Q. avoidance of smoking/alcohol/caffeine/drug abuse.
    R. chorion villus biopsy/nonstress testing/fetal monitoring (internal and external).
    S. amniocentesis/genetic counseling.
    T. contraception.
    U. tubal ligation/consent procedure/vasectomy.
    V. Doptone monitoring.
    W. Dental care.
    X. newborn care (formula preparation, breast-feeding, clothing, bathing, cord care, infant stimulation techniques, rest periods, immunizations, TB testing, clinic/M.D. appointments).

     Y. medication administration/adverse reactions.

     Z. follow-up M.D. appointments.

4. R.N. will provide M.D. with follow-up reports and discharge summary when case closes.

5. R.N. will notify client/spouse/father/significant others when case will close.

Breast-feeding Care Plan

I. NURSING DIAGNOSIS

1. Knowledge deficit related to:
   A. breast-feeding.
   B. care of breasts.
   C. fluid/dietary regimen.
   D. other_____

   _____

2. Breast pain related to:
   A. engorgement.
   B. poor fit of brassiere.
   C. poor positioning of infant.
   D. infected breast.
   E. poor fluid/dietary intake.
   F. other_____

   _____

3. Ineffective individual coping related to:
   A. irritability of infant.
   B. breast soreness.
   C. engorgement.
   D. cracked nipples.
   E. infection.
   F. mastitis.
   G. other_____

   _____

4. Potential fluid volume deficit related to poor fluid/caloric intake.

5. Alteration in bowel elimination (frequent, soft stools) related to breast-feeding.

6. Noncompliance with breast-feeding related to:
    A. infection.
    B. excessive demands of family.
    C. employment.
    D. other_____

7. Altered nutrition: more than body requirements related to:
    A. increased need for fluids and calories.
    B. frequent feedings.
    C. other_____

8. Potential impaired skin integrity related to:
    A. engorgement.
    B. nipple soreness.
    C. cracked nipples.
    D. infection.
    E. mastitis.
    F. blistered nipples.
    G. other_____

9. Potential anxiety related to:
    A. breast-feeding.
    B. inadequate milk supply.
    C. ineffective sucking reflex.
    D. letdown reflex.
    E. other_____

10. Sleep pattern disturbance related to:
    A. feeding demands.
    B. engorgement.
    C. breast pain.
    D. other_____

II. SHORT-TERM GOALS

1. Client/Spouse/Father will verbalize fears, anxieties, and concerns about breast-feeding after 1–2–3 R.N. visits.

2. Client will assume a suitable position for breast-feeding after 1–2 R.N. visits.
3. Client will wrap or clothe infant comfortably for breast-feeding after 1 R.N. visit.
4. Client will choose a quiet, suitable environment for breast-feeding after 1 R.N. visit.
5. Client will roll nipple between thumb and forefinger appropriately after 1 R.N. visit.
6. Client will assist infant with rooting reflex after 1–2 R.N. visits.
7. Client will fasten a safety pin to side of brassiere last used for feeding so alternate breasts may be used after 1 R.N. visit.
8. Client will offer water after feedings after 1 R.N. visit.
9. Client will burp infant after feeding after 1 R.N. visit.
10. Client will turn infant over quickly from prone to sitting position to provide stimulation for feeding after 1 R.N. visit.
11. Client will change wet diaper before initiating feeding after 1 R.N. visit.
12. Client will expose sore, tender breast/breasts to air for 10 minutes after feedings after 1–2 R.N. visits.
13. Client will apply light to assist with drying of nipples after feedings after 1–2–3 R.N. visits.
14. Client will use nipple shield as ordered after 1–2 R.N. visits.
15. Client will apply prescribed ointment/cream to sore or cracked nipples after 1–2 R.N. visits.
16. Client will use a breast pump (hand/electric) for engorgement after 1–2 R.N. visits.
17. Client will collect and freeze breast milk up to 1 month after 1 R.N. visit.
18. Client will prevent letdown reflex by crossing both arms firmly over nipples after 1–2 R.N. visits.
19. Client will consume fluids/diet as ordered after 1–2 R.N. visits.
20. Client will wear a properly fitted brassiere after 1 R.N. visit.
21. Client will cleanse nipples with water only after 1 R.N. visit.
22. Client will set up feeding schedule, if possible, after 1–2 R.N. visits.

III. LONG-TERM GOALS

1. Adequate nutritional status will be achieved during lactation.
2. Optimal level of health will be achieved for newborn and mother in 1–2 weeks.

IV. OUTCOME CRITERIA

1. Vital signs are normal in mother and child.
2. Nursing of infant is accomplished successfully.
3. Infant weight gain is appropriate.
4. Infant stools are normal.
5. Mother refrains from smoking and alcohol intake during breast-feeding.
6. Mother's weight gain is appropriate for height.
7. Intake and output are appropriate for mother and child.
8. Adequate sleep is obtained.
9. Menstrual cycle returns to normal.
10. Infant growth and development is appropriate.
11. Weaning is accomplished successfully.
12. Breasts return to normal size.
13. Normal maternal/paternal bonding occurs.
14. Skin integrity remains normal.
15. Client states she feels fine.

V. NURSING INTERVENTION/TREATMENT

1. R.N. will make arrangements for a home visit with family.
2. R.N. will instruct client/spouse/father on:
   A. breast-feeding, using leaflets, booklets, and audiovisual aids.
   B. care of breasts.
   C. importance of quiet, suitable environment for breast-feeding.
   D. comfortable wrapping or clothing of infant for breast-feeding.
   E. rolling of nipple for preparation of feeding.
   F. infant rooting reflex.
   G. alternate use of each breast for feedings.
   H. administration of water after each feeding.
   I. stimulation of infant during feedings.
   J. care of sore, cracked, or blistered nipples (appropriate cleansing, heat or light application for drying of nipples/medication administration/cream/ointment application/application of nipple shields).
   K. use of a breast pump.
   L. collection and freezing of breast milk.
   M. letdown reflex.
   N. fluid intake/dietary regimen as ordered.

    O. properly fitted brassiere.

    P. notification of M.D. of adverse reactions to medication or change in mother's or infant's condition.

    Q. observation of newborn stools.

    R. weaning.

    S. socialization.

    T. employment.

3. R.N. will provide M.D. with follow-up reports and discharge summary when case closes.

4. R.N. will notify client/family/significant others when case will close.

Family Planning
Care Plan

I. NURSING DIAGNOSIS

1. Anxiety related to:
   A. contraception/abortion/sterilization.
   B. wanted/unwanted pregnancy.
   C. rejection by significant others.
   D. fear of venereal disease.
   E. altered body image.
   F. male/female infertility.
   G. prenatal/postpartal care.
   H. complications of abortion.
   I. methods of delivery.
   J. genetic counseling.
   K. financial insecurity.
   L. single parenthood.
   M. marital discord.
   N. amniocentesis.
   O. chorion villus biopsy.
   P. other_____

2. Ineffective individual/family coping related to:
   A. poor understanding of contraception/abortion/sterilization.
   B. unwanted pregnancy.
   C. therapeutic/spontaneous/missed/elective abortion.
   D. financial insecurity.
   E. single parenthood.

    F. marital discord.

    G. male/female infertility.

    H. complications of abortion.

    I. need for genetic counseling.

    J. altered body image.

    K. amniocentesis.

    L. chorion villus biopsy.

    M. other _____

    _____

3. Altered family processes related to:

    A. poor understanding of contraception/abortion/sterilization.

    B. unwanted pregnancy.

    C. therapeutic/spontaneous/missed/elective abortion.

    D. financial insecurity.

    E. single parenthood.

    F. marital discord.

    G. complications of abortion.

    H. need for genetic counseling.

    I. other _____

    _____

4. Fear related to:

    A. contraception/abortion/sterilization.

    B. unwanted pregnancy.

    C. pregnancy testing/operative procedures.

    D. masturbation/frigidity.

    E. amniocentesis.

    F. chorion villus biopsy.

    G. other _____

    _____

5. Altered health maintenance related to:

    A. multiple abortions.

    B. multiple pregnancies.

    C. frequent pregnancies.

    D. maternal/paternal metabolic imbalance.

    E. maternal/paternal cardiopulmonary disorder.

    F. maternal/paternal respiratory disorder.

    G. maternal/paternal endocrine disorder.

    H. maternal/paternal reproductive disorder.

I. maternal/paternal renal disorder.

J. maternal/paternal mental disorder.

K. other _____

6. Knowledge deficit related to:

A. normal anatomy/physiology of male/female reproductive tracts.

B. menarche.

C. intercourse.

D. medication administration/oral contraception (hormonal steroids)/adverse reactions.

E. intrauterine devices/adverse reactions.

F. diaphragm/cervical cap/sponge/adverse reactions.

G. rhythm.

H. chemical contraceptives (foams/jellies/creams/foaming tablets/ suppositories)/adverse reactions.

I. douching.

J. latex condom application.

K. coitus interruptus.

L. therapeutic/threatened/spontaneous/incomplete/missed/elective abortion (morning-after pill/menstrual extraction/suction curettage/D&C/intraamniotic injection/hysterotomy).

M. complications of abortion.

N. genetic counseling for metabolic disorders/retardation/congenital anomalies/DES exposure.

O. infection/dysmenorrhea/premenstrual syndrome.

P. prevention/treatment of sexually transmitted disease.

Q. pregnancy testing/operative procedures (Pap test/D&C/cervical biopsy/culdoscopy/salpingogram/salpingectomy/oophorectomy/ hysterectomy/Rubin test/Sims-Huhner test).

R. methods of delivery/financial cost/insurance coverage.

S. newborn care.

T. amniocentesis.

U. chorion villus biopsy.

V. artificial insemination/gamete intrafallopian tube transfer/in vitro fertilization (husband versus donor).

W. other _____

7. Altered parenting related to:

A. unwanted pregnancy.

  B. male/female infertility.
  C. refusal of marital partner(s) to participate in contraception/abortion/sterilization.
  D. retardation/congenital anomalies of newborn.
  E. other _____

  _____

8. Self-esteem disturbance related to:
  A. marital infidelity.
  B. unwanted pregnancy.
  C. retardation/congenital anomalies of newborn.
  D. other _____

  _____

II. SHORT-TERM GOALS

1. Client/Spouse/Father will verbalize all fears, anxieties, and concerns after 1–2–3–4 R.N. visits.
2. Client/Spouse/Father will read recommended literature after 1–2 R.N. visits.
3. Client/Spouse/Father will safely administer oral contraceptives after 1–2 R.N. visits.
4. Client/Spouse/Father will state adverse reactions of oral contraceptives after 1–2 R.N. visits.
5. Client/Spouse/Father will immediately report adverse effects of oral contraceptives to M.D. after 1–2 R.N. visits.
6. Client/Spouse/Father will safely use diaphragm/cervical cap/sponge/foam/jelly/cream/foaming tablets/suppositories/morning-after pill/condom as ordered after 1–2 R.N. visits.
7. Client will seek menstrual extraction/D&C/suction curettage/intraamniotic injection/hysterotomy as ordered after 1–2 R.N. visits.
8. Client/Spouse/Father will immediately contact M.D. about signs/symptoms of infection/adverse reactions to contraception/abortion/sterilization after 1–2 R.N. visits.
9. Client/Spouse/Father will participate in pregnancy testing/infertility testing/operative procedures as ordered after 1–2 R.N. visits.
10. Client/Spouse/Father will seek genetic counseling as ordered after 1–2 R.N. visits.
11. Client/Spouse/Father will seek artificial insemination of spouse/donor after 6–12 months of M.D. visits.

12. Client/Spouse will seek in vitro fertilization after 6–12 months of M.D. visits.

III. LONG-TERM GOALS

1. Safe method of contraception will be used by client/spouse/father in 1–2 weeks.
2. Venereal disease will be eliminated/prevented in 1–2 weeks of counseling/treatment.
3. Delivery of normal, healthy newborn will occur in 9 months.
4. Safe method of abortion will be used by client in first to second trimester of pregnancy.

IV. OUTCOME CRITERIA

1. Vital signs are normal.
2. Male/Female reproductive organs function normally.
3. Client/Spouse/Father attend regularly scheduled M.D./clinic appointments.
4. Laboratory test results remain normal.
5. Bowel/Bladder elimination is normal.
6. Sexuality is normal.
7. Skin/Mucous membrane is healthy and intact.
8. Newborn is alert and healthy.

V. NURSING INTERVENTION/TREATMENT

1. R.N. will schedule convenient time for client interview in M.D. office/clinic/hospital.
2. R.N. will instruct client/spouse/father/H.H.A on:
   A. normal anatomy and physiology of male/female reproductive organs.
   B. menarche/body care/hygiene sprays/douching.
   C. intercourse.
   D. nutrition.
   E. medication administration/oral contraceptives (hormonal steroids)/adverse reactions.
   F. immediate notification of M.D. of adverse reactions or change in condition.
   G. intrauterine devices/adverse reactions.
   H. diaphragm/cervical cap/sponge/adverse reactions.

I. chemical contraceptives (foams/jellies/creams/foaming tablets/ suppositories) adverse reactions.

J. rhythm.

K. latex condom application.

L. coitus interruptus.

M. therapeutic/threatened/spontaneous/incomplete/missed/ elective abortion (morning-after pill/menstrual extraction/D&C/ suction curettage/intraamniotic injections/hysterotomy).

N. infection/dysmenorrhea/premenstrual syndrome/complications of abortion.

O. pregnancy testing/operative procedures (Pap test/D&C/cervical biopsy/culdoscopy/salpingogram/salpingectomy/Sims-Huhner test/Rubin test).

P. prevention/treatment of sexually transmitted disease.

Q. methods/locations of delivery/financial cost.

R. genetic counseling for metabolic disorders/retardation/ congenital anomalies.

S. amniocentesis.

T. chorion villus biopsy.

U. artificial insemination (husband versus donor)/gamete intrafallopian tube transfer/in vitro fertilization (husband versus donor).

V. care of the newborn.

3. R.N. will arrange for client/spouse/father to have access to additional educational materials (e.g., pamphlets, records, tapes, audiocassettes, slide presentations, movies, clubs, organizations, and parent groups).

4. R.N. will provide M.D. with follow-up reports and discharge summary when case closes.

5. R.N. will notify client/spouse/father/significant others when case closes.

Infant Stimulation
for the Retarded Newborn
Care Plan

I. NURSING DIAGNOSIS

1. Anxiety related to:
   A. developmental delay.
   B. seizure disorder.
   C. anomalies.
   D. irritability.
   E. lethargy.
   F. other_____

2. Knowledge deficit related to:
   A. retardation.
   B. infant stimulation techniques.
   C. laboratory testing.
   D. medication administration/adverse reactions.
   E. environmental stimulation.
   F. other_____

3. Ineffective individual/family coping related to:
   A. retardation.
   B. seizure disorder.
   C. anomalies.
   D. irritability.
   E. lethargy.

F. other_____
_____

4. Activity intolerance related to:
   A. anomalies.
   B. paralysis.
   C. weakness/fatigue.
   D. other_____
   _____

5. Altered nutrition: potential for more/less than body requirements related to:
   A. increased appetite.
   B. anorexia.
   C. obesity.
   D. other_____
   _____

6. Impaired home maintenance management related to:
   A. increased demands of the sick child.
   B. lengthy feeding periods.
   C. lack of support in the home.
   D. single parenthood.
   E. other_____
   _____

7. Altered family processes related to:
   A. sibling rivalry.
   B. increased demands of the sick child.
   C. marital discord.
   D. lack of support in the home.
   E. separation/divorce.
   F. grieving process.
   G. other_____
   _____

8. Altered parenting related to:
   A. sibling rivalry.
   B. lack of support in the home.
   C. excessive employment demands.
   D. anger.
   E. grieving stages.
   F. other_____
   _____

9. Grieving related to:
   A. birth of a retarded child.
   B. separation/divorce.
   C. other_____

   _____ _____

10. Noncompliance with therapy/infant stimulation related to:
    A. denial/disbelief of medical diagnosis.
    B. lack of support in the home.
    C. employment demands.
    D. other_____

    _____

II. SHORT-TERM GOALS

1. Parents will verbalize fears, anxieties, and concerns after 1–2–3 R.N. visits.
2. Parents will read literature on retardation after 1–2–3 R.N. visits.
3. Parents will join organizations or parent groups for children with similar conditions after 1–2–3 R.N. visits.
4. Parents will make stimulating toys for child after 1–2 R.N. visits.
5. Parents will use music or singing as stimulation after 1–2–3 R.N. visits.
6. Parents will stimulate child, using various colors, pictures, mobiles, odors, and textures after 1–2–3 R.N. visits.
7. Parents will feed child assorted foods as ordered after 1–2–3 R.N. visits.
8. Parents will encourage siblings to provide affection and stimulation to infant after 1–2 R.N. visits.
9. Parents will enroll child in infant stimulation/preschool program after 1–2 R.N. visits.
10. Parents will seek laboratory testing/M.D. appointments as ordered after 1–2 R.N. visits.

III. LONG-TERM GOALS

1. Paternal/Familial bonding will occur in 1–2 weeks.
2. Intelligence quotient will be developed by age 3.
3. Developmental milestones will be achieved by age 5 (and thereafter, appropriately for age).
4. Normal socialization will be achieved by age 3.
5. Mainstreaming will occur by age 5.

IV. OUTCOME CRITERIA

1. Vital signs are normal.
2. Fine/Gross motor coordination is normal.
3. Hearing/Vision is normal.
4. Weight and height are normal.
5. Appetite is normal.
6. Child is alert and playful and makes correct responses.

V. NURSING INTERVENTION/TREATMENT

1. R.N. will visit with parents as early after delivery as possible (will arrange visit before hospital discharge).
2. R.N. will assess parental acceptance of condition/normal grieving response.
3. R.N. will provide parents with:
   A. earliest intervention for psychologic support, along with aid of other parents with similar condition/parent groups.
   B. understanding of importance of early infant stimulation.
   C. encouragement to accept infant like any normal infant.
   D. understanding of importance of early sensory, motor, auditory, tactile, and verbal stimulation techniques.
   E. encouragement in promoting socialization of infant with other children.
   F. a list of toys that can be easily made. Expense can be minimal for stimulating toys (e.g., large, colored faces; finger or plate puppets; feel mitts; merry-go-round mobiles; rattles; wristbands; sound cans; wooden-spool necklaces; cooking extracts; food odors; fragrances; balls; rag dolls).
   G. exercises as ordered (sit-ups/waving bye-bye/reaching exercises/range-of-motion exercises, gently, for arms and legs). Infant is to be on a flat surface, preferably on abdomen.
   H. information on feedings: Face child during feedings. Never leave infant alone in room unstimulated for long periods. Speak to child frequently. Provide singing and music therapy.
   I. information on monitoring developmental progress in daily written record.
   J. encouragement to visit M.D. as ordered.
   K. enrollment in infant stimulation program or several programs after M.D. approval.
   L. foster care/adoption services.

    M. parental stimulation (e.g., reading good books out loud/asking and answering questions/going outdoors for exploration/holding and comforting when there is hurt/providing and enforcing clear and fair limits).

4. R.N. will provide M.D. with follow-up reports and discharge summary when case closes.

5. R.N. will notify client/family/significant others when case will close.

Postpartal and Newborn Care Plan

I. NURSING DIAGNOSIS

1. Anxiety related to:
   A. new addition to family.
   B. financial insecurity.
   C. contraception/sterilization.
   D. marital relations.
   E. dressing care for cesarean section.
   F. newborn care.
   G. other_____

   _____

2. Knowledge deficit related to:
   A. breast care/personal hygiene.
   B. fluid/dietary requirements.
   C. contraception/sterilization.
   D. marital relations.
   E. dressing care for cesarean section.
   F. newborn care (feeding/personal hygiene/cord care/rest).
   G. infant stimulation.
   H. care of the sick child/retarded child/child with congenital anomalies.
   I. infant safety.
   J. exercise/rest.
   K. immunization/TB testing.
   L. other_____

   _____

3. Self-care deficit: feeding/bathing/grooming/dressing/toileting related to:
   A. dependence on others for care.
   B. activity intolerance.
   C. fatigue/weakness.
   D. incisional pain (abdomen/episiotomy site).
   E. other_____

4. Potential impaired skin integrity related to:
   A. granulation of incision (abdomen/episiotomy site).
   B. soreness/cracking/bleeding of nipples.
   C. infection at nipples/episiotomy site.
   D. other_____

5. Altered nutrition: potential for more than body requirements related to:
   A. breast-feeding.
   B. anorexia.
   C. obesity.
   D. other_____

6. Fatigue related to:
   A. lack of/inadequate rest periods.
   B. other_____

7. Potential for infection related to:
   A. poor hand-washing technique.
   B. poor personal hygiene habits.
   C. other_____

8. Painful defecation related to:
   A. inadequate exercise regimen.
   B. constipated stools.
   C. inadequate fluid/dietary intake.
   D. other_____

9. Actual/Potential fluid volume deficit related to:
   A. poor intake.

    B. excessive newborn feeding schedule.

    C. other_____

    _____

10. Constipation/Diarrhea related to:

    A. insufficient/poor dietary intake.

    B. pain associated with episiotomy site/abdominal incision/ hemorrhoids/anal fissures.

    C. other_____

    _____

11. Impaired home maintenance management related to:

    A. excessive demands of infant.

    B. poor support from spouse/family members.

    C. poor time scheduling for homemaking chores.

    D. other_____

    _____

12. Altered parenting related to:

    A. fear of child care.

    B. overprotection/rejection of infant.

    C. abuse/neglect of infant.

    D. sibling rivalry.

    E. other_____

    _____

13. Ineffective individual/family coping related to:

    A. excessive demands of newborn.

    B. marital discord.

    C. poor support from spouse/family.

    D. financial insecurity.

    E. other_____

    _____

14. Sexual dysfunction related to:

    A. fear of conception.

    B. healing of episiotomy site.

    C. marital discord.

    D. other_____

    _____

II. SHORT-TERM GOALS

1. Client will maintain good personal hygiene after 1–2 R.N. visits.

2. Client/Spouse/Father will prepare meals from the 4 basic food groups after 1–2 R.N. visits.
3. Client will drink 2–3 qt of fluid daily after 1–2 R.N. visits.
4. Client will wear a firm, supportive brassiere after 1–2 R.N. visits.
5. Client will exercise and rest periodically throughout day after 1–2 R.N. visits.
6. Client will take supplemental vitamins after 1–2 R.N. visits.
7. Client will encourage spouse to participate in infant care after 1–2 R.N. visits.
8. Client will breast-feed infant appropriately after 1–2 R.N. visits.
9. Client/Spouse will demonstrate appropriate cord care after 1 R.N. visit.
10. Client/Spouse/Family will bathe infant daily after 1 R.N. visit.
11. Client/Spouse/Family will initiate daily individual infant schedule after 1–2 R.N. visits.
12. Client will use breast pump as ordered after 1–2 R.N. visits.
13. Client/Spouse will follow infant stimulation techniques after 1–2 R.N. visits.
14. Client/Spouse/Family will obtain immunizations/TB testing as ordered after 1–2 R.N. visits.
15. Client/Spouse/Family will follow infant safety instructions (e.g., appropriate-sized crib, side rails, appropriate infant seat, car seat, playpen, toys) after 1–2 R.N. visits.
16. Client/Spouse/Family will keep routine M.D. appointments after 1–2 R.N. visits.

III. LONG-TERM GOALS

1. Maternal/Paternal bonding will occur within the first 2 weeks after birth.
2. Appropriate developmental milestones will be reached within the first year of life.

IV. OUTCOME CRITERIA

1. Vital signs are normal for mother and child.
2. Mental health is normal for mother.
3. Apgar score is between 9 and 10 for infant.
4. Skin/Mucous membrane is normal, intact, and healthy in mother and infant.
5. Appetite is normal in mother and child.
6. Sleep pattern is normal for mother and child.

7. Elimination is normal for mother and child.

8. Urinary output is normal for mother and child.

9. Infant responds well to stimulation techniques.

10. Client states she feels better.

11. Breast-feeding occurs normally.

12. Marital/Family relationship remains normal.

V. NURSING INTERVENTION/TREATMENT

1. R.N. will contact client about appropriate time to visit home for instructions.

2. R.N. will allow client/spouse to verbalize all fears, anxieties, and concerns and will provide instructions.

3. R.N. will assess home environment, infant furniture, safety factors; will perform physical assessment of infant and mother; will assess nutritional factors.

4. R.N. will instruct client/spouse/family/H.H.A on:

   A. monitoring and recording of vital signs.

   B. proper hand-washing technique.

   C. infant safety.

   D. care of the mother (breast care/breast-feeding techniques/breast pump/episiotomy and abdominal dressing technique/postpartal M.D. appointments/nutrition/fluid needs/exercise/rest/ socialization/marital relations/formula preparation/lochia/ laundering and storage of infant clothing).

   E. infant care (personal hygiene/cord care/feeding schedule/rest periods/exercise/infant stimulation techniques/immunization/ TB testing/changes in stool/M.D. appointments).

   F. care of the sick child/retarded infant/child with congenital anomalies.

   G. genetic counseling.

   H. contraception/sterilization.

   I. laboratory testing if required.

   J. medication administration if required.

   K. sibling rivalry.

   L. normal integration of newborn into family; allowing other children to care for and play with infant.

5. R.N. will provide M.D. with follow-up reports and discharge summary when case closes.

6. R.N. will notify client/spouse/family/H.H.A./significant others when case will close.

Sterilization
Care Plan

I. NURSING DIAGNOSIS

1. Anxiety related to:
   A. permanent/reversible sterilization.
   B. postoperative complications.
   C. rejection by significant others.
   D. other _____

2. Knowledge deficit related to:
   A. types of surgical consents/procedures.
   B. cost/insurance coverage.
   C. postoperative complications.
   D. permanency/reversible effects.
   E. dressing care.
   F. postoperative ejaculation.
   G. sexual relations.
   H. exercise.
   I. seminalysis.
   J. contraception.
   K. other _____

3. Potential for infection related to:
   A. poor hand-washing technique.
   B. poor dressing technique.
   C. other _____

4. Pain related to:
   A. incisional healing.
   B. granulation of tissue.
   C. infection.
   D. nerve irritation from gas during laparoscopy.
   E. other _____
      _____

5. Impaired physical mobility related to:
   A. pain.
   B. other _____
      _____

II. SHORT-TERM GOALS

1. Client will verbalize fears, anxieties, and concerns after
   1–2–3–4 R.N. visits.
2. Client will wash hands properly before and after dressing changes
   after 1–2 R.N. visits.
3. Client will change abdominal dressings properly after
   1–2 R.N. visits.
4. Client will take medications as prescribed after 1–2 R.N. visits.
5. Client will notify physician of adverse effects of medication or
   impending secondary complications after 1–2 R.N. visits.
6. Client will ejaculate as ordered by physician after 1–2 R.N./
   M.D. visits.
7. Client will avoid excessive lifting or strenuous exercise after
   1–2 R.N. visits.
8. Client will return for postoperative seminalysis as ordered after
   1–2–3 R.N./M.D. visits.
9. Client will avoid intercourse as ordered after 1–2–3 R.N. visits.
10. Client will avoid strenuous exercise as ordered after
    1–2–3 R.N. visits.
11. Client will use an alternative form of birth control as ordered after
    1–2–3 R.N. visits.
12. Client will report any changes in postoperative menstrual flow
    after 1–2–3 R.N. visits.

III. LONG-TERM GOALS

1. Independent activities of daily living will be resumed in
   1–2 weeks.

2. Sterilization will occur in 4–6 weeks.

3. Optimum level of health will be achieved in 4–6 weeks.

IV. OUTCOME CRITERIA

1. Vital signs are normal.

2. Skin is healthy and intact.

3. Menses are normal.

4. Normal ejaculation is achieved.

5. Chest is clear.

6. Bowel/Bladder functions normally.

7. Contraception is achieved.

8. Ambulation is normal.

9. Client states he/she feels better.

10. Mental outlook is healthy.

V. NURSING INTERVENTION/TREATMENT

1. R.N. will instruct client on:

  A. cost of medical care/insurance coverage.

  B. proper hand-washing technique.

  C. aseptic dressing technique.

  D. types of surgery (e.g., vasectomy/spermatic duct injection/ laparoscopy/minilaparotomy/laparotomy/hysteroscopy).

  E. surgical consents.

  F. medication administration/adverse reactions.

  G. immediate notification of M.D. of adverse reactions or signs/ symptoms of secondary complications (e.g., pain/bleeding/ infection/uterine perforation/intestinal burns/abdominal soreness/sore neck/sore shoulder/epididymitis/sperm granuloma/hematoma.

  H. postoperative ejaculation.

  I. seminalysis.

  J. sexual relations.

  K. change in menses.

  L. avoidance of heavy lifting/excessive stair climbing.

  M. laboratory testing/M.D. appointments.

2. R.N. will provide M.D. with follow-up reports and discharge summary when case closes.

3. R.N. will notify client when case will close.

Threatened Abortion Care Plan

I. NURSING DIAGNOSIS

1. Fear related to threatened abortion.
2. Knowledge deficit related to:
   A. activity/strict bed rest.
   B. passage of tissue/fetal contents/blood/discharge/premature rupture of membranes.
   C. diet.
   D. sexual activity.
   E. medication regimen/adverse reactions.
   F. avoidance of emotional stress.
   G. other _____

   _____

3. Impaired physical mobility related to:
   A. pain.
   B. bleeding.
   C. strict bed rest.
   D. other _____

   _____

4. Ineffective individual/family coping related to fear of losing child.
5. Potential fluid volume deficit related to:
   A. bleeding.
   B. poor intake.
   C. other _____

   _____

6. Pain related to:
   A. threatened abortion.

   B. inadequate rest.

   C. failure to comply with medical orders.

   D. other _____

_____

7. Constipation/Diarrhea/Oliguria related to:

   A. poor fluid/dietary intake.

   B. strict bed rest/lack of exercise.

   C. pain.

   D. other _____

_____

8. Noncompliance with physician's orders related to denial.

9. Impaired home maintenance management related to confinement to bed.

10. Altered parenting related to:

   A. confinement to bed.

   B. weakness.

   C. other _____

_____

11. Anticipatory grieving related to fear of losing child.

12. Sleep pattern disturbance related to:

   A. pain.

   B. bleeding.

   C. other _____

_____

13. Self-esteem disturbance related to failure to carry to full term.

14. Self-care deficit: feeding/bathing/grooming/toileting/dressing related to:

   A. confinement to bed.

   B. pain.

   C. hemorrhage.

   D. other _____

_____

II. SHORT-TERM GOALS

1. Client/Family will notify M.D. of signs/symptoms of pain, bleeding, discharge, passage of tissue or fetal parts, or infection after 1 R.N. visit.

2. Client/Family will keep telephone and emergency telephone numbers within easy reach after 1 R.N. visit.

3. Client will consume a light diet/adequate fluids as ordered after 1–2 R.N. visits.
4. Client will adhere to strict bed rest after 1 R.N. visit as ordered.
5. Client will avoid emotional stress after 1–2 R.N. visits.
6. Client will avoid straining at stool after 1 R.N. visit.
7. Client/Family will keep a record of perineal pads used per 24 hours to estimate blood loss after 1 R.N. visit.
8. Client will use a bedpan at all times after 1 R.N. visit.
9. Client/Family will save all suspicious tissue passed vaginally after 1 R.N. visit.
10. Client/Family will administer medication as ordered after 1–2 R.N. visits.
11. Client/Family will make provisions to have other children cared for by family/relatives/friends after 1 R.N. visit.
12. Client/Family will seek laboratory testing/M.D. appointments as scheduled after 1–2–3 R.N. visits.
13. Client will seek nonstress testing/oxytocin challenge testing after 1–2–3 R.N. visits.
14. Client will wear external fetal monitor as ordered after 1–2–3 R.N. visits.

III. LONG-TERM GOALS

1. Client will carry pregnancy to term and deliver normal, healthy infant.
2. Independent activities of daily living will be resumed after threat of abortion has passed.
3. Optimal level of health will be achieved during and after pregnancy.

IV. OUCOME CRITERIA

1. Hemoglobin and hematocrit levels are within normal range.
2. Blood volume remains normal.
3. Vital signs remain normal.
4. Nutritional habits are normal.
5. Pain is relieved.
6. Bleeding ceases.
7. Mental health remains normal.
8. Bowel/Bladder functions normally.
9. Cardiac status remains normal.

10. Client carries pregnancy to term.
11. Chest remains clear.
12. Client states she feels better.
13. Delivery of normal, healthy infant is achieved.
14. Family bonding is achieved.

V. NURSING INTERVENTION/TREATMENT

1. R.N. will provide psychologic support to client/family; will allow client/family to verbalize all fears, anxieties, and concerns.
2. R.N. will monitor and record vital signs, fetal heart tones if possible, blood loss, location and duration of pain.
3. R.N. will instruct client/family/H.H.A. on:
   A. strict bed rest.
   B. use of a bedpad/call bell.
   C. immediate notification of M.D. of sudden change in condition; keeping emergency phone numbers at bedside at all times.
   D. medication administration (sedatives/antibiotics)/adverse reactions.
   E. immediate notification of M.D. of adverse reactions.
   F. recording of the number of perineal pads used in each 24-hour period.
   G. daily recording of intake and output.
   H. avoidance of emotional stress/placement of children with significant others.
   I. nonstress testing/oxytocin challenge testing.
   J. ultrasonography.
   K. application of external fetal monitor.
   L. laboratory testing/M.D. appointments.
   M. exercise/rest.
   N. diversional activity.
4. R.N. will visit daily/biweekly/triweekly/weekly/monthly as ordered for strict supervision of pregnancy to term.
5. R.N. will provide M.D. with follow-up reports and discharge summary when case closes.
6. R.N. will notify client/family/H.H.A./significant others when case will close.

Alcoholism
Care Plan

I. NURSING DIAGNOSIS

1. Anxiety related to:
   A. alcohol abuse.
   B. marital discord.
   C. financial instability.
   D. other _____

   _____

2. Potential for injury related to:
   A. alcoholism.
   B. altered levels of consciousness.
   C. falls/accidents.
   D. sensory/perceptual alterations.
   E. other _____

   _____

3. Knowledge deficit related to:
   A. adequate nutrition/meal preparation.
   B. adverse effects of alcohol.
   C. medication administration/adverse reactions.
   D. counseling.
   E. other _____

   _____

4. Ineffective individual/family coping related to:
   A. frequent altered levels of consciousness.
   B. irritability.
   C. violence.

   D. crime.
   E. child abuse/neglect.
   F. wife abuse.
   G. other _____

   _____

5. Self-care deficit: feeding/bathing/grooming/dressing/ambulating/
   toileting related to:
   A. altered levels of consciousness.
   B. mood swings.
   C. other _____

   _____

6. Impaired verbal communication related to:
   A. altered levels of consciousness.
   B. other _____

   _____

7. Sensory/perceptual alterations related to:
   A. altered levels of consciousness.
   B. other _____

   _____

8. Altered nutrition: potential for more than body requirements
   related to:
   A. alcohol abuse.
   B. poor dietary intake.
   C. other _____

   _____

9. Altered thought processes related to:
   A. inadequate rest.
   B. alcohol abuse.
   C. other _____

   _____

10. Ineffective breathing pattern related to:
    A. altered levels of consciousness.
    B. other _____

    _____

11. Powerlessness related to altered levels of consciousness.
12. Altered parenting related to:
    A. altered levels of consciousness.
    B. irritability.

    C. child abuse/neglect.

    D. violence.

    E. crime.

    F. other _____

    _____

13. Impaired physical mobility related to altered levels of consciousness.
14. Social isolation related to alcoholism.

II. SHORT-TERM GOALS

1. Client/Family will seek assistance for alcoholism after 2–3–4–5–6 R.N. visits.
2. Client will consume nutritionally sound meals after 1–2–3 R.N. visits.
3. Client will taper alcoholic intake after 1–2–3 R.N. visits.
4. Client will seek therapy/counseling services after 1–2–3–4–5–6 visits.
5. Client/Family will seek professional assistance in inpatient/ outpatient facility after 1–2–3 R.N. visits.
6. Client/Family will visit halfway house after 1–2–3 R.N. visits.
7. Client/Family will visit member of clergy for additional assistance after 1–2–3 R.N. visits.
8. Client/Family will visit community mental health center after 1–2–3 I..N. visits.
9. Client will seek vocational rehabilitation and skill training after 1–2–3 R.N. visits.
10. Client will participate in all independent activities of daily living after 1–2–3 R.N. visits.
11. Client will seek active employment after 1–2–3 R.N. visits.
12. Client will take prescribed medication/vitamins after 1–2–3 R.N. visits.
13. Client will visit alcoholism treatment center for teenagers after 1–2–3 R.N. visits.
14. Client will seek laboratory testing/M.D. appointments after 1–2 R.N. visits.
15. Client will budget financial resources after 2–3 R.N. visits.
16. Client will make provisions for appropriate child care after 1–2 R.N. visits.
17. Client will rest periodically throughout day after 1–2 R.N. visits.

18. Client will avoid socially stressful situations after 1–2–3 R.N. visits.

III. LONG-TERM GOALS

1. Adequate nutritional habits will be achieved in several weeks/months/years.
2. Independence will be achieved in several weeks/months/years.
3. A sense of trust/self-esteem will be developed after several months/years of treatment.
4. Effective parenting will occur in several months/years.
5. Optimal level of health will be achieved in several months/years.

IV. OUTCOME CRITERIA

1. Vital signs remain normal.
2. Laboratory testing results remain normal.
3. Weight is normal.
4. Client consumes nutritious meals.
5. Mental status remains stable and healthy.
6. Socialization remains normal.
7. Employment status remains productive.
8. Client participates in useful diversional activities and sports.
9. Client's spouse and children feel loved and accepted.
10. Financial status remains adequate.

V. NURSING INTERVENTION/TREATMENT

1. R.N. will proceed slowly with counseling for client and family; home visit should occur only with client consent and request. M.D. should discuss client's behavioral response before R.N. visits.
2. R.N. will respond to questions, fears, or anxieties expressed concerning counseling and treatment.
3. If client is unable to respond, R.N. will carefully assess who the primary caregiver will be and provide all instructions.
4. R.N. will instruct client/family/H.H.A. on:
   A. alcoholism and its effects on the body.
   B. fluid intake/dietary regimen/vitamin therapy.
   C. medication administration (Antabuse/tranquilizers/sedatives)/adverse reactions.

    D. immediate notification of M.D. of adverse reactions or change in condition.

    E. daily exercise/rest periods.

    F. diversional activities.

    G. provisions for child care.

    H. choices of individual or group therapy through community mental health center, alcoholism treatment center (detoxification unit), inpatient or outpatient facility, halfway house.

    I. family counseling.

    J. vocational rehabilitation, skill training, career counseling, college.

    K. financial planning/budgeting.

5. R.N. will provide additional services (e.g., medical social services, psychiatry, home attendant, homemaker, housekeeper).

6. R.N. will provide M.D. with follow-up reports and discharge summary when case closes.

7. R.N. will notify client/family/H.H.A./significant others when case will close.

Anorexia Nervosa
Care Plan

I. NURSING DIAGNOSIS

1. Anxiety related to:
   A. disturbed sense of body image.
   B. weight gain.
   C. amenorrhea.
   D. other _____

2. Constipation/Diarrhea related to:
   A. anxiety.
   B. excessive eating followed by induced vomiting.
   C. poor nutritional habits.
   D. other _____

3. Decreased cardiac output related to:
   A. electrolyte imbalance.
   B. extreme weight loss.
   C. poor fluid/dietary intake.
   D. other _____

4. Ineffective individual/family coping related to:
   A. disturbed sense of body image.
   B. marked anxiety about weight gain.
   C. overeating with induced vomiting.
   D. other _____

5. Potential fluid volume deficit related to:
   A. induced vomiting.
   B. poor fluid intake.
   C. other _____

   _____

6. Impaired home maintenance management related to:
   A. emotional stress.
   B. neurotic interactions with family members.
   C. extreme weakness.
   D. cachexia.
   E. other _____

   _____

7. Knowledge deficit related to:
   A. adequate diet.
   B. complications of poor nutritional habits (e.g., hypovolemia/
      electrolyte imbalance/hypotension/development of lanugo or
      frank hirsutism/edema/amenorrhea/death).
   C. other _____

   _____

8. Potential for violence: self-directed/directed at others related to:
   A. disturbed sense of body image.
   B. hormonal imbalance.
   C. other _____

   _____

9. Noncompliance with therapy (e.g., failure to obtain adequate
   nutrition) related to:
   A. denial of illness.
   B. disturbed sense of body image.
   C. anger.
   D. other _____

   _____

10. Altered nutrition: Potential for more than body requirements
    related to:
    A. anxiety.
    B. excessive eating followed by induced vomiting.
    C. extreme weight loss.
    D. cachexia.
    E. other _____

    _____

11. Altered parenting related to:
    A. child's/adolescent's/adult's manipulative behavior.
    B. tendency to deny illness.
    C. other _____

    _____

12. Potential for injury related to:
    A. excessive eating following by induced vomiting.
    B. poor fluid intake.
    C. refusal to eat.
    D. excessive exercise.
    E. other _____

    _____

13. Ineffective breathing pattern related to generalized physical decline
    (cachexia).
14. Body image disturbance related to severe emaciation.
15. Sexual dysfunction related to amenorrhea.
16. Altered thought process related to:
    A. disturbed sense of body image.
    B. preoccupation with food.
    C. excessive study of diets/calories.
    D. hoarding, concealing, wasting of food.
    E. preoccupation with collection of recipes.
    F. preparation of elaborate meals for others.
    G. other _____

    _____

17. Altered patterns of urinary elimination related to:
    A. poor fluid intake.
    B. vomiting.
    C. other _____

    _____

II. SHORT-TERM GOALS

1. Client/Family will verbalize fears, anxieties, and concerns after
   1–2–3–4 R.N. visits.
2. Client/Family will reduce environmental stress significantly after
   1–2 R.N. visits.
3. Client will avoid eating excessive amounts of food after 1–2 R.N.
   visits.

4. Client will stop inducing vomiting after 1–2 R.N. visits.
5. Client will state 2 reasons why he/she is concerned about weight gain after 1–2–3 R.N. visits.
6. Client will seek hospitalization after 1–2–3 R.N. visits.
7. Client will seek psychotherapy/counseling services after 1–2–3 R.N. visits.
8. Client will behave more maturely/independently after 4–5 R.N. visits.
9. Client will consume small, frequent feedings as ordered after 1–2 R.N. visits.
10. Client/Family will administer psychopharmacologic agents as ordered after 1–2–3 R.N. visits.
11. Client will seek behavior modification therapy as ordered after 1–2 R.N. visits.
12. Client/Family will seek laboratory testing/M.D. appointments as ordered after 1–2 R.N. visits.

III. LONG-TERM GOALS

1. Stable family relationship and environment will be developed in 1–2 months.
2. Adequate nutritional habits will be developed in 1–2 months.
3. Optimal mental/physical health will develop in 1–2 months.

IV. OUTCOME CRITERIA

1. Vital signs are normal.
2. Weight remains appropriate.
3. Appetite is normal.
4. Client consumes nutritious meals.
5. Family functions as a unit.
6. Emotional/Mental health is appropriate.
7. Menses are normal.
8. Bowels function normally.
9. Urinary output is of normal color and quantity.
10. Muscle mass is appropriate.
11. Laboratory test results are normal.
12. Moderate exercise is performed.
13. Client behaves maturely and independently.
14. Client states he/she feels better.

V. NURSING INTERVENTION/TREATMENT

1. R.N. will consult with community mental health clinic about working with anorexic client.
2. R.N. will make home visit on the basis of M.D./community referral, etc.; will allow client/family to ventilate and explore concerns about obesity, restriction of food, weight loss, intensive study of diets and calories, hoarding and wasting of food, collection of recipes, and elaborate meal preparation for others.
3. R.N. will instruct client/family on:
   A. monitoring and recording of vital signs.
   B. potential physical complications of excessive eating followed by induced vomiting: signs and symptoms of dehydration, electrolyte imbalance, cardiac problems, renal involvement, development of lanugo or frank hirsutism, edema.
   C. avoidance of family/environmental stress.
   D. laboratory testing.
   E. possible hospitalization.
   F. tube feedings/parenteral feedings.
   G. behavior modification therapy.
   H. psychotherapy.
   I. medication prescribed/adverse reactions.
   J. immediate notification of M.D. of adverse reactions or signs/symptoms of advance of condition.
   K. importance of small, frequent feedings, initially, eaten only when hungry; client should then progress to adequate meals.
   L. rest/exercise as ordered; client should avoid vigorous exercise as ordered.
4. R.N. will provide M.D. with follow-up reports and discharge summary when case closes.
5. R.N. will notify client/family/significant others when case will close.

Anxiety Reaction
Care Plan

I. NURSING DIAGNOSIS

1. Ineffective individual/family coping related to anxiety.
2. Increased cardiac output related to anxiety.
3. Ineffective breathing pattern related to anxiety.
4. Altered nutrition: potential for more than body requirements related to anxiety.
5. Altered parenting related to anxiety.
6. Feeding self-care deficit related to anxiety.
7. Bathing/Hygiene self-care deficit related to anxiety.
8. Dressing/Grooming self-care deficit related to anxiety.
9. Toileting self-care deficit related to anxiety.
10. Personal identity disturbance related to anxiety.
11. Sexual dysfunction related to anxiety.
12. Potential impaired skin integrity related to anxiety.
13. Sleep pattern disturbance related to anxiety.
14. Spiritual distress related to anxiety.
15. Altered thought processes related to anxiety.
16. Constipation related to anxiety.
17. Perceived constipation related to anxiety.
18. Colonic constipation related to anxiety.
19. Diarrhea related to anxiety.
20. Bowel incontinence related to anxiety.
21. Urge incontinence related to anxiety.
22. Altered patterns of urinary elimination related to anxiety.
23. Altered role performance related to anxiety.
24. Parental role conflict related to anxiety.

25. Body image disturbance related to anxiety.
26. Self-esteem disturbance related to anxiety.
27. Chronic low self-esteem related to anxiety.
28. Personal identity disturbance related to anxiety.
29. Impaired verbal communication related to anxiety.
30. Potential for violence: self-directed or directed at others related to anxiety.

II. SHORT-TERM GOALS

1. Client/Family will verbalize fears, anxieties, and concerns after 1–2–3–4–5–6 R.N. visits.
2. Client will state 5 items/situations/locations/persons that cause him/her to feel anxious after 1–2–3 R.N. visits.
3. Client will take appropriate measures to relax/meditate after 1–2–3–4–5–6 R.N. visits.
4. Client will seek spiritual aid/consolation after 1–2–3 R.N. visits.
5. Client/Family will administer prescribed medication as ordered after 1–2 R.N. visits.
6. Client/Family will immediately report adverse reactions/change in condition to M.D. after 1–2 R.N. visits.
7. Client will avoid excess sugar, tobacco, alcohol, and caffeine in diet after 1–2 R.N. visits.
8. Client will avoid known anxiety-provoking items, situations, locations, and people until anxiety is decreased/eliminated after 1–2–3 R.N. visits.
9. Client will seek professional therapy/counseling after 1–2–3 R.N. visits.
10. Client will deal with situations that cause anxiety, when appropriate, after 1–2–3 R.N. visits.
11. Client will seek career counseling/vocational training/college education after 1–2–3 R.N. visits.
12. Client will face major surgery after speaking with another person who has had a similar successful experience after 1–2 R.N. visits.
13. Client will join club/group/organization to work toward weight reduction after 1–2–3 R.N. visits.
14. Client will change careers after 1–2–3 R.N. visits.

III. LONG-TERM GOALS

1. Independent activities of daily living will be resumed in 1–2 weeks.

2. Healthy mental status will be achieved in 3–6 months.

3. Optimal level of health will be achieved in 3–6 months.

IV. OUTCOME CRITERIA

1. Vital signs are normal.
2. Skin is healthy and intact.
3. Appetite is normal.
4. Weight is appropriate for height.
5. Client is alert and well-adjusted and interacts well in society.
6. Client achieves appropriate goals/makes appropriate decisions.
7. Laboratory test results are normal.
8. Client seeks active employment.
9. Sleep pattern is normal.
10. Alcohol/Drug abuse is controlled/treated.
11. Child abuse/neglect is prevented.
12. Client states he/she feels better.

V. NURSING INTERVENTION/TREATMENT

1. R.N. will assess situations that are causing anxiety in client's life.
2. R.N. will offer explanations of and responses to any fears, concerns, or anxieties. If client is facing an anxiety-producing situation, R.N. will arrange for client to speak with a person with similar difficulty who has successfully resolved the problem.
3. R.N. will arrange for client to visit an M.D. office/mental health clinic/inpatient or outpatient facility/rehabilitation center/ detoxification unit for additional assistance.
4. R.N. will arrange for M.S.W./career counselor to meet with client for financial or employment assistance.
5. R.N. will encourage client to visit psychiatrist if necessary.
6. R.N. will provide M.D. with follow-up reports and discharge summary when case closes.
7. R.N. will notify client/family/H.H.A./significant others when case will close.

Child Abuse
Care Plan

I. NURSING DIAGNOSIS

1. Ineffective individual/family coping related to:
   A. unwanted pregnancy.
   B. familial history of child abuse.
   C. poor understanding of child care and development.
   D. history of alcoholism/drug abuse.
   E. battered wife syndrome.
   F. numerous children.
   G. history of prostitution.
   H. history of child molestation.
   I. overwhelming household/marital responsibilities.
   J. other _____

2. Knowledge of deficit related to:
   A. basic child care and development.
   B. child discipline.
   C. nutrition.
   D. other _____

3. Altered parenting related to:
   A. unwanted pregnancy.
   B. familial history of child abuse.
   C. poor understanding of child care and development.
   D. history of alcoholism/drug abuse.
   E. history of prostitution.

    F. history of child molestation.
    G. battered wife syndrome.
    H. numerous children.
    I. apathy.
    J. narcissism.
    K. overwhelming household/marital responsibilities.
    L. other _____

4. Impaired home maintenance management related to:
    A. overwhelming household/marital responsibilities.
    B. poor understanding of child care.
    C. lack of education.
    D. psychiatric history.
    E. lack of parental supervision in the home.
    F. other _____

5. Altered nutrition: potential for more than body requirements
   related to:
    A. poor meal preparation.
    B. abuse.
    C. neglect.
    D. ineffective parenting.
    E. failure to thrive.
    F. other _____

6. Fear related to:
    A. injuries sustained by child/children.
    B. violent behavior
    C. other _____

7. Potential for injury related to child abuse/neglect.
8. Sleep pattern disturbance related to:
    A. child abuse.
    B. neglect.
    C. ineffective parenting.
    D. other _____

9. Sexual dysfunction related to:
   A. child molestation.
   B. neglect.
   C. other _____

   _____

10. Impaired skin integrity related to:
    A. lice/scabies infestation.
    B. adult bites.
    C. welts.
    D. burns.
    E. bruises.
    F. hand-prints or impression of an instrument.
    G. fractures.
    H. other _____

    _____

11. Altered health maintenance related to child abuse/neglect.
12. Altered thought processes related to poor parental role model.
13. Social isolation related to:
    A. child abuse.
    B. child neglect.
    C. ineffective parenting.
    D. other _____

    _____

14. Self-esteem disturbance related to:
    A. child abuse.
    B. neglect.
    C. other _____

    _____

II. SHORT-TERM GOALS

1. Parent/Parents will provide a safe, clean home environment after 1–2–3 R.N. visits.
2. Parent/Parents will provide nutritionally sound meals for children after 1–2–3 R.N. visits.
3. Parent/Parents will administer necessary medications to family members after 1–2–3 R.N. visits.
4. Parent/Parents will seek professional counseling after 2–3–4–5–6 R.N./M.S.W. visits.

5. Parent/Parents will keep routine M.D. appointments for the entire family after 1–2 R.N. visits.

6. Parent/Parents will keep routine dental appointments for the whole family after 1–2–3 R.N. visits.

7. Parent/Parents will keep all family members clean and safe from physical injury after 1–2–3 R.N. visits.

8. Parent/Parents will dress all family members in clean, appropriate clothing after 1–2 R.N. visits.

9. Parent/Parents will obtain food stamps/additional financial income after 1–2 R.N. visits.

10. Parent/Parents will seek appropriate vocational counseling after 1–2–3 R.N./M.S.W. visits.

11. Parent/Parents will encourage daily attendance and completion of school activities after 1–2–3 R.N. visits.

12. Parent/Parents will provide appropriate recreation and diversional activities for family after 1–2–3 R.N. visits.

III. LONG-TERM GOALS

1. Normal family unit will be maintained in 1–2–3 months.
2. Effective parenting will occur in 1–2–3 months.
3. Optimal level of health will be achieved by all family members in 2–3 months.

IV. OUTCOME CRITERIA

1. Parents/Children are well-nourished.
2. Parents/Children are appropriately clothed.
3. Parents/Children are clean and healthy.
4. Parents/Children are sociable, responsible members of the community.
5. Home environment is safe and clean.
6. Parents/Children adapt well to new situations.
7. Financial resources are adequate.
8. Employment is maintained/obtained.

V. NURSING INTERVENTION/TREATMENT

1. R.N. will visit home and assess health status of all members.
2. R.N. will make arrangements for additional resource personnel in home (e.g., M.S.W., child psychiatrist, youth and family service workers, H.H.A., home attendant, homemaker, housekeeper).

3. R.N. will confer with staff and M.D. to determine if reporting to the appropriate authorities is necessary.
4. R.N. will instruct client/family/significant other/H.H.A./ homemaker/housekeeper/home attendant on:
   A. fluid and dietary preparation.
   B. bathing/personal hygiene (e.g., examine child for torn, stained, or bloody clothing, especially underwear/signs of genital bleeding/venereal disease, or urinary tract infection/thickening of labial skin and an enlarged vaginal opening/enlarged anal opening/failure to thrive/frequent upper respiratory infections/ difficulty walking or moving a limb).
   C. medication administration/adverse reactions.
   D. medical care.
   E. dental care.
   F. immunizations/TB testing.
   G. contraception/abortion/sterilization/adoption.
   H. financial planning/budgeting.
   I. career counseling/education.
   J. psychologic counseling/support groups/organizations/clubs.
   K. foster care/adoption services.
5. R.N. will provide M.D. with follow-up reports and discharge summary when case closes.
6. R.N. will notify parent/parents/H.H.A./significant others when case will close.

Depression
Care Plan

I. NURSING DIAGNOSIS

1. Anxiety related to:
   A. the unknown.
   B. the dying process.
   C. feelings of anger/hostility/rejection/inadequacy/guilt.
   D. suicidal tendencies.
   E. loneliness.
   F. dependence on others for care.
   G. financial insecurity.
   H. social isolation.
   I. alcoholism/drug abuse.
   J. promiscuity.
   K. incompatibility.
   L. ideas of self-depreciation.
   M. self-accusatory delusions.
   N. other _____

2. Ineffective individual/family coping related to:
   A. fear of the unknown.
   B. fear of death.
   C. feelings of anger/hostility/rejection/inadequacy/guilt.
   D. suicidal tendencies.
   E. loneliness.
   F. dependence on others for care.
   G. financial insecurity.
   H. social isolation.

    I. alcoholism/drug abuse.

    J. promiscuity.

    K. imcompatibility.

    L. ideas of self-depreciation.

    M. self-accusatory delusions.

    N. other _____

---

3. Altered thought processes related to:
   - A. fear of the unknown.
   - B. fear of death.
   - C. feelings of anger/hostility/rejection/inadequacy/guilt.
   - D. suicidal tendencies.
   - E. loneliness.
   - F. dependence on others for care.
   - G. financial insecurity.
   - H. social isolation.
   - I. alcoholism/drug abuse.
   - J. promiscuity.
   - K. adverse reactions to medications.
   - L. ideas of self-depreciation.
   - M. self-accusatory delusions.
   - N. other _____

---

4. Impaired adjustment related to:
   - A. fear of the unknown.
   - B. fear of death.
   - C. feelings of anger/hostility/rejection/inadequacy/guilt.
   - D. suicidal tendencies.
   - E. loneliness.
   - F. dependence on others for care.
   - G. financial insecurity.
   - H. social isolation.
   - I. alcoholism/drug abuse.
   - J. promiscuity.
   - K. incompatibility.
   - L. ideas of self-depreciation.
   - M. self-accusatory delusions.
   - N. other _____

5. Impaired home maintenance management related to:
   A. dependence on others for care.
   B. retarded thinking and action.
   C. weakness/immobility.
   D. financial insecurity.
   E. feeding problems.
   F. social isolation.
   G. other _____

   _____

6. Impaired verbal communication related to:
   A. inability to speak/limited speech.
   B. refusal to speak.
   C. other _____

   _____

7. Diversional activity deficit related to:
   A. lethargy.
   B. weakness.
   C. feelings of guilt.
   D. ideas of self-depreciation.
   E. self-accusatory delusions.
   F. other _____

   _____

8. Potential for injury related to:
   A. anorexia.
   B. immobility/lack of exercise.
   C. refusal to eat.
   D. insomnia.
   E. agitation.
   F. suicidal tendencies.
   G. other _____

   _____

9. Actual/Potential fluid volume deficit related to:
   A. refusal to drink.
   B. inability to perform activities of daily living.
   C. other _____

   _____

10. Altered nutrition: potential for more than body requirements related to:
    A. anorexia.
    B. refusal to eat.
    C. other _____
    _____

11. Constipation/Diarrhea/Incontinence related to:
    A. anorexia.
    B. poor fluid/dietary intake.
    C. refusal to eat.
    D. immobility.
    E. inability to perform activities of daily living.
    F. other _____
    _____

12. Ineffective breathing pattern related to:
    A. impending respiratory infection.
    B. other _____
    _____

13. Altered family processes related to:
    A. home confinement/hospitalization/institutionalization.
    B. total needs of client to carry out activities of daily living.
    C. alcoholism/drug abuse.
    D. other _____
    _____

14. Noncompliance with therapy related to:
    A. fear of the unknown.
    B. fear of death.
    C. feelings of anger/hostility/rejection/inadequacy/guilt.
    D. suicidal tendencies.
    E. loneliness.
    F. dependence on others for care.
    G. financial insecurity.
    H. social isolation.
    I. alcoholism/drug abuse.
    J. promiscuity.
    K. ideas of self-depreciation.
    L. self-accusatory delusions.
    M. other _____
    _____

15. Powerlessness related to:
    A. physical restraints (for suicidal tendencies)
    B. financial insecurity.
    C. alcoholism/drug abuse.
    D. ideas of self-depreciation.
    E. self-accusatory delusions.
    F. other _____

16. Altered patterns of urinary elimination related to:
    A. poor fluid intake.
    B. refusal to drink.
    C. infection.
    D. other _____

17. Potential for violence related to:
    A. agitation.
    B. feelings of hostility/rejection/guilt/inadequacy.
    C. alcoholism/drug abuse.
    D. ideas of self-depreciation.
    E. self-accusatory delusions.
    F. suicidal tendencies.
    G. other _____

18. Self-care deficit: feeding/bathing/dressing/grooming/toileting
    related to:
    A. retarded thinking and action.
    B. dependence on others for care.
    C. immobility.
    D. suicidal tendencies.
    E. other _____

19. Sleep pattern disturbance related to:
    A. fear of the unknown.
    B. fear of death.
    C. agitation.
    D. suicidal tendencies.
    E. loneliness.
    F. feelings of anger/hostility/rejection/inadequacy/guilt.
    G. alcoholism/drug abuse.

H. ideas of self-depreciation.

I. self-accustory delusions.

J. other _____

_____

II. SHORT-TERM GOALS

1. Client/Family will verbalize fears, anxieties, and concerns after 1–2–3–4–5–6–7–8 R.N. visits.
2. Client/Family will administer prescribed medication after 1–2–3–4 R.N. visits.
3. Client/Family will consume/administer nutritionally sound meals after 1–2–3–4–5–6–7–8 R.N. visits.
4. Client will bathe daily after 1–2–3–4–5–6 R.N. visits.
5. Client will perform daily exercise after 1–2–3–4–5–6 R.N. visits.
6. Client will seek employment after 5–10 R.N. visits.
7. Client/Family will take/administer warm, sedative tub baths as ordered after 1–2–3–4–5–6 R.N. visits.
8. Client/Family will take part in safe, diversional activities after 1–2–3–4–5–6 R.N. visits.
9. Client/Family will seek electroshock therapy as ordered after 1–2–3–4–5–6–7–8 M.D./R.N. visits.
10. Client/Family will seek hypnotherapy/hydrotherapy/ narcoanalysis/narcosynthesis/supportive psychotherapy/ expressive psychotherapy/brief psychotherapy/milieu therapy/ nurse-patient relationship therapy/nursing-group therapy/ psychoanalysis as ordered after 1–5–10 R.N. visits.
11. Client/Family will visit/attend recreation centers/foster homes/ adult day care centers/sheltered workshops/halfway houses/after-care clinics/hospitals/long-term care facilities as recommended by M.D. after 1–5–10 R.N. visits.
12. Client will seek religious counseling after 1–5–10 R.N. visits.

III. LONG-TERM GOALS

1. Client-nurse-physician therapeutic relationship will be developed in 1–6 months.
2. Client decision making/problem solving will be achieved in 6–12 months.
3. Independent activities of daily living will be resumed in 1–6 months.
4. Client interpersonal and intrapersonal relationships will be developed in 6–12 months.

IV. OUTCOME CRITERIA

1. Vital signs are normal.
2. CBC with differential/electrolyte level/BUN results are normal.
3. Urinary output is clear, yellow, and sufficient in quantity.
4. Bowel elimination is normal.
5. Weight is appropriate for height.
6. Skin is clear, intact, and healthy.
7. Vision is normal.
8. Hearing is normal.
9. Sleep pattern is normal.
10. Breathing is clear and unimpaired.
11. Ambulation is normal.
12. Thought processes are clear.
13. Client is cooperative, is willing to assist with all aspects of care, and expresses feelings in a positive manner.
14. Client communicates appropriately.
15. Client makes appropriate decisions/solves problems.
16. Client interacts with peers positively.
17. Client accepts self positively.
18. Client seeks housing/employment/recreation in community.

V. NURSING INTERVENTION/TREATMENT

1. R.N. will instruct client/family/H.H.A. on:
   A. daily routine schedule/limit setting.
   B. personal and environmental safety precautions.
   C. communication techniques.
   D. fluid intake/diet preparation.
   E. personal hygiene and performing activities of daily living.
   F. safe, diversional activities.
   G. bowel/bladder elimination habits.
   H. medication/injection administration/adverse reactions.
   I. immediate notification of M.D. of change in behavior or adverse reactions.
   J. monitoring and recording of vital signs.
   K. sleep pattern. Client may need warm fluids to drink; back rub; warm, sedative tub baths; hypnotics to reduce agitation.
   L. hypnotherapy/hydrotherapy/electroshock therapy/ narcoanalysis/narcosynthesis/supportive psychotherapy/

       expressive psychotherapy/brief psychotherapy/milieu therapy/
       nurse-patient relationship therapy/nursing-group therapy/
       psychoanalysis.

  M. recreation centers/foster homes/adult day care centers/sheltered
       workshops/halfway houses/after-care clinics/hospitals/long-
       term care facilities.

  N. additional services (e.g., H.H.A./home attendant/homemaker/
       housekeeper/P.T./O.T./S.T./M.S.W.).

2. R.N. will provide M.D. with follow-up reports and discharge
   summary when case closes.

3. R.N. will notify client/family/H.H.A./significant others when case
   will close.

Drug Abuse
Care Plan

I. NURSING DIAGNOSIS

  1. Anxiety related to:
    A. drug habituation.
    B. financial insecurity.
    C. signs/symptoms of withdrawal.
    D. other _____

    _____

  2. Knowledge deficit related to:
    A. habituation.
    B. signs/symptoms of drug abuse.
    C. treatment.
    D. other _____

    _____

  3. Altered thought processes related to:
    A. drug overdose.
    B. other _____

    _____

  4. Ineffective individual/family coping related to:
    A. financial insecurity.
    B. physical injury/death.
    C. mood swings.
    D. separation/divorce.
    E. other _____

    _____

5. Self-care deficit: feeding/bathing/grooming/dressing/toileting related to:
   A. altered levels of consciousness.
   B. dependence on others for care.
   C. other _____
   _____

6. Potential fluid volume deficit related to:
   A. nausea/vomiting.
   B. poor nutritional habits.
   C. other _____
   _____

7. Impaired home maintenance management related to:
   A. altered levels of consciousness.
   B. dependence on others for care.
   C. other _____
   _____

8. Impaired physical mobility related to altered levels of consciousness.

9. Noncompliance with withdrawal related to:
   A. pain.
   B. dependence.
   C. loss of control.
   D. peer pressure.
   E. other _____
   _____

10. Altered nutrition: potential for more than body requirements related to:
    A. poor dietary intake.
    B. nausea/vomiting.
    C. other _____
    _____

11. Altered parenting related to:
    A. neglect.
    B. altered levels of consciousness.
    C. other _____
    _____

12. Potential for injury related to:
    A. drug withdrawal.
    B. violence.
    C. crime.

   D. drug overdose.
   E. other _____

   _____

13. Ineffective breathing patterns related to:
   A. drug overdose.
   B. drug withdrawal.
   C. other _____

   _____

14. Self-esteem disturbance related to:
   A. feelings of isolation.
   B. unemployment.
   C. self-hate.
   D. anger.
   E. fear.
   F. grieving.
   G. other _____

   _____

15. Body image disturbance related to:
   A. weight loss/cachexia.
   B. poor personal hygiene.
   C. unkempt appearance.
   D. other _____

   _____

16. Sensory/Perceptual alterations related to:
   A. drug overdose.
   B. drug withdrawal.
   C. other _____

   _____

17. Actual/Potential impaired skin integrity related to:
   A. poor injection technique.
   B. break in aseptic technique.
   C. numerous injection sites.
   D. infection.
   E. other _____

   _____

18. Sleep pattern disturbance related to:
   A. drug withdrawal.
   B. other _____

   _____

II. SHORT-TERM GOALS

1. Client/Family will seek medical help for drug abuse after 1–2–3–4 R.N./M.S.W. visits.
2. Client/Family will seek psychologic counseling after 1–2–3–4 R.N./M.S.W. visits.
3. Client/Family will administer methadone as ordered after 1–2–3–4 R.N. visits.
4. Client will participate in group therapy after 1–2–3–4 R.N./M.S.W. visits.
5. Client/Family will keep emergency phone numbers readily available after 1 R.N. visit.

III. LONG-TERM GOALS

1. Drug dependence/abuse will be controlled within 6–12 months.
2. Optimal level of health will be achieved in 6–12 months.
3. Independent activities of daily living will be resumed in 3–4 weeks.
4. Education and employment will be sought after 6–12 months.
5. Reintegration into family and society will be achieved in 6–12 months.

IV. OUTCOME CRITERIA

1. Vital signs are normal.
2. Cardiovascular system functions appropriately.
3. Skin remains healthy and intact.
4. Neuromuscular system functions appropriately.
5. Vision is clear.
6. Bowel/Bladder elimination is normal.
7. Client is alert, sociable, and responsible.
8. Client functions appropriately at school/work/recreation.
9. Financial status remains adequate.
10. Client states he/she feels better.

V. NURSING INTERVENTION/TREATMENT

1. R.N. will assess client's willingness to accept help on the initial home visit.
2. R.N. will instruct client/family/H.H.A. on:

A. medical assistance with monitoring and recording of general health status/vital signs; laboratory testing; vision; assessment of cardiovascular/neuromuscular/renal systems.

B. administration of medication, especially methadone/adverse reactions.

C. immediate notification of M.D. of adverse reactions or change in condition.

D. tapering of narcotics.

E. individual therapy (detoxification/psychiatric care).

F. group therapy (inpatient and outpatient facilities).

G. family therapy.

H. vocational training/skill development/job training.

I. educational development (return to school/college).

J. getting assistance with housing/finances/child care.

K. parole/probation supervision.

L. prevention.

3. R.N. will assign additional personnel (e.g., M.S.W. or psychiatric social worker) to case if ordered.

4. R.N. will provide M.D. with follow-up reports and discharge summary when case closes.

5. R.N. will notify client/family/H.H.A./significant others when case will close.

Immigrant Assimilation Care Plan

I. NURSING DIAGNOSIS

1. Anxiety related to:
   A. communication deficit (language barrier).
   B. health problems.
   C. housing problems.
   D. social problems.
   E. financial problems.
   F. other _____

2. Fear related to living in a foreign country or extradition to home country.
3. Knowledge deficit related to:
   A. language barrier.
   B. living arrangements.
   C. job counseling.
   D. financial counseling.
   E. optimal health.
   F. cultural differences.
   G. practice of religion in a foreign country.
   H. meal preparation/purchase of ethnic food.
   I. other _____

4. Ineffective individual/family coping related to:
   A. stress of living in a new environment.
   B. lack of socialization.
   C. financial instability.

    D. inadequate food supply.

    E. poor housing/lack of utilities.

    F. poor dental/health care.

    G. schooling.

    H. poor communication.

    I. other _____

    _____

5. Diversional activity deficit related to:

    A. poor health.

    B. poor communication.

    C. isolation.

    D. fear.

    E. poor income.

    F. cultural changes.

    G. other _____

    _____

6. Impaired physical mobility related to:

    A. weakness.

    B. malnutrition.

    C. other _____

    _____

7. Potential fluid volume deficit related to:

    A. low intake.

    B. malnutrition.

    C. other _____

    _____

8. Impaired home maintenance management related to:

    A. numerous children/extended family/significant others (stress of overcrowding).

    B. malnutrition.

    C. unemployment.

    D. health problems.

    E. financial insecurity.

    F. other _____

    _____

9. Potential for injury related to:

    A. advance of illness/disease.

    B. poor supervision in the home.

    C. refusal to comply with medical advice.

   D. poor housing/plumbing/heating.
   E. other _____

10. Noncompliance with R.N. instructions related to:
    A. grieving.
    B. denial.
    C. social isolation.
    D. language barrier.
    E. fear.
    F. strict cultural/religious beliefs.
    G. other _____

11. Altered nutrition: potential for more than body requirements related to:
    A. lack of familiar ethnic foods.
    B. knowledge deficit pertaining to meal preparation.
    C. poor income.
    D. knowledge deficit pertaining to consumer buying.
    E. other _____

12. Self-care deficit: feeding/bathing/grooming/dressing related to:
    A. poor plumbing/housing condition.
    B. poor personal hygiene habits.
    C. inadequate grooming supplies.
    D. cultural habits.
    E. other _____

13. Self-esteem disturbance related to:
    A. cultural differences.
    B. loss of job.
    C. poor income.
    D. other _____

14. Potential impaired skin integrity related to:
    A. malnutrition.
    B. food allergies.
    C. other _____

15. Sleep pattern disturbance related to:
    A. anxiety.
    B. worry.
    C. poor housing.
    D. overcrowding.
    E. social isolation.
    F. loss of loved ones.
    G. other _____

    _____

16. Spiritual distress related to:
    A. cultural differences.
    B. loss of loved ones.
    C. social isolation.
    D. other _____

    _____

17. Altered patterns of urinary elimination related to:
    A. poor fluid/dietary intake.
    B. infection.
    C. malnutrition.
    D. stress.
    E. other _____

    _____

18. Constipation/Diarrhea related to:
    A. poor fluid/dietary intake.
    B. food allergy.
    C. anxiety.
    D. illness.
    E. other _____

    _____

II. SHORT-TERM GOALS

1. Client/Family will communicate appropriately (with/without aid of a translator) during 1 R.N. visit.
2. Client/Family will seek appropriate health care from M.D./clinic/hospital after 1–2 R.N. visits.
3. Client/Family will demonstrate adequate newborn care according to cultural norms after 1–2–3 R.N. visits.
4. Client/Family will consume nutritionally sound meals after 1–2–3 R.N. visits.

5. Client/Family will take prescribed medication after 1–2–3 R.N. visits.
6. Client/Family will notify M.D. immediately of adverse reactions after 1–2–3 R.N. visits.
7. Client/Family will seek assistance from social service agencies/ employment agencies/religious organizations/local board of health/ health unit after 1–2–3 R.N. visits.
8. Client/Family will seek appropriate schooling after 1–2–3 R.N. visits.

III. LONG-TERM GOALS

1. Adequate communication will be achieved in 1–2–3 weeks.
2. Adequate growth and development will be achieved in 3–6 months.
3. Immunization will be achieved in 1–2 months.
4. Adequate nutritional habits will be practiced in 1–2 months.
5. Adequate housing will be obtained in 1–2 months.
6. Schooling and employment will be obtained in 1–2 months.
7. Religious affiliation will be sought in 1–2 months.
8. Financial stability will be achieved in 1–2 months.

IV. OUTCOME CRITERIA

1. Vital signs are normal.
2. Appetite is appropriate.
3. Laboratory test results are normal.
4. Chest is clear.
5. Teeth and gums are normal, healthy.
6. Skin is intact, healthy.
7. Vision is clear, normal.
8. Hearing is normal.
9. Height and weight are appropriate.
10. Gait is normal.
11. Mental health is normal.
12. Client states he/she feels well.
13. Housing is obtained.
14. Employment is obtained.

V. NURSING INTERVENTION/TREATMENT

1. R.N. will make arrangements for interpreter to be of assistance in all matters if possible.
2. R.N. will instruct, within guidelines of cultural norms, client/family on:
   A. prenatal care.
   B. postpartal and newborn care.
   C. immunizations.
   D. medical care for entire family.
   E. dental care.
   F. financial assistance.
   G. housing assistance.
   H. religious assistance.
   I. schooling.
   J. meal preparation.
   K. consumer buying.
   L. medications/adverse reactions.
   M. immediate notification of M.D. of adverse reactions.
   N. personal hygiene.
   O. diversional activities.
3. R.N. will assign additional personnel (M.S.W., vocational counselor, clergy, or others) if ordered.
4. R.N. will provide M.D. with follow-up reports and discharge summary when case closes.
5. R.N. will notify client/family/H.H.A./significant others when case will close.

Learning Deficit Care Plan

I. NURSING DIAGNOSIS

1. Anxiety related to learning deficit.
2. Altered patterns of bowel/urinary elimination related to:
   A. adequate bowel regimen (administration of laxatives/enemas).
   B. adequate diet (meal preparation/consumer buying).
   C. adequate fluid intake.
   D. medication administration/adverse reactions.
   E. colostomy irrigation.
   F. catheter care.
   G. other _____

3. Increased/Decreased cardiac output related to:
   A. medication administration/adverse reactions.
   B. avoidance of stress.
   C. adequate rest/exercise/lifting/climbing stairs.
   D. avoidance of temperature extremes.
   E. pacemaker instructions.
   F. apical/radial pulse taking.
   G. fluid intake/diet as ordered.
   H. increased/decreased intake and output.
   I. other _____

4. Altered role performance related to learning deficit in:
   A. turning/positioning.
   B. prescribed exercises.
   C. injection therapy.

    D. dressing care.

    E. IV therapy/hyperalimentation procedures.

    F. respiratory care.

    G. fluid needs/diet therapy/meal preparation.

    H. medication administration/adverse reactions.

    I. personal hygiene/skin care/decubitus ulcer care.

    J. tracheostomy care.

    K. prenatal/postpartal/newborn care.

    L. catheter care.

    M. colostomy/ileostomy care.

    N. cast care.

    O. bowel regimen.

    P. other _____

    _____

5. Altered family processes related to learning deficit.
6. Self-care deficit related to learning deficit in:

    A. adequate fluid intake and meal preparation/consumer buying.

    B. injection therapy.

    C. medication administration/adverse reactions.

    D. proper hand-washing technique.

    E. dressing care.

    F. turning/positioning/ambulation/prescribed exercises.

    G. respiratory care.

    H. good personal hygiene/skin care/decubitus ulcer care.

    I. tracheostomy care.

    J. prenatal/postpartal/newborn care.

    K. catheter care.

    L. colostomy/ileostomy care.

    M. cast care.

    N. bowel regimen.

    O. other _____

    _____

7. Altered parenting related to learning deficit in child care.
8. Ineffective breathing pattern related to learning deficit in:

    A. medication regimen.

    B. breathing exercises.

    C. use of respiratory equipment.

    D. other _____

    _____

9. Potential impaired skin integrity related to learning deficit in:
   A. positioning/turning/exercise.
   B. medication/lotion/ointment administration.
   C. massage.
   D. dressing care.
   E. other _____

   _____

10. Impaired home maintenance management related to learning deficit.

II. SHORT-TERM GOALS

1. Client/Family will verbalize fears, anxieties, and concerns after 1–2–3 R.N. visits.
2. Client/Family will prepare a quiet, nonstressful atmosphere for learning after 1–2 R.N. visits.
3. Client/Family will have all necessary equipment available in the home for demonstration by the R.N. after 1–2 R.N. visits.
4. Client/Family will obtain necessary medication to be in the home for demonstration by the R.N. after 1–2–3 R.N. visits.
5. Client/Family will demonstrate/redemonstrate each procedure slowly to R.N. after 1–2–3 R.N. visits.
6. If client/family is unable to learn effectively, a responsible adult/friend will assist with procedure/medication to be administered after 1–2–3 R.N. visits.
7. Client/Family will seek the aid of an interpreter after 1 R.N. visit.
8. Client/Family will prepare nutritional meals after 1–2 R.N. visits.
9. Each session will be short enough for sufficient learning to be accomplished after 1–2–3 R.N. visits.
10. Sessions will last longer, depending on client's interest and comprehension, after 2–3 R.N. visits.

III. LONG-TERM GOALS

1. Adequate learning will be accomplished in 2–4 weeks.
2. Independent activities of daily living will be resumed in 1–2 weeks.
3. Optimal level of health will be achieved in 2–4 weeks.

IV. OUTCOME CRITERIA

1. Good personal hygiene habits are acquired.
2. Adequate growth and development occurs.
3. Intellectual growth occurs.
4. Adequate emotional growth occurs.
5. Disease prevention measures are achieved.
6. Effective contraception/reproduction is accomplished.
7. Comprehension of nursing/medical/dental procedures is demonstrated.
8. Appropriate nursing/medical/dental procedures are practiced.

V. NURSING INTERVENTION/TREATMENT

1. R.N. will consult with hospital discharge planner about treatment and rehabilitation for client; will discuss in preparation for home visiting all previous teaching done in hospital; will conduct remaining teaching in the home, if necessary.
2. R.N. will assess client/family recall as to what has been taught or demonstrated in the hospital; client/family will state or redemonstrate procedures in the home on initial nursing visit.
3. For any remaining teaching to be done in the home, R.N. will:
   A. select a quiet, nonstressful environment.
   B. instruct family to obtain/administer and assemble all medication/equipment necessary for care.
   C. demonstrate correct procedures.
   D. have client/family/significant other correctly redemonstrate what has been taught.
4. R.N. will provide M.D. with follow-up reports and discharge summary when case closes.
5. R.N. will notify client/family/H.H.A./significant others when case will close.

Senile Dementia (Alzheimer's Disease) Care Plan

I. NURSING DIAGNOSIS

1. Anxiety related to:
   - A. loss of concentration.
   - B. forgetfulness.
   - C. memory loss.
   - D. loss of self-identity.
   - E. disorientation.
   - F. confusion.
   - G. aphasia.
   - H. apraxia.
   - I. hallucinations.
   - J. delusions.
   - K. insomnia/sleep disturbances.
   - L. unsteadiness of gait.
   - M. slurred speech.
   - N. incontinence.
   - O. repeated falling.
   - P. other _____

2. Activity intolerance related to:
   - A. pain.
   - B. unsteadiness of gait and other movements.
   - C. slowing of gait.
   - D. weakness.
   - E. poor grasp of objects.
   - F. apraxia.

G. other _____

_____

3. Constipation/Bowel incontinence/Diarrhea/Fecal impaction related to:
   A. poor dietary habits.
   B. inability to arrange daily routine for evacuation.
   C. medication administration/adverse reactions.
   D. forgetfulness.
   E. confusion.
   F. other _____

_____

4. Altered patterns of urinary elimination (stress incontinence/ reflex incontinence/urge incontinence/functional incontinence/ total incontinence/urinary retention) related to:
   A. forgetfulness.
   B. confusion.
   C. inadequate toileting schedule.
   D. other _____

_____

5. Actual/Potential impaired skin integrity related to:
   A. incontinence.
   B. falls.
   C. scratching of skin.
   D. other _____

_____

6. Impaired verbal communication (aphasia/paraphasia/dysphasia/ slurred speech/perseveration/stereotypy/echolalia/verbigeration) related to:
   A. loss of concentration.
   B. confusion.
   C. hallucinations.
   D. delusions.
   E. other _____

_____

7. Altered oral mucous membrane: dryness/infection related to:
   A. inadequate fluid intake.
   B. vitamin deficiency.
   C. hyperorality.
   D. other _____

_____

8. Actual/Potential fluid volume deficit related to:
   A. poor intake.
   B. refusal to drink.
   C. forgetting to drink.
   D. other _____

9. Altered nutrition: more/less than body requirements related to:
   A. refusal to eat.
   B. forgetting to eat.
   C. bulimia.
   D. agitation during meals.
   E. wandering.
   F. other _____

10. Impaired home maintenance management related to:
    A. acalculia.
    B. agnosia.
    C. agraphia.
    D. alexia.
    E. apraxia.
    F. astereognosis.
    G. dyspraxia.
    H. dysphasia.
    I. wandering.
    J. confusion.
    K. disorientation.
    L. loss of consciousness.
    M. other _____

11. Altered family processes related to:
    A. dependence on others for care.
    B. need for constant safety monitoring.
    C. financial strain.
    D. rejection by significant others.
    E. other _____

12. Potential for injury related to:
    A. confusion.
    B. lack of supervision while preparing meals.

    C. gait disturbances.
    D. poor eyesight/blindness.
    E. deafness.
    F. hypermetamorphosis.
    G. hyperorality.
    H. wandering.
    I. occupational delirium.
    J. seizures.
    K. aggressive bouts.
    L. other _____

    _____

13. Altered thought processes related to:
    A. loss of short-term memory/forgetfulness.
    B. weakening of orientation in time.
    C. hiding of objects.
    D. mood swings.
    E. aphasia.
    F. acalculia.
    G. agnosia.
    H. alexia.
    I. astereognosis.
    J. mirror sign.
    K. confusion.
    L. disorientation.
    M. indifference to surroundings.
    N. unsociability.
    O. uncooperativeness.
    P. confabulation.
    Q. other _____

    _____

14. Altered health maintenance related to:
    A. poor nutritional habits.
    B. poor dental hygiene.
    C. difficulty keeping M.D./dental appointments.
    D. safety hazards in the home.
    E. deterioration of environment.
    F. lack of support by significant others in the home.
    G. other _____

    _____

15. Ineffective individual coping related to:
    A. embarrassment.
    B. depression.
    C. confusion.
    D. disorientation.
    E. rejection by significant others.
    F. inadequate finances.
    G. other _____

16. Sleep pattern disturbance related to:
    A. insomnia.
    B. wandering.
    C. confusion.
    D. disorientation.
    E. agitation.
    F. sundowning.
    G. other _____

17. Impaired physical mobility related to:
    A. weakness.
    B. pain.
    C. asterixis (myoclonic jerking).
    D. gait ataxia.
    E. gait apraxia.
    F. clasp knife gait.
    G. frontal lobe gait.
    H. other _____

18. Knowledge deficit related to:
    A. signs/symptoms of Alzheimer's disease.
    B. etiology.
    C. projected course of illness/long-term care.
    D. medication administration/adverse reactions.
    E. fluids/diet.
    F. safety precautions.
    G. finances/financial assistance.
    H. home care/institutionalization.
    I. routine medical/dental appointments.

    J. psychologic support.

    K. other _____

    _____

19. Self-care deficit: feeding/bathing/hygiene/dressing/grooming/ toileting related to:

    A. confusion.

    B. disorientation.

    C. mirror sign.

    D. agitation.

    E. occupational delirium.

    F. other _____

    _____

20. Altered role performance related to:

    A. memory loss.

    B. depression.

    C. disorientation.

    D. confusion.

    E. other _____

    _____

II. SHORT-TERM GOALS

1. Client/Spouse/Family/Significant others will verbalize all fears, anxieties, and concerns after 1–2 R.N. visits.

2. Client/Spouse/Family/Significant others will read recommended literature/attend family support groups after 1–2–3–4 R.N. visits.

3. Client/Spouse/Family/Significant others will safely administer prescribed medications after 1–2–3 R.N. visits.

4. Client/Spouse/Family/Significant others will state adverse reactions to medications after 1–2–3 R.N. visits.

5. Client/Spouse/Family/Significant others will immediately report adverse effects of medications to M.D. after 1–2–3 R.N. visits.

6. Client/Spouse/Family/Significant others will consume/administer nutritionally sound meals after 1–2–3 R.N. visits.

7. Client will bathe daily after 1–2–3 R.N. visits.

8. Spouse/Family/Significant others will decrease excessive stimuli and create a nonthreatening environment after 1–2–3 R.N. visits.

9. Spouse/Family/Significant others will not place excessive demands on client after 1–2–3 R.N. visits.

10. Spouse/Family/Significant others will utilize more than one sensory modality (visual/auditory/tactile, etc.) to communicate if necessary after 1–2–3–4 R.N. visits.
11. Spouse/Family/Significant others will avoid use of restraints, if possible, after 1–2–3–4 R.N. visits.
12. Spouse/Family/Significant others will provide meticulous oral hygiene after each meal after 1–2–3 R.N. visits.
13. Client/Spouse/Family/Significant others will dress appropriately throughout day after 1–2–3 R.N. visits.
14. Spouse/Family/Significant others will assist with/supervise ambulation after 1–2–3 R.N. visists.
15. Spouse/Family/Significant others will provide prescribed rest/exercise throughout day after 1–2–3 R.N. visits.
16. Spouse/Family/Significant others will use reality orientation and reality testing skills after 1–2–3 R.N. visits.
17. Spouse/Family/Significant others will encourage routine consistent toileting throughout day/night after 1–2–3 R.N. visits.
18. Spouse/Family/Significant others will change incontinence aids (e.g., adult diapers, Texas catheter) as needed after 1–2–3 R.N. visits.
19. Spouse/Family/Significant others will eliminate safety hazards in the home after 1–2–3 R.N. visits.
20. Spouse/Family/Significant others will keep scheduled M.D./dental appointments for client after 1–2–3 R.N. visits.

III. LONG-TERM GOALS

1. Open communication will be supported throughout course of illness.
2. Independent activities of daily living will be encouraged throughout course of illness.
3. Safety will be maintained throughout course of illness.
4. Optimal health maintenance level will be monitored throughout extent of illness.
5. Client/Family will be comforted and counseled in terminal stages.

IV. OUTCOME CRITERIA

1. Vital signs are normal.
2. Mental health remains stable.
3. Reality orientation is maintained.
4. Gait remains steady.

5. Ambulation is maintained.
6. Chest sounds are normal; chest x-ray film is clear.
7. Vision and hearing are normal.
8. CBC, electrolytes, and sedimentation rate are normal.
9. Liver function tests are normal.
10. Kidneys function normally; urinalysis and culture and sensitivity test results are normal.
11. EKG is normal.
12. EEG is normal.
13. Lumbar puncture is normal.
14. Syphilis serologic test result is normal.
15. Stool guaiac test result is normal.
16. CAT scan is normal.
17. Reflexes are normal.
18. Musculoskeletal system functions normally.
19. Endocrine system functions normally.
20. Client thrives in a healthful environment.

V. NURSING INTERVENTION/TREATMENT

1. R.N. will instruct client/spouse/family/significant others on:
   A. diagnosis/signs and symptoms of Alzheimer's disease memory loss/forgetfulness/dwelling on past events/ disorientation/confusion/hallucinations/delirium, etc.).
   B. causes (cerebrovascular accidents/tumors/infection/depression).
   C. medication administration (antipsychotics/tricyclic anti-depressants/vasodilators/monoamine oxidase inhibitors/ nootropics/lecithin/choline/physiostigmine, etc.)/adverse reactions. Tranquilizers are usually avoided. Use medication aids with supervision (e.g., 7-day pill dispensers, the Drink-A-Pill Cup, braille-labeled prescription vials, a reusable magnifying sleeve which slips over syringes, preprogrammed medication vial alarm system [MedTymer]).
   D. immediate notification of M.D. of adverse reactions or change in condition.
   E. environmental safety (use of nightlights/commonsense strategies [removal of automobile or house keys, scatter rugs, and breakable items])/protection from physical injury.
   F. fluids/dietary requirements (alcohol restriction)/food diary (recommend diet high in acetylcholine)/daily weights/educate guests about condition but not in front of client.

G. consistent toileting routine/use of incontinence aids/indwelling catheters/commode/raised toilet seat/bed padding.

H. bathing/dressing (use of Velcro instead of buttons).

I. daily rest/exercise (stretching and walking).

J. employment.

K. oral hygiene.

L. reality orientation (speak slowly and calmly and use short words and simple sentences; if possible, avoid pronouns use only nouns. Identify yourself and call client by name. Ask one question at a time. If you repeat a question, repeat it verbatim. Maintain eye contact and stand in front of client. Indicate phrases and nonverbal techniques that work with client on a chart. Simple mental status examinations include the following questions: time of day, month, year, counting backwards by 3s or 1s, repetition of 3 objects after 5 minutes. Ask client person, place, time, weather, colors, etc./reality-testing skills/listening techniques/nonverbal communication techniques (Alzheimer's disease clients avert their eyes, look down, back away, and increase hand gesturing when they don't understand).

M. structured milieu.

N. avoidance of translocation shock/isolation.

O. behavior modification techniques.

P. avoidance of infection.

Q. family support groups/group therapy sessions/voluntary Alzheimer's health organizations/respite care/adult day care/ mental health services/escort services/friendly visiting/resource libraries/resource directories/speaker's bureau/seminars and workshops.

R. loss of communicative skills (e.g., astereognosis/dysphasia/ paraphasia/perseveration/receptive aphasia/stereotypy/ verbigeration/acalculia/agnosia/agraphia/alexia).

S. use of restraints.

T. sleep pattern.

U. socialization.

V. M.D./dental appointments (shorter appointments and more frequent visits are encouraged along with sedation).

W. laboratory testing.

X. finances: federal, state, and local public assistance programs/ Medicare/Medicaid/a power of attorney/representative payee/ conservatorship/income/assets/private insurance carriers/ veteran's benefits/employer-sponsored health plans/SSI/social security/joint bank accounts/trusts.

    Y. in-home services (housekeeper/homemaker/H.H.A./home attendant)/alternative housing/residential placement.

    Z. institutionalization.

2. R.N. will follow up with M.D. regarding history and physical, neurologic exam, drug history, psychiatric testing, blood testing, chest x-rays, EKGs, EEGs, urinalyses with culture and sensitivity testing, stool guiac tests, syphilis serologic testing, CAT scans, lumbar punctures, brain biopsy, verbal/performance IQ on Wechsler Adult Intelligence Scale, and any other testing which is ordered.

3. R.N. will provide M.D. with follow-up reports and discharge summary when case closes.

4. R.N. will notify client/family/H.H.A./significant others when case will close.

Sudden Infant Death Syndrome Counseling Care Plan

I. NURSING DIAGNOSIS

1. Knowledge deficit related to SIDS.
2. Grieving related to SIDS.
3. Spiritual distress related to SIDS.
4. Potential for violence related to SIDS.
5. Altered thought processes related to SIDS.
6. Self-esteem disturbance related to SIDS.
7. Altered parenting related to SIDS.
8. Sleep pattern disturbance related to SIDS.
9. Impaired social interaction related to SIDS.
10. Ineffective individual/family coping related to SIDS.

II. SHORT-TERM GOALS

1. Client/Parents/Family will verbalize feelings of guilt, anger, hostility, or anxiety after 1–2–3–4–5–6 R.N. visits.
2. Client/Parents/Family will participate in group therapy if necessary after 1–2–3–4–5–6 R.N. visits.
3. Client/Parents/Family will develop rapport with R.N. after 1–2–3–4–5–6 R.N. visits.
4. Client/Parents/Family will maintain a safe environment after 1–2–3 R.N. visits.
5. Client/Parents/Family will provide appropriate care to other siblings after 1–2–3 R.N. visits.
6. Client/Parents/Family will administer prescribed medication after 1–2–3 R.N. visits.

7. Client/Parents/Family will sleep uninterruptedly after 1–2–3 R.N. visits.
8. Client/Parents/Family will keep M.D. appointments as scheduled after 1–2–3 R.N. visits.

III. LONG-TERM GOALS

1. Appropriate grieving will occur over the course of 1 year or longer.
2. Family unit will function normally in 6–12 months.

IV. OUTCOME CRITERIA

1. Client/Parents/Family resolve guilt feelings.
2. Client/Parents/Family are able to care for self/spouse/siblings.
3. Home maintenance management is normal.
4. Normal mental health is restored.
5. Normal socialization of all family members resumes in community.
6. Employment resumes.

V. NURSING INTERVENTION/TREATMENT

1. Before visiting client's home, R.N. will explain source of referral/ purpose of interview and set up date for interview.
2. R.N. will allow for adequate ventilation and reflection during visits.
3. R.N. will suggest support groups of those who have had similar experience.
4. R.N. will suggest additional assistance from clergy, social worker, psychotherapist, psychiatrist, mental health worker, or M.D.
5. R.N. will instruct client/parents/family in safe administration of medication if necessary.
6. R.N. will encourage client/parents/family to proceed with everyday activities as before death of child.
7. R.N. will encourage socialization in community when client/ parents/family are ready.
8. R.N. will provide M.D. with follow-up reports and discharge summary when case closes.
9. R.N. will inform client/parents/family of the importance of keeping appointments with M.D. as follow-up.
10. R.N. will notify client/parents/family when case will close.

Bibliography

ACOG Newsletter. CDC issues more AIDS guidelines for health care workers. October 1987, *31*(10), 9.

Adams, N. R. The nurse's role in systematic weaning from a ventilator. *Nursing 79,* August 1979, pp. 35–41.

Alzheimer's and related disorders. *Generations,* Fall 1982, pp. 6–45.

Alzheimer's disease: A scientific guide for health practitioners, NIH Pub. No. 81-2251. Office of Scientific and Health Reports, National Institute of Neurological and Communicative Disorders and Stroke, Bethesda, Md., November 1980, pp. 1–20.

Alzheimer's Disease and Related Disorders Association Newsletter, Spring 1985, pp. 4–5.

Household tips. Alzheimer's Disease and Related Disorders Association Newsletter, Summer 1985, pp. 6–7.

Alzheimer's Disease and Related Disorders Association Newsletter, Fall 1985, pp. 6–9.

Alzheimer's Disease and Related Disorders Association Newsletter, Winter 1985, pp. 1–7.

Amair, P., Khanna, R., Leibel, B., et al. Continuous ambulatory peritoneal dialysis in diabetics with end-stage renal disease. *New England Journal of Medicine,* March 1982, pp. 625–630.

Ament, M. E. Home total parenteral nutrition: An alternative approach to the management of children with severe chronic small bowel disease. *Journal of Pediatric Surgery,* 1977, No. 12, pp. 359–366.

Anderson, C. L. *Community health.* St. Louis: Mosby, 1973.

Anderson, D. AIDS: An update on what we know now. *R.N.,* March 1986, pp. 49–56.

Antenatal diagnosis of genetic disorders. *ACOG Technical Bulletin,* September 1987, No. 108, pp. 1–8.

Arnold, C. Why that liquid formula diet may not work (and what to do about it). *R.N.,* November 1981, pp. 34–39.

Aronson, M. K. Alzheimer's disease: An overview. *Generations*, Fall 1982, pp. 6–7.

AT&T Consumer Sales and Service booklet, *Products from the AT&T National Special Needs Center*, 2001 Route 46, Parsippany, N.J. 07054.

Atkins, J. M., and Oakley, C. W. A nurse's guide to TPN. *R.N.*, June 1986, pp. 20–24.

Ballantine, R., Fanning, J., Lawson, M., et al. Alternatives in outpatient chemotherapy administration. *The Cancer Bulletin*, 1980, *32*(5), pp. 173–176.

Banyard, S. G. New drug-free technique cuts post-op pain. *R.N.*, April 1982, pp. 31–33.

Barfoot, K. R., and Ross, K. L. Intravenous therapy at home: An overview. *Home Healthcare Nurse*, July/August 1988, pp. 11–13.

Baron, F. Should you infuse anything else through a TPN line? *R.N.*, October 1981, pp. 32–108.

Bast, C., and Hayes, P. PCA: A new way to spell pain relief. *R.N.*, August 1986, pp. 18–20.

Beebe, W. K., and Gomez, K. Amyotrophic lateral sclerosis. *Home Healthcare Nurse*, May/June 1985, pp. 8–17.

Beneson, A. S. (Ed.). *Control of communicable diseases in man* (13th ed.). Washington, D.C.: American Public Health Association, 1981.

Berger-Apuzzo, D. AIDS: Could you be at risk? *R.N.*, February 1983, pp. 67–78.

Berkow, R. *The Merck manual of diagnosis and therapy* (14th ed.). Rahway, N.J.: Merck, Sharp & Dohme Research Laboratories, 1982.

Binkley, L. S. Keeping up with peritoneal dialysis. *American Journal of Nursing*, June 1984, pp. 729–733.

Biosearch Medical Products, Inc. *Procedure for insertion and maintenance of the Entriflex feeding tubes* (Pamphlet No. DG 005-881). Somerville, N.J.

Biosearch Medical Products, Inc. *Procedure for insertion and maintenance of the Hydromer-Dobbhoff enteral feeding tube* (Pamphlet No. DG 005-881). Somerville, N.J.

Bjeletich, J., and Hickman, R. O. The Hickman indwelling catheter. *American Journal of Nursing*, 1980, *80*, 62–65.

Bleyer, W. A. Current status of intrathecal chemotherapy for human meningeal neoplasms, in *Modern Concepts in Brain Tumor Therapy* (Monograph No. 46). Bethesda, Md.: National Cancer Institute, 1977, pp. 171–178.

Bontempo, Sister T., and Eggland, E. T. Nursing implications for home parenteral therapy. *Home Healthcare Nurse*, July/August 1988, pp. 14–19.

Brown, S. L. Avoiding post-op pitfalls with hip fracture patients. *R.N.*, May 1982, pp. 49–54.

Brunner, L. S., Emerson, C. P. Jr., Ferguson, L. K., et al. *Textbook of medical-surgical nursing*. Philadelphia: J. B. Lippincott, 1970.

Burnside, I. M. Alzheimer's disease: An overview. *Journal of Gerontological Nursing*, July/August 1979, pp. 14–20.

Bushman, M. C. Treatment of renal osteodystrophy with Dialume recipes. *Home Healthcare Nurse*, November/December 1983, pp. 42–45.

Bushnell, S. S. *Respiratory intensive care nursing*. Boston: Little, Brown, 1973.

Byrne, W. J., Halpin, T. C., Asch, M. J., et al. Home total parenteral nutrition: An alternative approach to the management of children with severe chronic small bowel disease. *Journal of Pediatric Surgery*, 1977, *12*, 359–366.

Campbell, C. *Nursing diagnosis and intervention in nursing practice* (2nd ed.). New York: John Wiley, 1984.

Campese, V., Easterling, R. E., Finkelstein, F., et al. Renal osteodystrophy and the status of aluminum and other trace metals in CAPD patients: A panel review. *Peritoneal Dialysis Bulletin*, July/September 1984, pp. 129–135.

CAPD and you, helping hands: A guide for home hemodialysis assistants, and home hemodialysis & you. Des Moines, Ia.: National Kidney Foundation of Iowa, Inc., 1981.

Carr, P. When the patient needs TPN at home. *R.N.*, June 1986, pp. 25–27.

Casey, C. A. When a patient has novel-syndrome diabetes. *R.N.*, September 1986, p. 78.

Castaldo, P. Respiratory home care from the DME point of view. *Home Healthcare Nurse*, March/April 1985, pp. 32–35.

Centers for Disease Control. Sexually transmitted diseases treatment guidelines 1982. *Morbidity and Mortality Weekly Report*, August 20, 1982, Vol. 31, No. 25, pp. 37S–58S.

Chekryn, J. Support for the family of the dying patient. *Home Healthcare Nurse*, May/June 1985, pp. 18–24.

Clausen, J. P. *Maternity nursing today*. McGraw-Hill, 1973.

Coleman, D. A. How to care for an AIDS patient. *R.N.*, July 1986, pp. 16–21.

Communicable disease summary. Trenton: New Jersey State Department of Health, 1982.

Crow, S. Tips for successful respiratory suctioning. *R.N.*, April 1986, pp. 31–33.

D'Agostino, J. S. You can breathe new life into your COPD patients. *Nursing 83*, September 1983, pp. 72–77.

Dangel, R. B. How to use an implantable infusion pump. *R.N.*, September 1985, pp. 40–43.

Denniston, D., and Burns, K. T. Home peritoneal dialysis. *American Journal of Nursing*, November 1980, pp. 2022–2026.

Dolbee, S. F., and Creason, N. S. Outcome criteria for the patient using intravenous antibiotic therapy at home. *Home Healthcare Nurse*, July/ August 1988, pp. 22–29.

Dolinger, R. How radiation complicates stoma care. *R.N.*, September 1986, pp. 32–34.

Esparza, D. M., and Weyland, J. B. Nursing care for the patient with an Ommaya Reservoir. *Oncology Nursing Forum*, 1982, 9(4), 17–20.

Even moderate drinking may be hazardous to maturing fetus. *JAMA Medical News*, 1977, *237*, 2585–2587.

Facts about kidney diseases and their treatment and diabetes and the kidneys. Bethesda, Md.: American Kidney Fund, 1981.

FDA Drug Bulletin, September 1987, *17*(2), 14–24.

Fodor, J. T., and Dalis, G. V. *Health instruction: Theory and application* (2nd ed.). Philadelphia: Lea & Febiger, 1974.

Fuerst, E. V., and Wolff, L. *Fundamentals of nursing* (4th ed.). Philadelphia: J. B. Lippincott, 1969.

Gallo, A. M., Edwards, J., and Vessey, J. Little refugees with big needs. *R.N.*, December 1980, pp. 44–48.

Greifzu, S. Colorectal cancer: When a polyp is more than a polyp. *R.N.*, September 1986, pp. 23–29.

Guidelines for venereal disease education. Trenton: New Jersey Department of Education, Division of Curriculum and Instruction, 1975.

Hamilton, H. K. *Procedures: Nurse's reference library*. Springhouse, Pa.: Springhouse, 1985, pp. 277–286.

Heart defects accompanying fetal alcohol syndrome. *JAMA Medical News*, 1976, *235*, 2073.

Heimbach, D. M., and Ivey, T. D. Technique for placement of a permanent home hyperalimentation catheter. *Surgery, Gynecology and Obstetrics*, 1976, *143*, 634–636.

Henderson, S., Leung, A. C. T., and Shenkin, A. Vitamin status in continuous ambulatory peritoneal dialysis. *Peritoneal Dialysis Bulletin*, July/September 1984, pp. 143–145.

Hickman, R. O., Buckner, C. D., Clift, R. A., et al. A modified right atrial catheter for access to the venous system in marrow transplant recipients. *Surgery, Gynecology and Obstetrics*, 1979, *148*, 871–875.

Hirsch, J., and Hannock, L. *Mosby's manual of clinical nursing procedures*. St. Louis: C. V. Mosby, 1981.

Hoffman, L. A., and Maszkiewicz, R. C. CE airway management, the specifics of suctioning. *American Journal of Nursing*, January 1987, pp. 44–53.

Hollingsworth, A. O., Brown, L. P., and Brooton, D. A. The refugees and childbearing: What to expect. *R.N.*, November 1980, pp. 44–48.

How to treat glaucoma. *R.N.*, June 1986, p. 73.

Ingram, N. M. Stanching nosebleeds: Your guide to all the measures available. *R.N.*, September 1982, pp. 51–53, 115.

Iorio, J. *Principles of obstetrics and gynecology for nurses* (2nd ed.). St. Louis: C. V. Mosby, 1971.

Irwin, B. C. Now––peritoneal dialysis for chronic patients, too. *R.N.*, June 1981, pp. 49–52, 98.

Jacobs, A., Clifford, P., and Kay, H. E. M. The Ommaya Reservoir in chemotherapy for malignant disease of the CNS. *Clinical Oncology*, 1981, 7, 123–129.

Jensen, T. G. Home enteral nutrition. *Ross Timesaver, Dietetic Currents*, 1982, 9(4), 15–20.

Johnson, S. A safer gastrostomy for the high-risk patient. *R.N.*, March 1986, pp. 29–32.

Jones, D. A. *Nursing Diagnosis Newsletter*, 1988, 14(4), 1–3.

Jones, D. A. *Nursing Diagnosis Newsletter*, 1988, 15(1), 1–3.

Juliani, L. M. Keep this quick flow-rate calculator handy. *R.N.*, October 1981, pp. 64–65.

Keiffer, E. Premenstrual syndrome. *Family Circle*, Apr. 6, 1982, pp. 28–37.

Kiely, M. A. Alzheimer's disease: Making the most of the time that's left. *R.N.*, March 1985, pp. 34–41.

Kim, M. J., and Moritz, D. A. *Classification of nursing diagnosis* (Proceedings of the Third and Fourth National Conferences). New York: McGraw-Hill, 1982, pp. 281–314.

Kosier, J. H. and Thompson, A. Supervising the hemodialysis client in self medication in the home. *Home Healthcare Nurse*, May/June 1985, pp. 31–36.

Krachenfels, M. Home tube feedings: Gastrointestinal complications. *Home Healthcare Nurse*, January/February 1987, pp. 41–42.

LaMonica, E. *The nursing process: A humanistic approach*. Reading, Mass.: Addison-Wesley, 1979.

Latham, H. C., and Heckel, R. V. *Pediatric nursing* (2nd ed.). St. Louis: C. V. Mosby, 1972.

Lent-Wunderlich, E., and Ott, M. J. Helping your patient through eye surgery. *R.N.*, June 1986, pp. 43–47.

Letherland, J. Do you know child abuse when you see it? *R.N.*, November 1986, pp. 28–30.

Levine, Z. Care of the renal patient. Philadelphia: W. B. Saunders, 1983.

Levitt, D. Z. Cancer chemotherapy—those dreaded side effects and what to do about them. *R.N.*, December 1980, pp. 33–37, 112.

Lilly, Eli and Co. *Diabetes mellitus* (7th ed.). Indianapolis: Lilly Research Laboratories, 1967.

Lokich, J. J., Perri, J., Bothe, A., et al. Cancer chemotherapy via ambulatory infusion pump. *American Journal of Clinical Oncology* (CCT), 1983, 6, 355–363.

Masoorlie, S. T. Trouble-free IV starts. *R.N.*, February 1981, pp. 20–27.

McKinstry, D. W. Diagnosis, cause and treatment of Alzheimer's disease. *Research Resources Reporter*, 1(6), DHHS-PHS Pub., National Institutes of Health, June 1982.

Mereness, D. *Essentials of psychiatric nursing*, 13th ed. St. Louis: C. V. Mosby, 1970.

Miller, L., Roy, C., and Atcherson, E. Home peritoneal training and the community nurse. *Home Healthcare Nurse*, May/June 1985, pp. 26–30.

Miller, S. An effervescent flush for clogged feeding tubes. *R.N.*, April 1986, p. 87.

Mims, B. C. Back surgery: Helping your patient get through it. *R.N.*, May 1985, pp. 26–34.

Mitchell, H. S., Rynbergen, H. J., Anderson, L., et al. *Cooper's nutrition in health and disease* (15th ed.). Philadelphia: J. B. Lippincott, 1968.

Miyares, M. U. Medication aids your elderly patients will love. *R.N.*, November 1985, pp. 44–45.

Moser, K. M., Archibald, C., Hansen, P., et al. *Better living and breathing* (2nd ed.). St. Louis: C. V. Mosby, 1980.

Moses, R. M., and Steinberg, S. Does the MA-1 respirator make you nervous? *R.N.*, April 1979, pp. 2–11.

The Mount Sinai Medical Center. *Newsletter of The Gerald and May Ellen Ritter Department of Geriatrics and Adult Development*, Fall 1985, 2(3), 2–3.

Mundinger, M. O., and Javron, G. D. Developing a nursing diagnosis. *Nursing Outlook*, February 1975, pp. 94–98.

National resource directory. Newton Upper Falls, Mass.: National Spinal Cord Injury Foundation, 1979.

Neurogenic bladder/catheterization policies. New York: Nursing and Urology Departments, New York University Medical Center, 1983.

Nursing guidelines for patients with arteriovenous fistula and A-V shunt. New York: Rogosin Kidney Center, 1981.

N.Y. State Department of Health. *AIDS Institute Newsletter*, May 1984, 1(1), 1–4.

Ommaya, A. K. Subcutaneous reservoir and pump for sterile access to ventricular cerospinal fluid. *Lancet*, 1963, 2, 983–984.

Operational manual for the Robert Wood Johnson, Jr., Renal Treatment Center. New York: The Mount Sinai Medical Center, 1984.

Paradiso, C. The dialysis patient, the family and the home health nurse. *Home Healthcare Nurse*, July/August 1986, pp. 26–34.

Persons, C. Why risk TPN when tube feeding will do? *R.N.*, January 1981, pp. 34–41.

Pollack, P. F., Kadden, M., Byrne, W. J., et al. 100 patient years' experience with the Broviac silastic catheter for central venous nutrition. *Journal of Parenteral and Enteral Nutrition*, 1981, 5, 32–36.

Pool, F., and Kohn, I. What to tell patients about sterilization. *R.N.*, May 1986, pp. 55–61.

Posner, J. B. Reservoirs for intraventricular chemotherapy. *New England Journal of Medicine*, 1973, 288, 212.

Potential problems of mechanical ventilation. *American Journal of Nursing*, December 1980, pp. 2206–2213.

Rabyne, R. Helpful hints: On dealing with caregiving stresses. *Alzheimer's Disease and Related Disorders Association Newsletter*, Fall 1984, p. 6.

Ratcheson, R. A., and Ommaya, A. K. Experience with the subcutaneous cerebrospinal-fluid reservoir. *New England Journal of Medicine*, 1968, 279, 1025–1031.

Read, D. A., and Greene, W. H. *Creative teaching in health* (2nd ed.). New York: Macmillan, 1975.

Reisberg, B. The clinical syndrome. The Martin Steinberg Memorial Symposium on Alzheimer's Disease and Related Disorders, The Hebrew Home for the Aged, Riverdale, N.Y., 1983, pp. 7–17.

Reisberg, B., Ferris, S. H., deLeon, M. J., et al. The global deterioration scale for assessment of primary degenerative dementia. (See Table 1: Global deterioration scale for age associated cognitive decline and Alzheimer's disease.) *American Journal of Psychiatry*, 1982, 139, 1136–1139.

Reisberg, B., London, E., Ferris, S. H., et al. The Brief Cognitive Rating Scale: Language, Motoric, and Mood Concomitants in Primary Degenerative Dementia (See Table 5). *Psychopharmacology Bulletin*, 1983, 19, 702–708.

Riella, M. C., and Scribner, B. H. Five years' experience with a right atrial catheter for prolonged parenteral nutrition at home. *Surgery, Gynecology and Obstetrics*, 1976, 143, 205–208.

Ross Laboratories. *Home tube feeding instruction kit: Suggestions for patient home tube feeding instruction; Home tube feeding instructions;* and *Home tube feeding instruction cards.* Columbus, Ohio: Ross Medical Nutritional Systems, 1982.

Sager, C. J. Recognizing alcoholism as a teratogen. *Medical Tribune, Sexual Medicine Today,* Apr. 27, 1977, pp. 16–21.

Salyer, J., Waters, H., and Yow, P. AIDS: Holistic home care. *Home Healthcare Nurse,* March/April 1987, pp. 10–21.

Sanderson, R. G. *The cardiac patient.* Philadelphia: W. B. Saunders, 1972.

Santopietro, M. C. S. How to get through to a refugee patient. *R.N.,* January 1981, pp. 42–48.

Schmeck, A. M., Jr. New prenatal test raises concern for fetus. *The New York Times,* May 27, 1984, p. 35.

Schrock, T. R. *Handbook of surgery* (6th ed.). Greenbrae, Cal.: Jones Medical Publications, 1978.

Schwarz, T. Is it acute abdomen? *R.N.,* July 1982, pp. 29–31, 94, 96.

Secor, J. *Patient studies in medical-surgical nursing.* Philadelphia: J. B. Lippincott, 1967.

Segal, M. *From birth to one year.* Rolling Hills Estates, Ca.: B. L. Winch, 1974.

Simmons, D. A. *Nurse planning information series no. 14: A classification scheme for client problems in community health nursing,* Health Manpower Reference, DHHS Pub. No. HRA 80-16. Springfield, Va.: National Technical Information Service, 1980.

Slawson, M., and Slawson, S. Problem ingredients in OTCs. *R.N.,* April 1985, pp. 53–61.

Smith, J. B. The patient who can't remember to take her meds. *R.N.,* September 1986, pp. 38–41.

Starkey, J. F., Jefferson, P. A., and Kirby, D. F. Taking care of percutaneous endoscopic gastrostomy. *American Journal of Nursing,* January 1988, pp. 42–45.

Sterilization, *ACOG Technical Bulletin,* February 1988, No. 113, pp. 1–8.

Storch, M. Cramps: How to relieve them and other menstrual problems. *Family Circle,* Feb. 15, 1983, pp. 62–66.

Stuckey, P. A., and Waters, H. Oncology alert for the home care nurse: Spinal cord compression. *Home Healthcare Nurse,* March/April 1987, pp. 29–31.

The PMS Newsletter, Fall/Winter, 1987, Vol. 1, No. 1, pp. 1–4.

Travenol Laboratories, Inc. *Continuous ambulatory peritoneal dialysis kit: An introduction to continuous ambulatory peritoneal dialysis; An introduction to peritoneal dialysis; Going home with confidence procedure guide for the Travenol CAPD ultraviolet germicidal* exchange system with UV-XD; CAPD: A new alternative in dialysis; Simplifying the CAPD exchange; Travenol home patient training; All CAPD solutions are not created equal; An advanced line of blood sets designed to simplify and improve dialysis therapy; SPS 450 series; CF capillary flow dialyzers; Trav-X-Change connection device training procedure guide; and Peritoneal automated cycler with X-connector set. Deerfield, Ill.: Travenol Artificial Organs Division, 1984.

Urinary incontinence. ACOG Technical Bulletin, January 1987, No. 100, pp. 1–6.

vanLoveran-Huyben, C. M. S., Engelaar, H. F. W. J., Hermans, M. B. M., et al. Double-blind clinical and psychologic study of ergoloid mesylates (Hydergine) in subjects with senile mental deterioration. Journal of the American Geriatrics Society, 1984, 32(8), 584–588.

Ventilators and how they work. American Journal of Nursing, December 1980, pp. 2202–2205.

Votava, M., Cleveland, T., and Hiltunen, K. Home care of the patient dependent on mechanical ventilation. Home Healthcare Nurse, March/April 1985, pp. 18–25.

Walters, J. Birth defects and adolescent pregnancies. Journal of Home Economics, November 1975, pp. 23–29, 56.

Weaning patients from mechanical ventilation. American Journal of Nursing, December 1980, pp. 2214–2217.

Weinstein, S. M. Biohazards of working with antineoplastics. Home Healthcare Nurse, January/February 1987, pp. 30–34.

What everyone should know about kidneys and kidney diseases, and CAPD: A new alternative in dialysis. New York: National Kidney Foundation, Inc., 1984.

Wilson, V. How to make a feeding tube go down easy. R.N., November 1986, pp. 40–42.

Woodland, C. How to make infusion control devices work for you. R.N., November 1981, pp. 58–63.

Woods, M. E. Nursing Diagnosis Newsletter, 1983, 10(2), 6–8.

Woods, M. E., and Griffin, P. A. Nursing Diagnosis Newsletter, 1983, 10(1), 1–2.

Ziai, M., Janeway, C. A., and Cooke, R. E. Pediatrics. Boston: Little, Brown, 1969.